FALK SYMPOSIUM 78

Cytokines and the Liver

EDITED BY

W. Gerok

Medizinische Universitätsklinik
Hugstetter Str. 55
D-79106 Freiburg-im-Breisgau
Germany

K. Decker

Biochemisches Institut der Universität
Herrmann-Herder-Str. 7
D-79104 Freiburg-im-Breisgau
Germany

T. Andus and V. Gross

Klinik und Poliklinik für Innere Medizin I
Klinikum der Universität Regensburg
Franz-Josef-Strauss-Allee 11
D-9305 Regensburg
Germany

Proceedings of the 78th Falk Symposium (Part II of the Gastroenterology Week Freiburg 1994), held in Freiburg-im-Breisgau, Germany, June 15–16, 1994

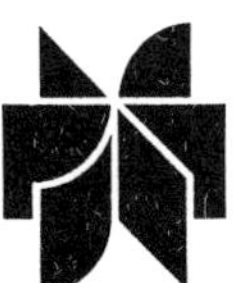

KLUWER ACADEMIC PUBLISHERS
DORDRECHT / BOSTON / LONDON

Distributors

---

for the United States and Canada: Kluwer Academic Publishers, PO Box 358,
Accord Station, Hingham, MA 02018-0358, USA
for all other countries: Kluwer Academic Publishers Group, Distribution
Center, PO Box 322, 3300 AH Dordrecht, The Netherlands

A catalogue record for this book is available from the British Library

ISBN 0-7923-8878-X

Copyright

Published in the United Kingdom by Kluwer Academic Publishers,
PO Box 55, Lancaster, UK.

Kluwer Academic Publishers BV incorporates the publishing programmes of
D. Reidel, Martinus Nijhoff, Dr W. Junk and MTP Press.

Typeset by Lasertext Ltd., Stretford, Manchester, UK
Printed and bound in Great Britain by Hartnolls Ltd., Bodmin, Cornwall.

Contents

List of Principal Authors ix

Introduction xi

Part A: CYTOKINES AND THEIR RECEPTORS IN THE LIVER

Section I: REGULATION OF SYNTHESIS

1 Interleukin-8 and other chemokines: new perspectives in inflammation
M. Baggiolini, M. Uguccioni and M. D'Apuzzo 5

2 IL-6 signal transduction from the plasma membrane to the nucleus
F. Horn, C. Lütticken, U. Wegenka, J. Yuan and P. C. Heinrich 14

Section II: SIGNAL TRANSDUCTION PATHWAYS AND EFFECTS

3 Activation of NH-κB and AP-1 in rat Kupffer cells
T. A. Tran-thi, K. Decker and P. A. Baeuerle 31

4 Cytokines and adhesion molecules in the liver
K. Tanikawa 37

Part B: CELL BIOLOGICAL ASPECTS

Section III: INFLAMMATION AND FIBROGENESIS

5 Role of sinusoidal endothelial cells in liver fibrosis
G. Ramadori and K. Neubauer 57

6 The contribution of hepatocytes to cytokine-directed activation of fat-storing cells – a pathogenetic key mechanism in liver fibrogenesis
A. M. Gressner, C. Hoffmann, M. G. Bachem, G. Schüftan, B. Lahmer and A. Brenzel 58

Section IV: FUNCTION OF STELLATE CELLS AND GROWTH REGULATION

7   On the contraction and relaxation of stellate cells induced by Kupffer cell-derived vasoactive substances
N. Kawada and K. Decker   83

8   The initiation of liver regeneration and the regulation of liver growth by transforming growth factor alpha (TGF-α)
N. Fausto   93

9   Role of HGF in liver regeneration
G. K. Michalopoulos, W. M. Mars and M.-L. Liu   103

Part C: CLINICAL IMPLICATIONS

Section V: HEPATITIS AND CIRRHOSIS

10   Kupffer cell processing of bacterial lipopolysaccharide
E. S. Fox and P. Thomas   115

11   Cytokines in alcoholic liver cirrhosis
J. Dévière, O. le Moine, M. Goldman and E. Dupont   127

12   Autoimmune hepatitis and cytokines
C. Trautwein and M. P. Manns   138

13   Cytokine profiles in primary biliary cirrhosis: an approach to define the underlying immunoreactivity
P. A. Berg, R. Klein, M. Leuschner and U. Leuschner   145

Section VI: RESPONSES OF THE CHALLENGED LIVER

14   Growth factors in liver disease
W. E. Fleig   157

15   Cytokine regulation of hepatic acute phase protein expression
Z. Xing, C. D. Richards, T. Braciak, V. Thibault and J. Gauldie   164

16   Cytokine-induced alterations in hepatic lipid metabolism
K. R. Feingold, I. Hardardóttir and C. Grunfeld   172

CONTENTS

Section VII: LIVER TRANSPLANTATION

17   Cytokines in liver transplantation and alcoholic liver disease
      R. G. Thurman, E. Savier, Y. Adachi, S. I. Shedlofsky,
      J. J. Lemasters, W. Gao, B. U. Bradford, Z. Zhong, K. T. Knecht,
      W. Qu, R. T. Currin, S. Lichtmman, J. Wang and M. Goto   185

18   Role of cytokines in the regulation of cell – cell and cell – matrix
      adhesion molecules in human liver transplants
      G. Steinhoff   204

19   Cytokines in liver allograft rejection
      A. S. Gaweco and W. J. Hofmann   213

      Index   221

List of Principal Authors

T. Andus
Klinik und Poliklinik für Innere Medizin I
Klinikum der Universität Regensburg
D-93053 Regensburg
Germany

M. Baggiolini
Theodor-Kocher-Institut der Universität
  Bern
Freiestr. 1
CH-3000 Bern 9
Switzerland

P. A. Berg
Abteilung Innere Medizin II
Medizinische Universitätsklinik
Otfried-Müller-Str. 10
D-72076 Tübingen
Germany

K. Decker
Biochemisches Institut der Universität
Hermann-Herder-Str. 7
D-79104 Freiburg
Germany

J. Dévière
Department of Gastroenterology
ULB Erasmus Hospital
808 route de Lennik
B-1070 Brussels
Belgium

N. Fausto
Department of Pathology
University of Washington
Seattle
WA 98185
USA

K. R. Feingold
Department of Veterans Affairs Medical
  Center
Metabolism Section (111F)
4150 Clement St
San Francisco
CA 94121
USA

W. E. Fleig
Klinik und Poliklinik für Innere Medizin I
Martin-Luther-Universität Halle-Wittenberg
Ernst-Grube-Str. 40
D-06097 Halle-Saale
Germany

J. Gauldie
Department of Pathology
McMaster University
1200 Main St West
Hamilton
Ontario L8N 3Z5
Canada

W. Gerok
Medizinische Universitätsklinik und
  Poliklinik
Hugstetter Str. 55
D-79106 Freiburg
Germany

A. M. Gressner
Abteilung Klinische Chemie und
  Zentrallaboratorium
Klinikum der Phillips-Universität
Baldingerstr.
D-35033 Marburg
Germany

V. Gross
Klinik und Poliklinik für Innere Medizin I
Klinikum der Universität Regensburg
Franz-Josef-Strauss-Allee 11
D-93053 Regensburg
Germany

LIST OF PRINCIPAL AUTHORS

P. C. Heinrich
Institut für Biochemie der RWTH Aachen
Ncuklinikum
Pauwelsstr. 30
D-52057 Aachen
Germany

W. F. Hofmann
Institute of Pathology, INF 220-221
University of Heidelberg
D-69120 Heidelberg
Germany

N. Kawada
Department of Biochemistry
Osaka City University Medical School
1-4-54, Asahi-machi
Abeno-ku
Osaka 545
Japan

M. P. Manns
Abteilung für Gastroenterologie und
  Hepatologie
Medizinische Hochschule Hannover
Konstanty-Gutschow-Str. 8
D-30625 Hannover
Germany

G. K. Michalopoulos
University of Pittsburgh Medical Center
Department of Pathology
Pittsburgh PA 15261
USA

G. Ramadori
Abteilung für Gastroenterologie und
  Endokrinologie
Universitat Göttingen
Zentrum für Innere Medizin
Robert-Koch-Str. 40
D-37075 Göttingen
Germany

G. Steinhoff
Klinik für Herz- und Gefäßchirurgie
Klinikum der Universität Kiel
Arnold-Heller-Str. 7
D-24105 Kiel
Germany

K. Tanikawa
The 2nd Department of Internal Medicine
Kurume University School of Medicine
67 Asahi-machi
Kurume-shi 830
Japan

P. Thomas
Laboratory of Cancer Biology
Department of Surgery
New England, Deaconess Hospital
Harvard Medical School
50 Binney Street
Boston
MA 02115
USA

R. G. Thurman
Laboratory of Hepatobiology and
  Toxicology
Department of Pharmacology, CB# 7365
University of North Carolina at Chapel Hill
Chapel Hill
NC 27599-7365
USA

T. A. Tran-Thi
Biochemisches Institut der Universität
Hermann-Herder-Str. 7
D-79104 Freiburg
Germany

Introduction

W. Gerok

Cytokines may be defined as a group of soluble protein mediators secreted by one cell and acting on one or more other cells. Most cytokines were initially identified by analysing mediator molecules responsible for the multiple changes occurring during immunological reactions and inflammation. Cytokines represent the signal substances causing inflammatory responses such as fever, leukocytosis, immune response and hepatic secretion of acute phase proteins. Molecular cloning allowed the effects of pure cytokines to be studied in simple experimental systems, in isolated cells, in organs and in the whole organism. These studies gave insight into the physiological function of cytokines.

Interactions between cytokines and the liver can be classified into three main areas. First, extrahepatically produced cytokines enter the liver via the portal or arterial blood and cause changes in hepatic metabolism. This effect of cytokines on the intermediary metabolism of the liver affects many metabolic reactions: a classic example is the alteration of amino acid uptake and the regulation of synthesis and secretion of acute phase proteins. Second, cytokines can be produced within the liver by different cell types, including hepatocytes, endothelial cells, Kupffer cells and fat storing cells. Cytokines produced by one hepatic cell type can act on other cells within the liver in an autocrine or paracrine way. For instance, during liver regeneration after partial hepatectomy, the synthesis and secretion of some cytokines (hepatic growth factor, transforming growth factor α) by fat storing cells are increased. These cytokines induce the division of hepatocytes as a prerequisite for liver regeneration. Cytokines can also be secreted by the liver, reaching extrahepatic targets via the blood-stream. An example is the interaction of cytokines with classical hormones such as glucocorticoids. Third, the liver is the main organ for clearance of circulating cytokines. IL-5 binds preferentially to the surface of periportal hepatocytes, while EGF has been found to bind to hepatocytes, followed by its rapid internalization and degradation. The rapid hepatic clearance of circulating cytokines may constitute an important mechanism limiting the systemic action of cytokines. On the other hand, variation of degradation may modify the intrahepatic action of cytokines. In the regenerating liver, for instance, the lysosomal degradation of EGF is reduced and the cytokine is shifted to hepatocyte nuclei, followed by stimulation of DNA synthesis.

There are, therefore, many aspects to the interactions of cytokines and the liver, and the whole field cannot be discussed in the 2 days of our symposium. We therefore propose to concentrate and focus on two main aspects: new results of basic science on the interaction of cytokines with their target cells, the main topics of which are structure and function of receptors, intracellular signal transduction and signal response, and new results of clinical investigation. The main topics are here the significance of various cytokines in the pathogenesis of hepatitis and cirrhosis, and the function of cytokines in liver regeneration, the acute phase response and liver transplantation.

Karl Decker and myself hope that this symposium will be informative with respect to novel observations, and will stimulate thoughtful hypotheses. Last but not least the symposium should give the opportunity for new contacts between scientists in this area.

Finally, on behalf of the organizers I wish to express our thanks to Dr Herbert Falk, the Falk Foundation and his coworkers behind the scenes for generous support and perfect organization of our symposium.

Part A
Cytokines and their receptors in the liver

Section I
Regulation of synthesis

1
Interleukin-8 and other chemokines: new perspectives in inflammation

M. BAGGIOLINI, M. UGUCCIONI and M. D'APUZZO

INTRODUCTION

Inflammation is a protective response to disturbances of homeostasis induced by a wide variety of exogenous or endogenous agents, and is characterized by the accumulation and activation of leukocytes in the affected tissue. The mechanism of leukocyte recruitment has been studied since leukocyte diapedesis was first observed. A breakthrough came about in recent years with the discovery of interleukin-8 (IL-8) and several related chemotactic cytokines, which are now collectively called chemokines. Decades ago, the characterization of chemotactic agonists, such as anaphylatoxin C5a, microbial N-formylmethionyl peptides, leukotriene B_4 and platelet-activating factor, helped elucidate how leukocytes, and neutrophils in particular, are activated. The properties of these classical chemoattractants, however, did not explain adequately some important aspects of the inflammatory reaction, namely the selectivity for certain leukocytes and the relatively long duration of the recruitment process in vivo. In addition, the generation of chemoattractants in the affected tissue seemed to be conditioned by the import of foreign elements such as bacteria, and/or the extravasation of plasma and leukocytes. IL-8 and related cytokines can arise from the tissues, have higher target cell selectivity, and are long acting, which makes them particularly suited as mediators of inflammation. For this reason many laboratories became interested in chemokines, and progress in the field has been very rapid.

The chemokines[1] are small proteins (70–80 amino acids) with four conserved cysteines linked to disulphide bonds, which are essential for biological activity, a short amino-terminus and a relatively long carboxyl-terminal domain. Two subfamilies are distinguished according to the arrangement of the first two cysteines which are either separated by one amino acid (CXC chemokines) or adjacent (CC chemokines). CXC chemokines act mainly on neutrophil leukocytes, while CC chemokines stimulate monocytes, and, as shown more recently, also basophilic and eosinophilic leukocytes and T lymphocytes. The genes of the two chemokine subfamilies are clustered on different chromosomes, chromosome 4 for the CXC and 17 for the CC chemokines.

CXC CHEMOKINES

IL-8 is generated as a 99 amino acid precursor, and is secreted after cleavage of a leader sequence of 20 residues. The mature protein is processed extracellularly at the amino-terminus leading to a considerable increase in specific activity[2]. Nuclear magnetic resonance spectroscopy shows that IL-8 forms dimers in solution[3]. The monomer has a conformationally disordered amino-terminal domain which is anchored by the disulphide bonds to the core of the molecule, consisting of three antiparallel β-strands followed by a prominent C-terminal α-helix[3]. The disulphide bonds keep the molecule in its active conformation, and the biological activity is immediately lost when the bonds are cleaved by chemical reduction. Until recently, the dimer was believed to be the active form of IL-8. To test this hypothesis, we compared the activity of natural IL-8 and a derivative with an *N*-methylated leucine in position 25 that does not dimerize. This derivative was as active as natural IL-8, showing that dimerization is not necessary, and indicating that IL-8 acts as a monomer[4].

Several analogues of IL-8 were identified in rapid succession: neutrophil-activating protein-2 (NAP-2), which arises from the N-terminal processing of platelet basic protein; three GRO proteins (GROα, GROβ and GROγ) and an epithelial cell-derived neutrophil-activating protein, ENA-78[1]. These are all CXC chemokines and share with IL-8 the properties of neutrophil chemoattractants. They induce a shape change, chemotaxis, a transient rise in intracellular free Ca^{2+} concentration, release of granule contents, up-regulation of adhesion proteins, formation of bioactive lipids, and a respiratory burst[5]. IL-8 and other CXC chemokines were also tested in vivo. After intradermal injection in animals and man, IL-8 induces plasma exudation and the accumulation of massive numbers of neutrophils[6]. Its duration of action in vivo is unusually long, presumably because of resistance to inactivation and binding to matrix glycosaminoglycans. Intravenous administration of IL-8 in baboons led to a rapid, marked neutropenia followed by a rebound granulocytosis, due to demargination[7]. IL-8 is weakly chemotactic for basophils in vitro, but not for monocytes or eosinophils[8–10]. The ability of IL-8 to attract lymphocytes, as reported some years ago[11] is disputed by most laboratories[12], and is not supported by experiments in human volunteers[13]. All other CXC chemokines are less potent than IL-8, and do not appear to act on cells other than neutrophils.

IL-8 receptors

Selective receptors for IL-8 were demonstrated by binding studies with human neutrophils, and shown to be coupled to GTP-binding proteins. In general agreement with other reports, we found that human neutrophils possess approximately $64\,500 \pm 14\,000$ receptors with an apparent K_{d} of $0.18 \pm 0.07\,nM$[14,15]. Radiolabelled IL-8 is displaced by cold IL-8, but also by NAP-2 and GROα. The displacement curve of IL-8 by NAP-2 or GROα is bimodal, revealing the existence of two types of receptors on neutrophils: one with high affinity for all three ligands (K_{d} $0.1-0.3\,nM$), and the other with high affinity for IL-8, but low affinity for NAP-2 and GROα (K_{d} $100-130\,nM$)[14,15].

Desensitization experiments showed that all CXC chemokines share the receptors on neutrophils[1]. The receptor which is selective for IL-8 is termed IL-8R1 or IL-8RA, and the other IL-8R2 or IL-8RB[1].

The cDNAs of two receptors for IL-8 was cloned and shown to code for seven transmembrane domain receptors[16,17]. These results confirmed the evidence provided by functional studies that IL-8 and other CXC chemokines act via rhodopsin-type receptors like all other neutrophil chemotaxins known[1]. The expression of the IL-8-selective and the promiscuous receptors was studied by Northern analysis and reverse transcriptase PCR. The mRNA for the IL-8-selective receptor was found in all white blood cells and related cell lines, as well as, in low copy numbers, in melanoma, melanocyte and fibroblast cell lines, while the mRNA for the promiscuous receptor was detectable in neutrophils and some other myeloid cells only[18]. These results are in agreement with the observation that all CXC chemokines which bind with high affinity to the promiscuous receptor only are even more selective for neutrophils than IL-8[1].

Structural requirements for receptor interaction

The conspicuous carboxyl-terminal α-helix revealed by NMR spectroscopy was originally suggested as the receptor binding domain. Using chemically synthesized analogues, we found that removal of the entire carboxyl-terminal sequence after the fourth cysteine decreased but did not suppress the biological activity of IL-8. In contrast, receptor binding and neutrophil activation were abrogated by deletion[2] or substitution[19] of the amino-terminal sequence Glu-Leu-Arg (ELR) indicating that this motif is essential for receptor recognition and signalling. Interestingly, the ELR motif is common to all CXC chemokines that activate and attract neutrophils, but is not found in other chemokines. A direct demonstration that the ELR motif is essential for CXC chemokine activity on neutrophils was obtained by substituting ELR for the natural DLQ sequence in platelet factor 4 (PF4). ELR-PF4 competes for IL-8 binding, and induces chemotaxis and enzyme release responses in neutrophils similar to those observed with IL-8. On the other hand, the truncated form of PF4 (DLQ-PF4) and IL-8 with ELQ in place of ELR were inactive[20].

After recognition of the importance of the N-terminus, several analogues of the amino-terminally truncated IL-8 were synthesized as potential IL-8 receptor antagonists. Deletions or amino acid replacements in the ELR region led to the envisaged goal. The most potent antagonists identified so far are R-IL-8 and AAR-IL-8, which inhibit IL-8 receptor binding, exocytosis ($IC_{50} = 0.3\,m$M), chemotaxis and the respiratory burst. Inhibition is restricted to responses elicited by IL-8, GROα or NAP-2, and no effect is observed when the unrelated agonists fMet-Leu-Phe or C5a are used as stimuli, demonstrating that they are selective for IL-8 receptors[21].

CC CHEMOKINES

One of the first CC chemokines to be identified and extensively characterized biologically was the monocyte chemotactic protein MCP-1[22]. Several other CC chemokines were identified by cloning and/or purification and sequence analysis, namely LD78[23], Act-2[24], which are generally termed human MIP-1α and MIP-1β, respectively, because of their high degree of amino acid sequence identity with the murine proteins MIP-1α and MIP-1β[25], I-309[26], RANTES[27], HC14[28] which is also termed MCP-2[29], and MCP-3[29]. The structures of most known CC and CXC chemokines are presented in a recent review[1]. The deduced cDNA sequences consist of 92–99 amino acids with characteristic putative leader sequences of 20–25 amino acids. The sequence identities of the mature (biologically active) forms of the CC chemokines with MCP-1 are between 29 and 71%. Computer modelling on the basis of the NMR-derived structure of IL-8 suggests that IL-8 and MCP-1 have a high degree of folding analogy[30].

We have recently compared the activities of the six best known CC chemokines, MCP-1, MCP-2, MCP-3, RANTES, MIP-1α and MIP-1β, on human blood monocytes[31]. All six chemokines elicited a bimodal chemotaxis response in vitro. Highest numbers of migrating cells were obtained with the monocyte chemotactic proteins (MCPs), somewhat lower numbers with RANTES and MIP-1α, and only weak migration with MIP-1β. The most potent attractants were MCP-1 and MIP-1α, which reached maximum efficacy at 0.1 - 1 nM. All CC chemokines also induced the release of granule enzymes from cytochalasin B-pretreated monocytes. Here too, the MCPs were most effective, RANTES and MIP-1α showed moderate activity (about 25% of that of MCP-1), and MIP-1β had only a minimal effect.

Cytosolic free Ca^{2+} changes and exocytosis were used to monitor receptor desensitization. Marked cross-desensitization was observed among MCP-1, MCP-2 and MCP-3 on the one hand, and RANTES, MIP-1α and MIP-1β on the other, indicating receptor sharing within these two subgroups. The responses to RANTES, MIP-1α and MIP-1β were also significantly desensitized by pretreatment with MCP-1, MCP-2 or MCP-3, while the responses to the MCPs were unaffected by pretreatment with RANTES, MIP-1α and MIP-1β. These patterns of desensitization prove the existence of two distinct CC chemokine receptors in monocytes, one recognizing the MCPs, and the other recognizing RANTES, MIP-1α and MIP-1β, as well as the MCPs. There is an interesting difference in the ability of MCP-1 and MCP-3 to desensitize monocytes toward RANTES (or MIP-1α and MIP-1β). While MCP-3 virtually abrogates responsiveness to RANTES, desensitization by MCP-1 reaches only about 50%. These results suggest that RANTES, MIP-1α , MIP-1β and MCP-3 share two distinct receptors, only one of which also recognizes MCP-1. The RANTES receptors, however, are presumably of minor importance in monocyte activation by the MCPs since the responses to MCP-1, MCP-2 or MCP-3 are not appreciably affected by the pretreatment of the monocytes with RANTES.

Actions on basophil and eosinophil leukocytes

In contrast to CXC chemokines, which act almost exclusively on neutrophils, CC chemokines have been shown to exhibit marked effects on basophil and eosinophil leukocytes as well as lymphocytes[32]. Basophil and eosinophil leukocytes bear functional IL-8 receptors as shown by binding studies and $[Ca^{2+}]_i$

changes after stimulation with IL-8[10,33]. The action of IL-8 on basophils, however, is barely detectable unless the cells are primed with hematopoietic growth factors such as GM-CSF or IL-3[34]. The effects of CC chemokines were documented most recently by studies showing that MCP-1 is nearly as effective as C5a and much more potent than IL-8 as a stimulus of exocytosis for human basophils[35–37]. MCP-1 induces high levels of histamine release from normal (i.e. non-primed) cells. After priming with IL-3, IL-5 or GM-CSF, the release of histamine is markedly enhanced, and abundant production of leukotriene C_4 is observed in addition[35,37]. Histamine release was also shown to occur after stimulation with RANTES and MIP-1α, but not with MIP-1β[38–40]. MCP-1 and RANTES elicit mediator release as well as chemotaxis, but differ considerably in their action: MCP-1 is a strong inducer of release and only a moderate chemoattractant, while RANTES is a highly effective chemoattractant and a weak stimulus of release[38]. We recently found that MCP-3 combines the properties of MCP-1 and RANTES toward basophil leukocytes since it is as effective as MCP-1 in inducing mediator release, and as effective as RANTES in inducing chemotaxis. The finding that MCP-3 is a strong stimulus of release was not unexpected given its sequence identity of over 70% with MCP-1. It was surprising, however, to find that MCP-3 has the same chemoattractant properties as RANTES which has only 25% sequence identity.

CC chemokines also activate eosinophil leukocytes. RANTES is a powerful chemoattractant: it compares well with C5a and is 2- to 3-fold more effective than MIP-1α[41,42]. As shown for basophils, however, RANTES is a relatively weak stimulus of exocytosis and leukotriene formation even when the eosinophils are primed[42]. Eosinophils are also activated by MCP-3, which is highly effective as a stimulus of chemotaxis and release (as in basophils), but do not respond to MCP-1[42].

Pathophysiological implications

IL-8 was originally identified in cultures of human blood monocytes and it was then found that most tissue cells and leukocytes, including neutrophils, can express and release IL-8 following appropriate stimulation. IL-1 and TNF induce IL-8 expression in virtually all types of cells. Mononuclear phagocytes, which are a major source of chemokines, respond to a multitude of proinflammatory agents in addition to IL-1 and TNF, including IL-7, GM-CSF and IL-3, lectins, immune complexes and bacteria. Even adherence to plastic, or changes in oxygen partial pressure trigger the production of IL-8[1].

It is well documented that several CXC chemokines are expressed together with IL-8 in a variety of different cells in response to IL-1, TNF, tissue growth factors and viral infection. More selective, differential expression independent of the tissue and the stimulus has been reported, however, and the conditions for the selective expression of a given chemokine will have to be investigated in different pathophysiological processes. The same situation is expected to occur with CC chemokines, where selective expression may well be the basis for differences in the composition of the cellular infiltrate. The existence of so many different chemokines with often redundant chemotactic and activating properties toward leukocytes and lymphocytes indicates that this family of cytokines is essential in the pathophysiology of inflammation and inflammation-related conditions.

In view of the prominence of the chemokine family, future research must consider the possibility that some chemokines may have biological properties in addition to leukocyte activation. If we consider IL-8, which has been studied most thoroughly, we realise that it was recognized early on as a potential mediator of inflammation owing to its ability to attract and activate neutrophils. This role is meanwhile firmly established on the basis of overwhelming evidence documenting activity and mode of action on neutrophils, activity in vivo, expression in disease, etc.[1]. IL-8, in common with other CXC and CC chemokines, has all the essential properties of a mediator of leukocyte recruitment and inflammation. As a product of different types of cells IL-8 can arise focally in any tissue as a result of infection, ischaemia, trauma and other disturbances of tissue homeostasis. Thanks to its resistance to inactivation and its tendency to bind to matrix glycosaminoglycans, IL-8 is cleared only slowly from the tissues, and can thus persist in active form for longer periods of time within the immediate environment of the cells from which it is released.

Considerable effort has been put into the study of potential functions of CXC and CC chemokines on cells other than leukocytes. Since GROα was originally described as the product of a growth-related gene[43], and reported to be mitogenic for melanocytes[44], activities of chemokines on the proliferation of normal and transformed tissue cells were often investigated. It is interesting that tumour cells constitutively produce chemokines which could act in auto- or paracrine fashion[1]. Chemokines have also been studied in the context of tissue repair and remodelling, a process related to growth and inflammation. GROα and IL-8, but no CC chemokines, were shown to inhibit collagen expression in synovial fibroblasts rheumatoid joints[45]. Enhanced expression of CXC chemokines was reported in wounds, tumours and around implants in rats[46] and chickens[47], where tissue repair and neovascularization takes place. Human IL-8 was reported to be angiogenic in the rat cornea[48]. CXC chemokines were reported to attract umbilical vein endothelial cells[48], epidermal cells[49] or melanocytes[50] in vitro. Of obvious interest is the potential action of CXC and CC chemokines on the maturation of white cells. Murine MIP-1α and MIP-1β were reported to act as co-stimulators of committed granulocyte–macrophage progenitor cells together with GM-CSF or CSF-1[51]. MIP-1α, on the other hand was shown to inhibit the proliferation of less mature, IL-3 dependent progenitor cells[52,53], an effect that is prevented by MIP-1β[54]. Some of these effects could eventually turn out to be important. Until now, however, the results are more suggestive than conclusive.

REFERENCES

1. Baggiolini M, Dewald B, Moser B. Interleukin-8 and related chemotactic cytokines – CXC and CC chemokines. Adv Immunol. 1994;55:97–179.
2. Clark-Lewis I, Schumacher C, Baggiolini M, Moser B. Structure-activity relationships of interleukin-8 determined using chemically synthesized analogs. Critical role of NH_2-terminal residues and evidence for uncoupling of neutrophil chemotaxis, exocytosis, and receptor binding activities. J Biol Chem. 1991;266:23128–34.

3. Clore GM, Gronenborn AM. NMR and X-ray analysis of the three-dimensional structure of interleukin-8. In: Baggiolini M, Sorg C, editors. Cytokines Vol. 4. Interleukin-8 (NAP-1) and related chemotactic cytokines. Basel: Karger; 1992:18–40.

4. Rajarathnam K, Sykes BD, Kay CM et al. Neutrophil activation by monomeric interleukin-8. Science. 1994;264:90–2.

5. Baggiolini M, Imboden P, Detmers P. Neutrophil activation and the effects of interleukin-8/neutrophil-activating peptide 1 (IL-8/NAP-1). In Baggiolini M, Sorg C, editors. Cytokines. Vol. 4. Interleukin-8 (NAP-1) and related chemotactic cytokines. Basel: Karger; 1992:1–17.

6. Colditz I, Zwahlen R, Dewald B, Baggiolini M. In vivo inflammatory activity of neutrophil-activating factor, a novel chemotactic peptide derived from human monocytes. Am J Pathol. 1989;134:755–60.

7. Van Zee KJ, Deforge LE, Fischer E et al. IL-8 in septic shock, endotoxemia, and after IL-1 administration. J Immunol. 1991;146:3478–82.

8. Yoshimura T, Matsushima K, Tanaka S et al. Purification of a human monocyte-derived neutrophil chemotactic factor that has peptide sequence similarity to other host defense cytokines. Proc Natl Acad Sci USA. 1987;84:9233–7.

9. Leonard EJ, Skeel A, Yoshimura T, Noer K, Kutvirt S, Van Epps D. Leukocyte specificity and binding of human neutrophil attractant/activation protein-1. J Immunol. 1990;144:1323–30.

10. Krieger M, Brunner T, Bischoff SC et al. Activation of human basophils through the IL-8 receptor. J Immunol. 1992;149:2662–7.

11. Larsen CG, Anderson AO, Appella E, Oppenheim JJ, Matsushima K. The neutrophil-activating protein (NAP-1) is also chemotactic for T lymphocytes. Science. 1989;243:1464–6.

12. Fraser CM. Site-directed mutagenesis of beta-adrenergic receptors. Identification of conserved cysteine residues that independently affect ligand binding and receptor activation. J Biol Chem. 1989;264:9266–70.

13. Leonard EJ, Yoshimura T, Tanaka S, Raffeld M. Neutrophil recruitment by intradermally injected neutrophil attractant/activation protein-1. J Invest Dermatol. 1991;96:690–4.

14. Moser B, Schumacher C, von Tscharner V, Clark-Lewis I, Baggiolini M. Neutrophil-activating peptide 2 and *gro*/melanoma growth-stimulatory activity interact with neutrophil-activating peptide 1/interleukin 8 receptors on human neutrophils. J Biol Chem. 1991;266:10666–71.

15. Schumacher C, Clark-Lewis I, Baggiolini M, Moser B. High- and low-affinity binding of GROα and neutrophil-activating peptide 2 to interleukin 8 receptors on human neutrophils. Proc Natl Acad Sci USA. 1992;89:10542–6.

16. Holmes WE, Lee J, Kuang W-J, Rice GC, Wood WI. Structure and functional expression of a human interleukin-8 receptor. Science. 1991;253:1278–80.

17. Murphy PM, Tiffany HL. Cloning of complementary DNA encoding a functional human interleukin-8 receptor. Science. 1991;253:1280–3.

18. Moser B, Barella L, Mattei S et al. Expression of transcripts for two interleukin 8 receptors in human phagocytes, lymphocytes and melanoma cells. Biochem J. 1993;294:285–92.

19. Hébert CA, Vitangcol RV, Baker JB. Scanning mutagenesis of interleukin-8 identifies a cluster of residues required for receptor binding. J Biol Chem. 1991;266:18989–94.

20. Clark-Lewis I, Dewald B, Geiser T, Moser B, Baggiolini M. Platelet factor 4 binds to interleukin 8 receptors and activates neutrophils when its N terminus is modified with Glu-Leu-Arg. Proc Natl Acad Sci USA. 1993;90:3574–7.

21. Moser B, Dewald B, Barella L, Schumacher C, Baggiolini M, Clark-Lewis I. Interleukin-8 antagonists generated by N-terminal modification. J Biol Chem. 1993;268:7125–8.

22. Yoshimura T, Leonard EJ. Human monocyte chemoattractant protein-1: Structure and function. In: Baggiolini M, Sorg C, editors. Cytokines. Vol. 4. Interleukin-8 (NAP-1) and related chemotactic cytokines. Basel: Karger; 1992:131–52.

23. Obaru K, Fukuda M, Maeda S, Shimada K. cDNA clone used to study mRNA inducible in human tonsillar lymphocytes by a tumor promoter. J Biochem (Tokyo). 1986;99:885–94.

24. Lipes MA, Napolitano M, Jeang KT, Chang NT, Leonard WJ. Identification, cloning, and characterization of an immune activation gene. Proc Natl Acad Sci USA. 1988;85:9704–8.

25. Wolpe SD, Davatelis G, Sherry B et al. Macrophages secrete a novel heparin-binding protein with inflammatory and neutrophil chemokinetic properties. J Exp Med. 1988;167:570–81.

26. Miller MD, Hata S, De Waal Malefyt R, Krangel MS. A novel polypeptide secreted by activated human T lymphocytes. J Immunol. 1989;143:2907–16.

27. Schall TJ, Jongstra J, Dyer BJ et al. A human T cell-specific molecule is a member of a new gene family. J Immunol. 1988;141:1018–25.

28. Chang HC, Hsu F, Freeman GJ, Griffin JD, Reinherz EL. Cloning and expression of a gamma-interferon-inducible gene in monocytes: a new member of a cytokine gene family. Int Immunol. 1989;1:388–97.

29. Van Damme J, Proost P, Lenaerts J-P, Opdenakker G. Structural and functional identification of two human, tumour-derived monocyte chemotactic proteins (MCP-2 and MCP-3) belonging to the chemokine family. J Exp Med. 1992;176:59–65.

30. Gronenborn AM, Clore GM. Modeling the three-dimensional structure of the monocyte chemo-attractant and activating protein MCAF/MC-1 on the basis of the solution structure of interleukin-8. Protein Eng. 1991;4:263–9.

31. Uguccioni M, D'Apuzzo M, Loetscher M, Dewald B, Baggiolini M. Action of the chemotactic cytokines MCP-1, MCP-2, MCP-3, RANTES, MIP-1α and MIP-1β on human monocytes. Eur J Immunol. 1995;(in press).

32. Baggiolini M, Dahinden CA. CC chemokines in allergic inflammation. Immunol Today. 1994;15:127–33.

33. Kernen P, Wymann MP, von Tscharner V et al. Shape changes, exocytosis, and cytosolic free calcium changes in stimulated human eosinophils. J Clin Invest. 1991;87:2012–7.

34. Dahinden CA, Kurimoto Y, De Weck AL, Lindley I, Dewald B, Baggiolini M. The neutrophil-activating peptide NAF/NAP-1 induces histamine and leukotriene release by interleukin 3-primed basophils. J Exp Med. 1989;170:1787–92.

35. Kuna P, Rddigari SR, Rucinski D, Openheim JJ, Kaplan AP. Monocyte chemotactic and activating factor is a potent histamine-releasing factor for human basophils. J Exp Med. 1992;175:489–93.

36. Alam R, Lett-Brown MA, Forsythe PA et al. Monocyte chemotactic and activating factor is a potent histamine-releasing factor for basophils. J Clin Invest. 1992;89:723–8.

37. Bischoff SC, Krieger M, Brunner T, Dahinden CA. Monocyte chemotactic protein 1 is a potent activator of human basophils. J Exp Med. 1992;175:1271–5.

38. Bischoff SC, Krieger M, Brunner T et al. RANTES and related chemokines activate human basophil granulocytes through different G protein-coupled receptors. Eur J Immunol. 1992;23:761–7.

39. Kuna P, Reddigari SR, Schall TJ, Rucinski D, Viksman MY, Kaplan AP. RANTES, a monocyte and T lymphocyte chemotactic cytokine releases histamine from human basophils. J Immunol. 1992;149:636–42.

40. Alam R, Forsythe PA, Stafford S, Lett-Brown MA, Grant JA. Macrophage inflammatory protein-1α activates basophils and mast cells. J Exp Med. 1992;176:781–6.

41. Kameyoshi Y, Dörschner A, Mallet AI, Christophers E, Schröder J-M. Cytokine RANTES released by thrombin-stimulated platelets is a potent attractant for human eosinophils. J Exp Med. 1992;176:587–92.

42. Rot A, Krieger M, Brunner T, Bischoff SC, Schall TJ, Dahinden CA. RANTES and macrophage inflammatory protein 1α induce the migration and activation of normal human eosinophil granulocytes. J Exp Med. 1992;176:1489–95.

43. Anisowicz A, Bardwell L, Sager R. Constitutive overexpression of a growth-related gene in transformed Chinese hamster and human cells. Proc Natl Acad Sci USA. 1987;84:7188–92.

44. Richmond A, Thomas HG. Melanoma growth stimulatory activity: Isolation from human melanoma tumours and characterization of tissue distribution. J Cell Biochem. 1988;36:185–98.

45. Unemori EN, Amento EP, Bauer EA, Horuk R. Melanoma growth-stimulatory activity/GRO decreases collagen expression by human fibroblasts. Regulation by C-X-C but not C-C cytokines. J Biol Chem. 1993;268:1338–42.

46. Iida N, Grotendorst GR. Cloning and sequencing of a new *gro* transcript from activated human monocytes: Expression in leukocytes and wound tissue. Mol Cell Biol. 1990;10:5596–9.

47. Martins-Green M, Bissell MJ. Localization of 9E3/CEF-4 in avian tissues: expression is absent in Rous sarcoma virus-induced tumours but is stimulated by injury. J Cell Biol. 1990;110:581–95.

48. Koch AE, Polverini PJ, Kunkel SL et al. Interleukin-8 as a macrophage-derived mediator of angiogenesis. Science. 1992;258:1798–801.

49. Michel G, Kemény L, Peter RU, Beetz A, Ried C, Arenberger P, Ruzicka T. Interleukin-8 receptor-mediated chemotaxis of normal human epidermal cells. FEBS Lett. 1992;305:241–3.

50. Wang JM, Taraboletti G, Matsushima K, Van Damme J, Mantovani A. Induction of haptotactic migration of melanoma cells by neutrophil activating protein/interleukin-8. Biochem Biophys Res Commun. 1990;169:165–70.

51. Broxmeyer HE, Sherry B, Lu L et al. Myelopoietic enhancing effects of murine macrophage inflammatory proteins 1 and 2 on colony formation in vitro by murine and human bone marrow granulocyte/macrophage progenitor cells. J Exp Med. 1989;170:1583–94.
52. Broxmeyer HE, Sherry B, Lu L et al. Enhancing and suppressing effects of recombinant murine macrophage inflammatory proteins on colony formation in vitro by bone marrow myeloid progenitor cells. Blood. 1990;76:1110–6.
53. Graham GJ, Wright EG, Hewick R et al. Identification and characterization of an inhibitor of haemopoietic stem cell proliferation. Nature. 1990;344:442–4.
54. Broxmeyer HE, Sherry B, Cooper S et al. Macrophage inflammatory protein (MIP)-1β abrogates the capacity of MIP-1α to suppress myeloid progenitor cell growth. J Immunol. 1991;147: 2586–94.

2
IL-6 signal transduction from the plasma membrane to the nucleus

F. HORN, C. LÜTTICKEN, U. WEGENKA, J. YUAN and
P. C. HEINRICH

THE ACUTE PHASE RESPONSE OF THE LIVER

The response of the organism to disturbances of its physiological homeostasis by tissue injury and infection consists of a number of complex defence reactions. Besides the activation of the endocrine and immune systems, the liver responds with an altered synthesis and secretion of a group of proteins, the so called acute phase proteins[1]. Cytokines, in particular interleukin (IL)-6 and IL-1, and glucocorticoids have been found to be the mediators responsible for the regulation of acute phase proteins in hepatocytes[2]. Two classes of acute phase proteins seem to exist[3]. As shown in Table 1 class I acute phase proteins are regulated by IL-1 and/or IL-6, whereas class II acute phase proteins are regulated by IL-6 and glucocorticoids.

Table 1 Classification of acute phase proteins

Class I acute phase protein genes (induced by IL-1 or IL-1 and IL-6)
α_1-acid glycoprotein
angiotensinogen
C-reactive protein (only in the human system)
haptoglobin
haemopexin
complement factor B
complement factor C
serum amyloid A

Class II acute phase protein genes (induced mainly by IL-6)
α_1-antichymotrypsin
α_2-macroglobulin (only in the rat)
α-fibrinogen
β-fibrinogen
γ-fibrinogen
T-kininogen (only in the rat)

IL-6 AND ITS RECEPTOR

IL-6 is produced by many different cells, particularly monocytes/macrophages, endothelial cells and fibroblasts[4,5]. Although hepatocytes are major target cells for IL-6, the cytokine shows a pleiotropic spectrum of action. As a differentiation and growth factor it is involved in the immune response, haematopoiesis and neural differentiation. IL-6 belongs to a family of the so called α-helical cytokines, the members of which are characterized by a high α-helix content and four antiparallel helices[6].

IL-6 exerts its action via a plasma membrane receptor complex consisting of an IL-6 binding subunit (gp80)[7], which after limited proteolysis also exists as a soluble form[8], and a signal transducing protein (gp130)[9]. After binding of IL-6 to gp80, the complex of IL-6 and gp80 interacts with gp130 and leads to its dimerization[10] and signalling. gp80 alone is not capable of eliciting a signal to the cell nucleus[8]. A soluble form of gp80 also exists but, in contrast to many other soluble cytokine receptors which show an antagonistic action, soluble IL-6 receptor/IL-6 complexes bind to gp130 and act agonistically[11].

ACUTE PHASE RESPONSE FACTOR (APRF)

The acute phase response element (APRE) in the promoter of the rat α_2-macroglobulin gene was identified by several laboratories[12–14]. This element is characterized by two homologous sequence motifs, CTGGAA and CTGGGA. We used a synthetic oligonucleotide containing the proximal motif, CTGGGA, as a probe in gel retardation assays in order to identify IL-6-activated transcription factors. Lipopolysaccharide (LPS) from *Escherichia coli* was injected i.p. into rats, and nuclear extracts were prepared from livers at different times thereafter. Gel retardation experiments showed the transient activation of a novel nuclear factor which we call the acute phase response factor, APRF[15]. Maximal APRF activation occurred 1 h after LPS injection. Injection of IL-6 also resulted in the activation of APRF but in this case the activation was faster: active APRF was detected within 15 min. IL-6-induced activation of APRF was also demonstrated in human hepatoma cells (HepG2) in vitro[15], as well as in many other cells which are target cells for IL-6, e.g. fibroblasts, monocytes, myeloma cells and hepatocytes[16]. This observation indicates that the IL-6-dependent activation of APRF is a ubiquitous phenomenon. Since the receptors for IL-11, leukaemia inhibitory factor (LIF), oncostatin M (OSM) and ciliary neurotrophic factor (CNTF) share the signal transducer gp130 with the IL-6 receptor[17–19], and since these cytokines have been found to also induce acute phase protein synthesis in liver cells[20–22], we examined whether these 'IL-6-type' cytokines are also capable of activating APRF. Indeed, all four cytokines induced the rapid APRF activation in rat hepatocytes[16]. Binding of APRF was also demonstrated for IL-6 response elements of various other acute phase protein genes[15]. From comparison of the identified APRF binding sites, a palindromic consensus binding sequence $TT^C/_ACNG^G/_TAA$, was deduced (Fig. 1). Furthermore, based on this consensus we demonstrated binding of APRF also to IL-6 response elements of several IL-6-induced immediate early genes, including the intercellular adhesion molecule-1 (ICAM-1), interferon regulatory

T	C	C	T	T	C	T	G	G	G	A	A	T	T	C		rat α_2M, -175/-161
C	A	G	T	A	A	C	T	G	G	A	A	A	A	T		rat α_2M, -198/-184
C	T	C	T	T	A	C	G	G	G	A	A	T	G	G		human α_2M, -229/-215
G	C	T	G	T	A	C	G	G	T	A	A	A	A	G		human α_2M, -249/-234
G	G	C	T	T	C	T	G	G	G	A	A	A	A	A		rat α_1-acid glycoprotein ("C")
T	T	G	T	T	A	C	T	G	G	A	A	A	A	G		human haptoglobin ("B")
C	A	T	G	T	A	C	T	G	G	A	A	G	A	A		human γ-fibrinogen, -293/-279
A	A	T	T	T	C	T	G	G	T	A	A	T	A	G		human α_1-antichymotrypsin, -114/-128

Palindromic consensus: T T $\frac{C}{A}$ C N G $\frac{G}{T}$ A A — palindromic consensus

Fig. 1 Sequence comparison of APRF binding sites in different promoters. APRF binding sites defined by gel retardation assays in the 5′-flanking regions of the rat α_2-macroglobulin (α_2M) and α_1-acid glycoprotein genes, and of the human genes for α_2-macroglobulin, haptoglobin, γ-fibrinogen, and α_1-antichymotrypsin were aligned[15]. The shaded boxes indicate the homology to a palindromic consensus sequence derived from these sites

factor-1 (IRF-1), and junB[23]. These findings suggest a more general role of APRF in the regulation of IL-6 target genes.

Purification of APRF

In order to further characterize APRF we purified the transcription factor from rat liver nuclei obtained from rats treated with LPS. Nuclear protein (100 mg) was subjected to heparin–Sepharose and subsequent affinity chromatography. The affinity resin was obtained by coupling multimerized, biotinylated oligonucleotides containing palindromic APRF binding sites to streptavidin–agarose. The purified protein was homogeneous upon SDS-PAGE and silver staining and exhibited a molecular mass of 87 kDa[16]. After cleavage with cyanogen bromide, two peptides separated by HPLC were sequenced: peptide 1: MLEQHLQNVRKRVQDLE; peptide 2: MKVVENLQD. These sequences were not found in protein data banks, indicating that APRF represents a new transcription factor.

Recently, Zhong et al.[24] published the cDNA cloning of murine Stat3. Interestingly, both of our APRF peptide sequences are present in the Stat3 sequence indicating that APRF is identical to Stat3. Cloning of an APRF cDNA by Akira et al.[25] also confirmed the identity of Stat3 and APRF.

Activation of APRF occurs in the cytoplasm and is a post-translational event

The rapid activation of APRF suggested that de novo synthesis may not be necessary for the IL-6-induced APRF activation. Indeed, a 1 h preincubation of HepG2 cells with the protein synthesis inhibitor cycloheximide did not affect IL-6-induced APRF activation[15]. We concluded from this observation that APRF exists in a latent inactive form and that its activation occurs post-translationally. We also demonstrated that APRF activation in HepG2 cells is likely to occur in the cytoplasm and to be followed by nuclear translocation[15]. Many transcription factors are regulated by protein phosphorylation/dephosphorylation processes. In order to test whether APRF is also phosphorylated we incubated nuclear extracts from livers of LPS-treated rats with alkaline phosphatase. Binding of APRF to the APRE was completely abolished by this treatment[15]. Furthermore, preincubation of HepG2 cells with the tyrosine phosphatase inhibitor orthovanadate caused a stronger and longer lasting activation of APRF by IL-6[15]. These results strongly suggest that phosphorylation events are involved in APRF activation.

Tyrosine phosphorylation of APRF

The question of which protein kinases are involved in the IL-6-induced APRF activation was addressed using a panel of protein kinase inhibitors. While various inhibitors of serine/threonine kinases did not prevent APRF activation the protein tyrosine kinase inhibitors genistein and tyrphostin, and staurosporin at high concentrations, blocked IL-6-dependent APRF activation in HepG2 cells[16]. To analyse whether APRF itself is a substrate for protein tyrosine kinases we incubated activated APRF with monoclonal antibodies to phosphotyrosine. This treatment inhibited APRF binding to DNA as shown by a gel retardation experiment[26], showing that phosphotyrosine residues are present in the APRF molecule.

Binding of interferon-γ activated factor (GAF) to the APRE

We and others have found that interferon-γ (IFN-γ) is also capable of stimulating α_2-macroglobulin synthesis in rat hepatocytes and HepG2 cells[23,27]. We therefore examined whether IFN-γ can also induce the α_2M promoter fused to the reporter gene CAT in transiently transfected HepG2 cells. As shown in Figure 2, a 4-fold increase in CAT expression was observed. Deletion of the APRE led, as in the case of IL-6, to a loss of CAT induction by IFN-γ indicating that this element is also responsible for the effect of IFNγ on the α_2M promoter.

To determine whether APRF is also activated by IFN-γ or whether another IFN-γ-activated factor binds to the APRE, nuclear extracts from IFN-γ-treated HepG2 cells were incubated with the proximal IL-6-responsive element of the α_2M promoter and subjected to a gel retardation experiment. As shown in Figure 3A a retarded band with slightly higher mobility than the APRF-DNA complex was detected. Compared to the APRF activation by IL-6 the kinetics of activation was different: as in the case of APRF the activation was rapid, but the signal remained high for at least 4h (Fig. 3B). Similar experiments to those described above for APRF showed that cycloheximide does not affect the activation of this factor and that a tyrosine kinase is involved in its activation[23].

IFN-γ has been described as activating a transcription factor called IFN-γ-activated factor (GAF) in fibroblasts and HeLa cells[28]. GAF is formed by a homodimer of the Stat91 protein which is phosphorylated at tyrosine in response to IFN-γ[29]. Using antibodies to Stat91, we could show that the APRE-binding

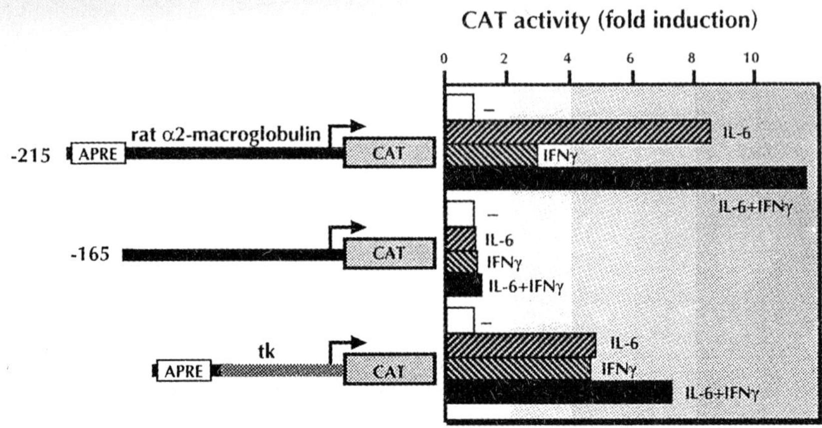

Fig. 2 Stimulation of the α_2-macroglobulin promoter by IFN-γ. HepG2 cells were transiently transfected by the calcium phosphate co-precipitation method with 15 μg of the plasmids pα_2M-215CAT, pα_2M-165CAT, or pα_2M-APREtkCAT and 2 μg of the β-galactosidase expression vector pCH110 as internal control for transfection efficiency. pα_2M-215CAT and pα_2M-165CAT contain 215 and 165 base pairs, respectively of the 5′-flanking region of the rat α_2-macroglobulin gene fused to the bacterial chloramphenicol acetyl transferase (CAT) gene. pα_2M-APREtkCAT contains the APRE of the same promoter fused to the herpes virus thymidine kinase (tk) promoter and the CAT gene. One day post-transfection, the cells were treated with either IL-6 (100 units/ml) or IFN-γ (500 units/ml) and incubation was continued for another 24h. Then the cells were harvested and β-galactosidase and CAT activities were determined in the protein extracts. CAT activities were normalized to β-galactosidase. The induction of CAT activity in cytokine-treated over untreated control cells is shown[23]

factor activated by IFN-γ in HepG2 cells is identical to GAF/Stat91[23]. We corroborated this observation by purifying the factor by affinity chromatography[23].

The observation that GAF/Stat91 binds to the APRE of the α_2M promoter raised the question whether there exists an accidental overlap in binding specificities for GAF and APRF or whether both transcription factors recognize similar sequences. We therefore carried out gel retardation experiments with various known IL-6 and IFN-γ-responsive elements of acute phase protein and IFN-γ target genes. As summarized in Figure 4, APRF and GAF exhibit essentially identical sequence specificities, except that GAF showed a slightly higher preference in binding to the IFP53 and GBP-GAS elements[23].

IL-6-INDUCED TYROSINE PHOSPHORYLATION OF APRF AND Stat91

The nearly identical sequence specificities and similarities in their activation mechanisms suggested that APRF and GAF/Stat91 may be closely related transcription factors. We tested several antisera raised against Stat91 for a cross-reactivity with APRF. While most antisera did not cross-react, antibodies recognizing the N-terminus of Stat91 gave rise to supershift formation with APRF-DNA complexes in gel retardation experiments[16]. Furthermore, APRF

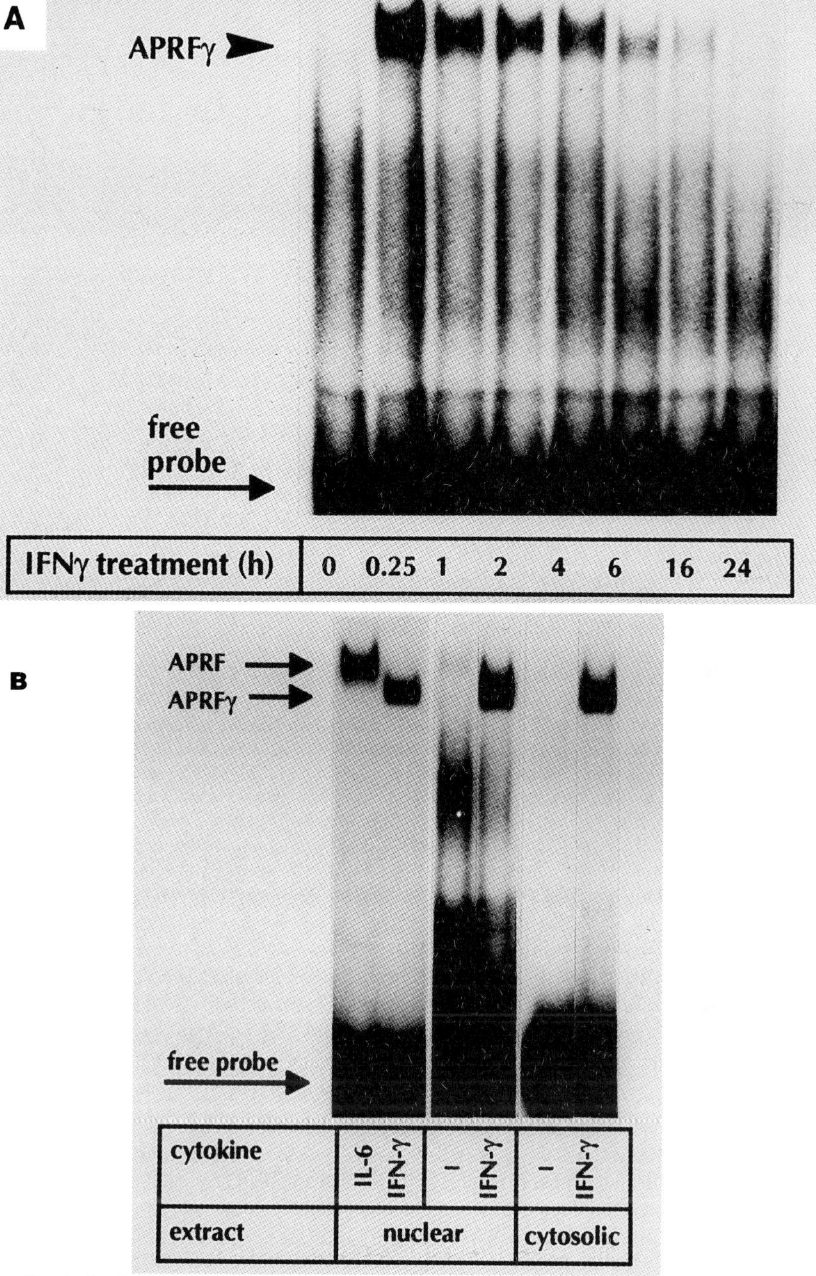

Fig. 3 Activation of an APRE-binding protein by IFN-γ in HepG2 cells. (**A**) HepG2 cells were treated with IFN-γ (500 units/ml medium). After the time indicated, the cells were harvested and nuclear extracts prepared. 5 μg of nuclear protein were incubated with the double-stranded ^{32}P-labelled α_2-macroglobulin APRE 'CTGGGA' probe. Subsequently, the DNA–protein complexes formed were separated on a native 4% polyacrylamide gel. After drying, the gel was exposed overnight to X-ray film. The complex formed by an IFN-γ-activated factor is indicated as APRFγ. This factor was later identified as GAF[23]. (**B**) HepG2 cells were treated for 15 min with IL-6 (100 units/ml medium) or IFN-γ (500 units/ml). Nuclear and cytosolic extracts were prepared and subjected to a gel retardation assay as described in (**A**)

															palindromes	binding of APRF	GAF
			T	T	C	C		G	G	A	A				palindromes		
			T	T	A	C	N	G	T	A	A						
			T	T	C	T		A	G	A	A						
T	C	C	T	T	C	T	G	G	G	A	A	T	T	C	rat α_2M, IL-6RE	+	+
C	A	G	T	A	A	C	T	G	G	A	A	A	G	T	human α_2M, IL-6RE	+	+
C	T	C	T	T	A	C	G	G	G	A	A	T	G	G	human α_2M, IL-6RE	+	+
G	C	T	G	T	A	C	G	G	T	A	A	A	A	G		+	+
G	G	C	T	T	C	T	G	G	G	A	A	A	A	A	rat α_1-AGP, distal IL-6RE	+	+
T	T	G	T	T	A	C	T	G	G	A	A	A	A	G	human haptoglobin, IL-6RE	+	ND
C	A	T	G	T	A	C	T	G	G	A	A	G	A	A	human γ-fibrinogen, IL-6RE	+	+
A	A	T	T	T	C	T	G	G	T	A	A	T	A	C	human α_1-ACT, IL-6RE	+	ND
C	A	C	T	G	T	C	A	G	G	A	A	G	C	G	murine junB, IL-6RE	+	ND
	G	T	T	A	C	G	G	G	A	A	T	A	T		human Ly-6E/A, IFN-γRE	+	+
T	G	T	T	T	C	T	G	A	G	A	A	T	C	T	human IFP 53, IFN-γRE	+	+
G	G	T	T	T	C	C	G	G	G	A	A	A	G	C	human ICAM-1, IFN-γRE	+	+
C	A	T	T	T	C	G	G	G	G	A	A	A	T	C	human IRF-1, IFN-γRE	+	+
C	T	T	T	T	C	T	G	G	G	A	A	A	T	A	human FcγRI, IFN-γRE	ND	+
G	A	T	T	T	A	G	A	G	T	A	A	T	A	T	human GBP, GAS	(+)	+
T	C	T	T	T	C	C	G	A	G	A	A	A	T	C	human ICSBP, IFN-γRE	ND	+
G	A	T	T	G	A	C	G	G	G	A	A	C	T	G	human c-fos, sis-ind. element	+	+

Fig. 4 Sequence comparison of APRF and GAF binding sites present in the promoters of various IL-6- or IFN-γ-inducible genes. APRF and GAF binding sites in IL-6 response elements (IL-6RE) and IFN-γ response elements (IFN-γRE) of the rat α_2-macroglobulin (α_2M) and α_1-acid glycoprotein (α_1-AGP) genes, of the human genes for α_2M, haptoglobin, γ-fibrinogen, α_1-antichymotrypsin (α_1-ACT), guanylate binding protein 1 (GBP), Ly6E/A, interferon consensus sequence binding protein (ICSBP), Fcγ receptor I (FcγRI) and IFP 53/tryptophanyl tRNA synthetase, and of the murine *junB* promoter were aligned[23]. Also shown is the c-*fos* gene sis-induced element which also binds both factors[23]. The shaded boxes indicate the homology to the palindromic motifs shown at top. ND: not determined

purified to homogeneity from ^{32}P-labelled IL-6-stimulated HepG2 cells was immunoprecipitated with this anti-Stat91 antiserum[16]. These findings demonstrated a cross-reactivity of this antiserum with APRF and indicated for the first time that APRF is likely to be a new member of the STAT family. Using the cross-reacting antiserum we immunoprecipitated APRF and Stat91 from ^{32}P-labelled IL-6-stimulated HepG2 cells. Phosphoamino acid analysis of APRF showed the presence of phosphotyrosine and phosphoserine, but no phosphothreonine in activated APRF. Immunoblots using antibodies to phosphotyrosine demonstrated that both APRF and Stat91 are tyrosine phosphorylated in response to IL-6 in HepG2 cells[26].

Association of APRF with the IL-6 receptor subunit gp130

As shown by Murakami et al.[30] the signal transducing subunit gp130 of the IL-6 receptor is rapidly phosphorylated at tyrosine after binding of IL-6. We observed the co-precipitation of a tyrosine phosphorylated 145 kDa protein when APRF was immunoprecipitated from IL-6-treated HepG2 cells. As shown in Figure 5A,

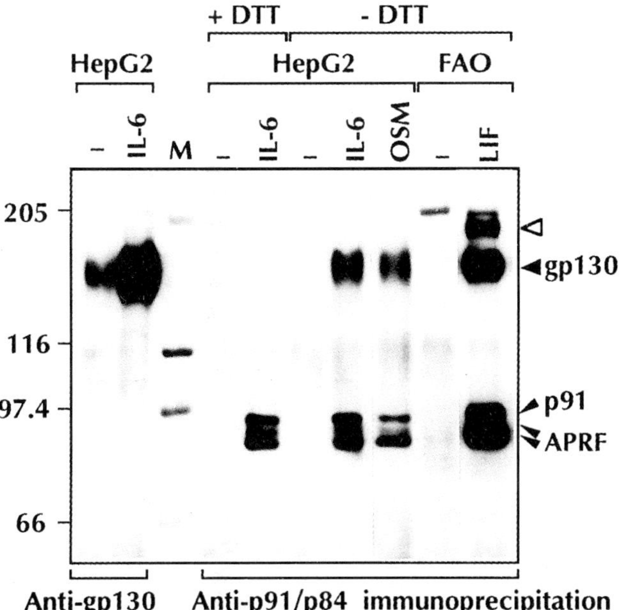

Fig. 5 IL-6-induced association of APRF and gp130. (**A**) HepG2 or FAO (rat hepatoma) cells were incubated for 10 min with IL-6 (200 U/ml), oncostatin M (20 ng/ml) or LIF (25 ng/ml). Lysates were prepared either in the absence or presence of 1 mM dithiothreitol (DTT). Immunoprecipitation was performed with monoclonal antibodies to gp130 or anti-Stat91/84. After SDS–PAGE immunoblotting with phosphotyrosine antibodies was carried out. The open arrow head marks a 190 kDa phosphoprotein which probably corresponds to the LIF receptor[26]. (**B**) Since the gp130 antibodies did not recognize the denatured protein on membranes, indirect proof of the identity of the co-precipitated 145 kDa band with gp130 was necessary. An anti-Stat91/84 immunoprecipitate from IL-6-precipitated HepG2 cells (see A) was bound to protein A-Sepharose and subsequently washed with lysis buffer first without (lane 3) and then with 1 mM DTT (lane 4). The supernatants of both washes were then immunoprecipitated with an anti-gp130 antibody and after SDS–PAGE analysed by anti-phosphotyrosine immunoblotting. For comparison anti-gp130 (lane 1) or anti-Stat91/84 (lane 2) immunoprecipitates from IL-6-stimulated HepG2 cells were applied directly[26]

this protein exhibited the same mobility upon SDS-PAGE as tyrosine-phosphorylated gp130[26]. Co-precipitation of APRF and the 145 kDa phosphoprotein was only observed when the immunoprecipitation was carried out under non-reducing conditions, whereas addition of dithiothreitol to the lysis buffer abolished the co-precipitation. To unambiguously demonstrate an association of APRF with gp130, we first immunoprecipitated the lysate of IL-6-stimulated HepG2 cells under non-reducing conditions with antiserum to Stat91. The immunoprecipitate was then treated with dithiothreitol to remove gp130 from the complex. From the supernatant tyrosine phosphorylated gp130 was then immunoprecipitated by antibodies to gp130 (Fig. 5B).

Since no gp130 was co-precipitated from unstimulated cells, we conclude that the association of APRF with gp130 is ligand-induced. The same observation was made with oncostatin M-treated HepG2 as well as with LIF-treated rat hepatoma cells (Fao cells). In the latter case the LIF-receptor was also co-precipitated in addition to gp130 (Fig. 5A, open arrowhead)[26].

IL-6-induced tyrosine phosphorylation of protein tyrosine kinases of the JAK family

A protein tyrosine kinase activity is known to be co-immunoprecipitated with gp130 from IL-6-stimulated cells[31]; however, the nature of this kinase was unknown. A new class of protein tyrosine kinases, the so-called JAK family, has recently been discovered to be involved in the signal transduction of IFN-α and -γ[32,33]. Based on the similarities of the activation of STAT factors by IFN-γ and of APRF by IL-6, we investigated the role of members of the JAK family in IL-6 signalling. There was a rapid activation of tyrosine phosphorylation of Jak1 and Tyk2 in IL-6-treated HepG2 cells (Fig. 6)[26].

Since the IL-6-type cytokines oncostatin M, LIF, IL-11 and CNTF all signal via gp30 and activate APRF[23], it was of interest to examine whether these cytokines also activate Jak1 by tyrosine phosphorylation. In fact, tyrosine phosphorylation of Jak1 was observed in response to OSM, CNTF, LIF, IL-11 and also IFN-γ, although to rather different extents (Fig. 7).

Association of Jak1 with gp130

The IL-6-induced activation of JAK kinases suggested a role for these enzymes in IL-6 signalling. Co-precipitation of Jak1 and gp130 with corresponding antibodies was observed, although the signals were rather weak. We therefore used a membrane-permeable cleavable cross-linker (dithio-succinimidyl-propionic acid) to covalently link the proteins. After immunoprecipitation and cleavage by 2-mercaptoethanol an association of Jak1 and gp130 could clearly be demonstrated by immunoblotting (Fig. 8). It is remarkable that even in the absence of IL-6 the association of Jak1 with gp130 was evident[26]. Jak1 is, therefore, constitutively associated with gp130.

A Anti-JAK1 immunoprecipitation

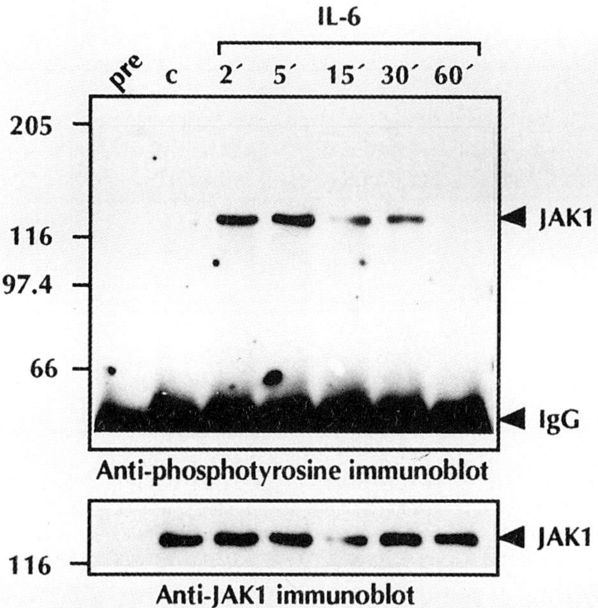

B Anti-tyk2 immunoprecipitation

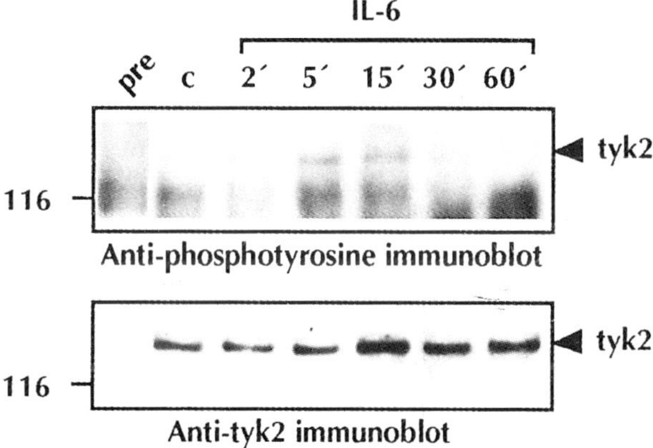

Fig. 6 IL-6-induced tyrosine phosphorylation of Jak1 and Tyk2. HepG2 cells were incubated with IL-6 (200 U/ml) for the times indicated, and all lysates were immunoprecipitated with antibodies against Jak1 (**A**) or Tyk2 (**B**). After SDS–PAGE phosphotyrosine immunoblots were performed. Immunoprecipitations with pre-immune serum ('pre', left lane) served as controls. The membranes were subsequently immunoblotted with anti-Jak1 or anti-Tyk2 to control equal protein loading[26]

Anti-phosphotyrosine immunoblots

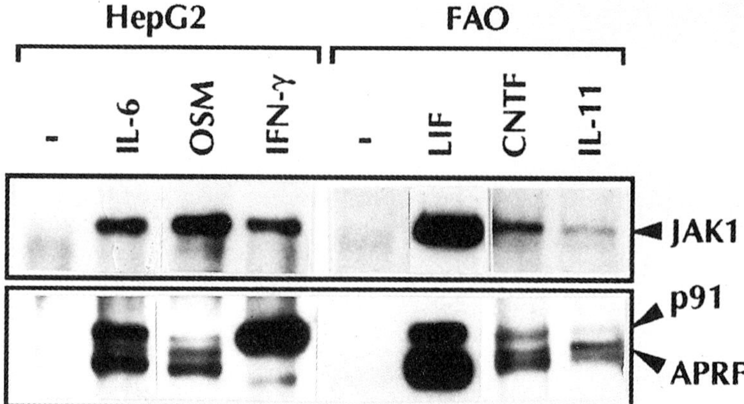

Fig. 7 Tyrosine phosphorylation of Jak1, APRF and Stat91 by different cytokines. HepG2 or FAO cells were stimulated with IL-6 (200 U/ml), oncostatin M (20 ng/ml), IFN-γ (25 ng/ml), LIF (25 ng/ml), CNTF (20 ng/ml) or IL-11 (50 ng/ml) and lysed. Lysates were immunoprecipitated with anti-Jak1 (upper part) or anti-Stat91/84 (lower part) and analysed by immunoblotting with phosphotyrosine antibodies[26]

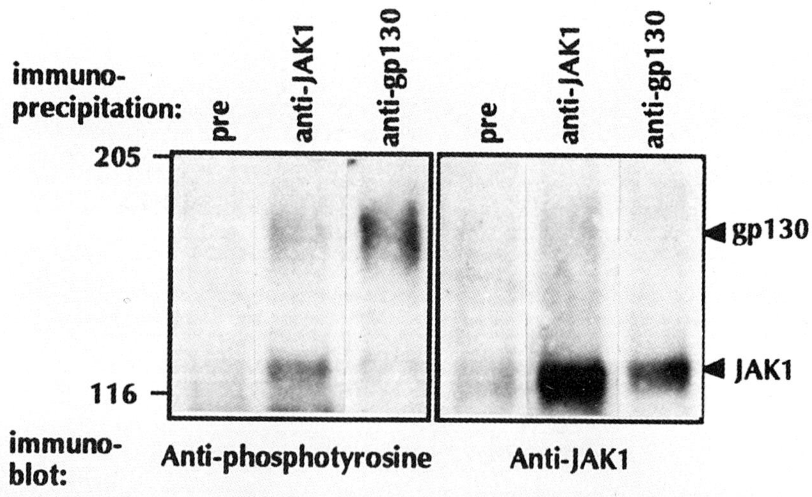

Fig. 8 Association of Jak1 and gp130. Unstimulated HepG2 cells (right panel) or HepG2 cells incubated with IL-6 (200 U/ml) for 5 min (left panel) were washed with ice-cold phosphate buffered saline and incubated at 4°C for 30 min with the cross-linker dithiobis-succinimidylpropionate (0.5 mM). Cell lysates were subsequently either immunoprecipitated with pre-immune serum ('pre'), anti-Jak1 or anti-gp130 antiserum. The cross-linker was cleaved by boiling in SDS-sample buffer with 2-mercaptoethanol. The proteins separated by SDS–PAGE were analysed by immunoblotting with anti-phosphotyrosine (left) or anti-Jak1 (right) antisera[26]

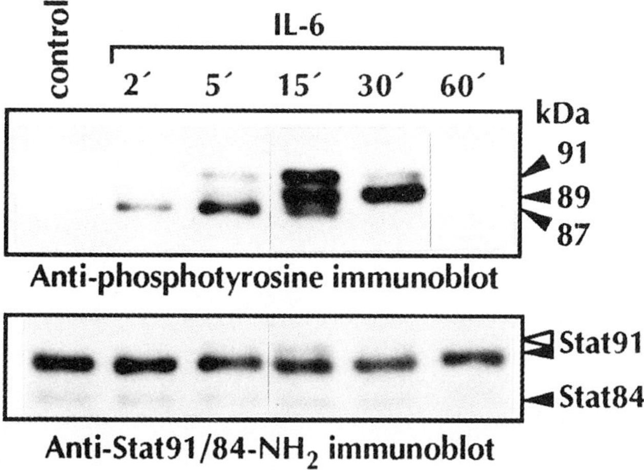

Fig. 9 Time course of APRF tyrosine phosphorylation and activation. HepG2 cells were treated with IL-6 (200 U/ml) for various periods and lysed. The lysates were immunoprecipitated with anti-Stat91/84, the immune complexes separated by SDS–PAGE on a 6% gel, electroblotted to polyvinyldifluoride membrane, and analysed with antibodies to phosphotyrosine (upper panel) and with anti-Stat91/84 to control equal protein loading (lower panel)[16]

ROLE OF PROTEIN SERINE/THREONINE KINASES DURING THE INDUCTION OF IL-6 TARGET GENES

Serine/threonine kinase inhibitors did not affect the IL-6-induced tyrosine phosphorylation and DNA-binding of APRF[16]. However, phosphoamino acid analysis of APRF after IL-6 stimulation of HepG2 cells had clearly shown a serine phosphorylation of the factor. We therefore investigated a possible role of serine phosphorylation in the induction of IL-6 target genes. In transient transfection experiments in HepG2 cells, the induction of reporter genes from various IL-6-responsive promoters, i.e. the promoters of the α_2-macroglobulin, ICAM-1 and junB genes, was blocked by the serine/threonine-kinase inhibitor H7 (unpublished results). This observation indicates that in addition to the APRF binding to its enhancer an H7-sensitive process plays an important role in the transactivation of IL-6 target genes.

IL-6 induces serine phosphorylation of APRF

When the time course of the IL-6-induced APRF activation in HepG2 cells was studied by immunoprecipitation of APRF a mobility shift of the APRF band from 87 kDa to a slower migrating form (89 kDa) was found to occur between 10 and 15 min (Fig. 9). This mobility shift is due to an IL-6-induced serine phosphorylation of APRF which is prevented by preincubation of HepG2 cells with H7. Furthermore, the 89 kDa-form of APRF was transformed into the 87 kDa-form by phosphatase 2 A (unpublished results). We therefore propose that the serine phosphorylation of APRF, although not needed for its activation,

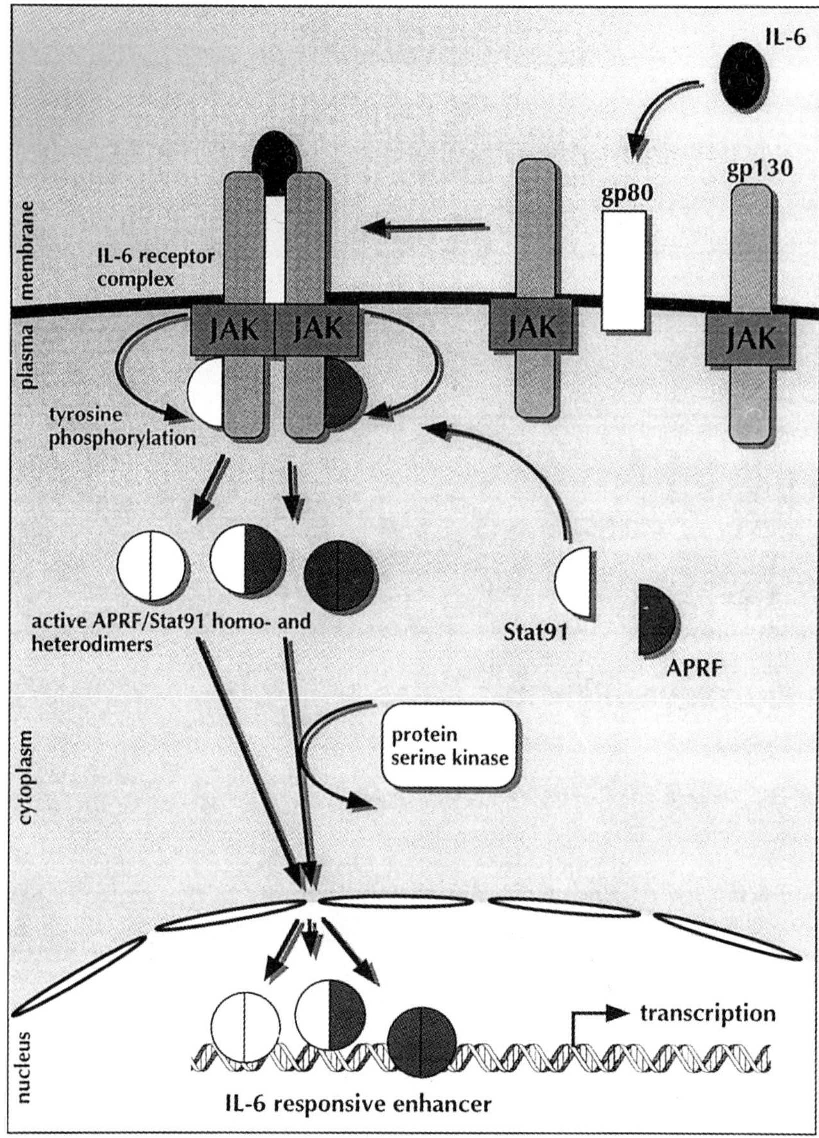

Fig. 10 Schematic representation of IL-6 signal transduction via Jak protein tyrosine kinases, APRF and Stat91

translocation to the nucleus and binding to DNA, may be required for the nuclear functions of the factor and may thus represent the H7-sensitive step necessary for the activation of IL-6 target genes.

Figure 10 summarizes the results of our studies on the mechanisms involved in IL-6 signalling.

ACKNOWLEDGEMENTS

We thank C. Schindler (New York) for the gift of antisera to Stat proteins, A. Ziemiecki (Bern) for antisera to Jak1, S. Pellegrini (Paris) for anti-Tyk2, and K. Yasukawa (Kanagawa, Japan) for anti-gp130. We also acknowledge the help of M. Robbertz with artwork and S. Cottin with the preparation of the manuscript. Experiments described herein were supported by the Deutsche Forschungsgemeinschaft (Bonn) and the Fonds der Chemischen Industrie (Frankfurt).

References

1. Koj A. Liver response to inflammation and synthesis of acute phase plasma proteins. Part III. In: Gordon AH, Koj A, editors. The acute phase response to injury and infection. Amsterdam: Elsevier; 1985:139–232.
2. Heinrich PC, Castell J, Andus T. Review article. Interleukin-6 and the acute phase response. Biochem J. 1990;265:621–36.
3. Baumann H, Prowse KR, Marinkovic S, Won KA, Jahreis GP. Stimulation of hepatic acute phase response by cytokines and glucocorticoids. Ann NY Acad Sci. 1989;557:280–95.
4. Hirano T, Kishimoto T. Interleukin-6. In: Sporn MB, Roberts AB, editors. Handbook of experimental pharmacology: peptide growth factors and their receptors. I. Berlin: Springer; 1990:633–65.
5. Van Snick J. Interleukin-6: An overview. Annu Rev Immunol. 1990;8:253–79.
6. Bazan JF. Haemopoietic receptors and helical cytokines. Immunol Today. 1990;11:350–4.
7. Taga T, Hibi M, Hirata Y et al. Interleukin-6 triggers the association of its receptor with a possible signal transducer, gp130. Cell. 1989;58:573–81.
8. Müllberg J, Schooltink H, Stoyan T et al. The soluble interleukin-6 receptor is generated by shedding. Eur J Immunol. 1993;23:473–80.
9. Hibi M, Murakami M, Saito M, Hirano T, Taga T, Kishimoto T. Molecular cloning and expression of an IL-6 signal transducer, gp130. Cell. 1990;63:1149–57.
10. Murakami M, Hibi M, Nakagawa N et al. IL-6-induced homodimerization of gp130 and associated activation of a tyrosine kinase. Science. 1993;260:1808–10.
11. Mackiewicz A, Schooltink H, Heinrich PC, Rose-John S. Complex of soluble human IL-6-receptor/IL-6 up-regulates expression of acute-phase proteins. J Immunol. 1992;149:2021–7.
12. Kunz D, Zimmermann R, Heisig M, Heinrich PC. Identification of the promoter sequences involved in the interleukin-6 dependent expression of the rat α_2-macroglobulin gene. Nucleic Acids Res. 1989;17:1121–38.
13. Ito T, Tanahashi H, Misumi Y, Sakaki Y. Nuclear factors interacting with an interleukin-6 responsive element of rat alpha 2-macroglobulin gene. Nucleic Acids Res. 1989;17:9425–35.
14. Hattori M, Abraham LJ, Northemann W, Fey GH. Acute-phase reaction induces a specific complex between hepatic nuclear proteins and the interleukin 6 response element of the rat alpha 2-macroglobulin gene. Proc Natl Acad Sci USA. 1990;87:2364–8.
15. Wegenka UM, Buschmann J, Lütticken C, Heinrich PC, Horn F. Acute-phase response factor, a nuclear factor binding to acute-phase response elements, is rapidly activated by interleukin-6 at the posttranslational level. Mol Cell Biol. 1993;13:276–88.
16. Wegenka UM, Lütticken C, Buschmann J et al. The interleukin-6-activated acute-phase response factor is antigenically and functionally related to members of the signal transducer and activator of transcription (STAT) family. Mol Cell Biol. 1994;14:3186–96.
17. Gearing DP, Comeau MR, Friend D et al. The IL-6 signal transducer, gp130: an oncostatin M receptor and affinity converter for the LIF receptor. Science. 1992;255:1434–7.
18. Ip NY, Nye SH, Boulton TG et al. CNTF and LIF act on neuronal cells via shared signaling pathways that involve the IL-6 signal transducing receptor component gp130. Cell. 1992;69:1121–32.
19. Yin T, Taga T, Tsang ML, Yasukawa Y, Kishimoto T, Yang YC. Involvement of IL-6 signal transducer gp130 in IL-11-mediated signal transduction. J Immunol. 1993;151:2555–61.

20. Baumann H, Schendel P. Interleukin-11 regulates the hepatic expression of the same plasma protein genes as interleukin-6. J Biol Chem. 1991;266:20424–7.

21. Baumann H, Won KA, Jahreis GP. Human hepatocyte-stimulating factor-III and interleukin-6 are structurally and immunologically distinct but regulate the production of the same acute phase plasma proteins. J Biol Chem. 1989;264:8046–51.

22. Richards CD, Brown TJ, Shoyab M, Baumann H, Gauldie J. Recombinant oncostatin M stimulates the production of acute phase proteins in HepG2 cells and rat primary hepatocytes in vitro. J Immunol. 1992;148:1731–6.

23. Yuan J, Wegenka UM, Lütticken C et al. The signaling pathways of interleukin-6 and interferon-γ converge by the activation of different transcription factors which bind to common responsive DNA elements. Mol Cell Biol. 1994;14:1657–68.

24. Zhong Z, Wen Z, Darnell JE Jr. Stat3: a STAT family member activated by tyrosine phosphorylation in response to epidermal growth factor and interleukin-6. Science. 1994;264:95–8.

25. Akira S, Nishio Y, Inoue M et al. Molecular cloning of APRF, a novel IFN-stimulated gene factor 3 p91-related transcription factor involved in the gp130-mediated signaling pathway. Cell. 1994;77:63–71.

26. Lütticken C, Wegenka UM, Yuan J et al. Association of transcription factor APRF and protein kinase JAK1 with the IL-6 signal transducer gp130. Science. 1994;263:89–92.

27. Magielska-Zero D, Bereta J, Gzuba-Pelech B, Pajdak W, Gauldie J, Koj A. Inhibitory effect of human recombinant interferon gamma on synthesis of acute phase proteins in human hepatoma HepG2 cells stimulated by leukocyte cytokines, TNF alpha and IFN beta 2/BSF-2/IL-6. Biochem Int. 1988;17:17–23.

28. Decker T, Lew DJ, Mirkovitch J, Darnell JE Jr. Cytoplasmic activation of GAF, an IFN-γ-regulated DNA-binding factor. EMBO J. 1991;10:927–32.

29. Shuai K, Schindler C, Prezioso VR, Darnell JE Jr. Activation of transcription by IFN-γ tyrosine phosphorylation of a 91-kD-DNA binding protein. Science. 1992;258:1808–12.

30. Murakami M, Narazaki M, Hibi M et al. Critical cytoplasmic region of the interleukin 6 signal transducer gp130 is conserved in the cytokine receptor family. Proc Natl Acad Sci USA. 1991;88:11349–53.

31. Murakami M, Hibi M, Nakagawa N et al. IL-6-induced homodimerization of gp130 and associated activation of a tyrosine kinase. Science. 1993;260:1808–10.

32. Velazquez L, Fellous M, Stark G, Pellegrini S. A protein tyrosine kinase in the interferon α/β signaling pathway. Cell. 1992;70:313–22.

33. Müller M, Briscoe J, Laxton C et al. The protein tyrosine kinase JAK1 complements defects in interferon-α/β and -γ signal transduction. Nature. 1993;366:129–35.

Section II
Signal transduction pathways and effects

3
Activation of NF-κB and AP-1 in rat Kupffer cells

T. A. TRAN-THI, K. DECKER and P. A. BAEUERLE

INTRODUCTION

Nuclear transcription factors are required for gene expression in eukaryotic cells. The activation of these factors may accelerate or retard the transcriptional rate, and induction and transcription of many genes requires an interplay of distinct transcription factors. NF-κB is an ubiquitous transcription factor which is activated by different stimuli including lipopolysaccharide (LPS), viruses, cytokines such as TNF-α and IL-1β, u.v. irradiation and oxidative stress (for a review see ref. 1). Since LPS derived from the gut is cleared in vivo by Kupffer cells[2,3] and these cells are also the site of production of cytokines in the liver[4-6], we were interested to know whether LPS and cytokines activate NF-κB in primary cultures of Kupffer cells. To test the specificity of activation of NF-κB in response to different stimuli the activation of another transcription factor, AP-1[7], was also assessed.

MATERIALS AND METHODS

Kupffer cells from male Wistar rats (350–400 g) were isolated according to the method of Brouwer[8], modified by Eyhorn[9]. Three-day-old cultures were used for all experiments.

Electrophoretic mobility shift assay

After exposure of Kupffer cells to different stimuli, they were washed twice with Hank's buffer and suspended in 1.5 ml buffer. After 15 s centrifugation at 18 000 g cell pellets were lysed with 35 μl 20 mM Hepes, pH 7.9 containing 0.35 M NaCl, 20% glycerol, 1% Nonidet P-40, 1 mM MgCl$_2$, 0.1 mM EGTA, 0.5 mM EDTA, 5 mM dithiothreitol (DTT), 1 mM phenylmethyl sulphonyl-fluoride (PMSF), 0.1% aprotinin. After 30 min incubation on ice, cell lysates

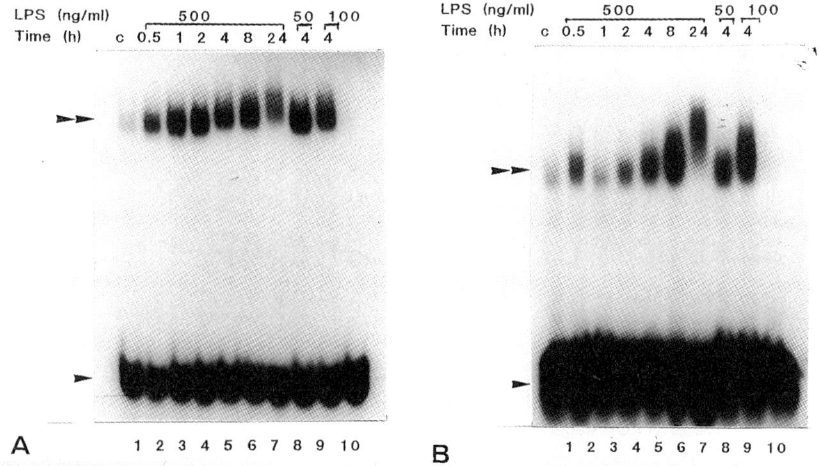

Fig. 1 Kinetics and dose response of NF-κB and AP-1 activation after LPS treatment. LPS, at concentrations given in the figure, was added to primary cultures of Kupffer cells. At indicated times cells were harvested and the total cell extraction was performed as described in Materials and methods. DNA binding activity of NF-κB **(A)** and AP-1 **(B)** were monitored in electrophoretic mobility shift assays. Double arrow indicates the position of NF-κB-DNA complex, single arrow the position of the unbound DNA probe. c: control without LPS. In lane 10, the same sample as in lane 5 was incubated in the presence of an excess of 0.5 pmol unlabelled oligonucleotides with binding site for either NF-κB or AP-1

were centrifuged for 5 min at 10 000 g at 4°C. The supernatants containing the total cell extracts were aliquoted and stored at −80°C. Binding assays were performed for 15–30 min at room temperature with 19 μg protein (from total cell extract) in 20 μl volume containing 4 μl 5× binding buffer (20 mM Hepes pH 7.9, 60 mM KCl, 2 mM DTT, 4% Ficoll), 2 μg bovine serum albumin, 2 μg poly(dI-dC) and 30 000 cpm of ^{32}P-labelled oligonucleotides with binding sites for either NF-κB or AP-1. Labelling of oligonucleotides was performed as described by Meyer et al.[10]. DNA–protein complexes were separated from unbound DNA probe on native 4% polyacrylamide gels at 220 V in 45 mM Tris-borate, pH 8.0 containing 1 mM EDTA. The cytotoxic activity of TNF-α was measured according to Flick and Gifford[11]. Protein was measured according to Bradford[12].

RESULTS AND DISCUSSION

NF-κB was very rapidly activated by LPS in Kupffer cells. DNA-binding activity occurred as early as 30 min and persisted for at least 24 h (Fig. 1A). LPS at a concentration of 50 ng/ml was sufficient to cause maximal activation. In contrast to NF-κB, activation of AP-1 seemed to be biphasic. A transient activation occurred at 30 min and a long-lasting one at 4 h after stimulation with LPS. The activation of AP-1 persisted for at least 24 h (Fig. 1B). To assess the specificity of NF-κB and AP-1 binding to DNA, cell extracts were incubated with an excess of the respective unlabelled oligonucleotides. Under these

Table 1 Modulation of TNF-α production elicited by LPS with different agents

Conditions	TNF-α activity (%)
LPS	100
LPS + TGF-β	52 ± 10 (3)
LPS + dexamethasone	8 ± 5 (3)
LPS + IL-4	88 ± 17 (3)
LPS + IL-10	33 ± 12 (3)
LPS + PDTC	3 ± 1 (3)
LPS + PGE$_2$	5 ± 2 (3)

Kupffer cells were pretreated for 90 min with 100 μM PDTC or 2 μM PGE$_2$ before LPS addition (500 ng/ml). Incubation was performed for further 90 min. TGF-β (20 ng/ml), 2 μM dexamethasone, IL-4 (10 U/ml), IL-10 (66 ng/ml) were given 60 min prior to LPS addition. Cells were incubated in the presence of LPS for a further 4h. 100% represents the activity of TNF-α released in the medium in the presence of LPS alone. It was 740 ± 480 U/10^6 KC ($n = 5$) and 885 ± 469 U/10^6 KC ($n = 4$) after 4h and 90 min, respectively

conditions, binding of NF-κB as well as of AP-1 to DNA was competitively inhibited (lane 10, Fig. 1A, B).

As the activation of NF-κB and the production and release of TNF-α by Kupffer cells[13] are both very rapid, we tested whether activation of NF-κB is involved in the new production of TNF-α. In the presence of 100 μM pyrrolidinedithiocarbamate (PDTC), an inhibitor of NF-κB activation[10], the production of TNF-α elicited by LPS was completely suppressed (Table 1). TNF-α synthesis was also inhibited by dexamethasone, PGE$_2$, TGF-β and IL-10 (Table 1), PDTC, PGE$_2$ and dexamethasone being the most efficient inhibitors. The anti-inflammatory cytokine IL-10 also reduced activity of TNF-α to one-third and that of TGF-β to 50% of the control. IL-4, which was reported to inhibit TNF-α production in human monocytes[14] inhibited just 10% of TNF-α production (Table 1).

Among the agents inhibiting TNF-α production, only PDTC inhibited activation of NF-κB. At the same time, the compound activated AP-1 in untreated cells as well as in cells stimulated with LPS (Fig. 2A,B). IL-10, TGF-β and PGE$_2$ did not affect activation of NF-κB and AP-1 at all (Fig. 2A,B), indicating that they may act at a post transcriptional step. In line with these findings, Bogdan et al.[15] reported that TGF-β inhibited the production of TNF-α by suppressing translation while IL-10 promoted the degradation of cytokine mRNA. Dexamethasone inhibited the activation of AP-1 but had no effect on NF-κB activation. This implies that this corticosteroid may exert its action at the transcriptional level of TNF-α. In agreement with this idea Grewe et al.[16] found a partial inhibition of the expression of mRNA for TNF-α after treatment of Kupffer cells with LPS and dexamethasone. These results indicate that different mechanisms are involved in down-regulating the production of TNF-α; the most rapid and efficient appears to be inactivation of NF-κB.

As different cytokines, including TNF-α and IL-1β, have been reported to activate NF-κB[1], we wanted to test whether they also activate this transcription factor in Kupffer cells. Figure 3A shows that only TNF-α and macrophage

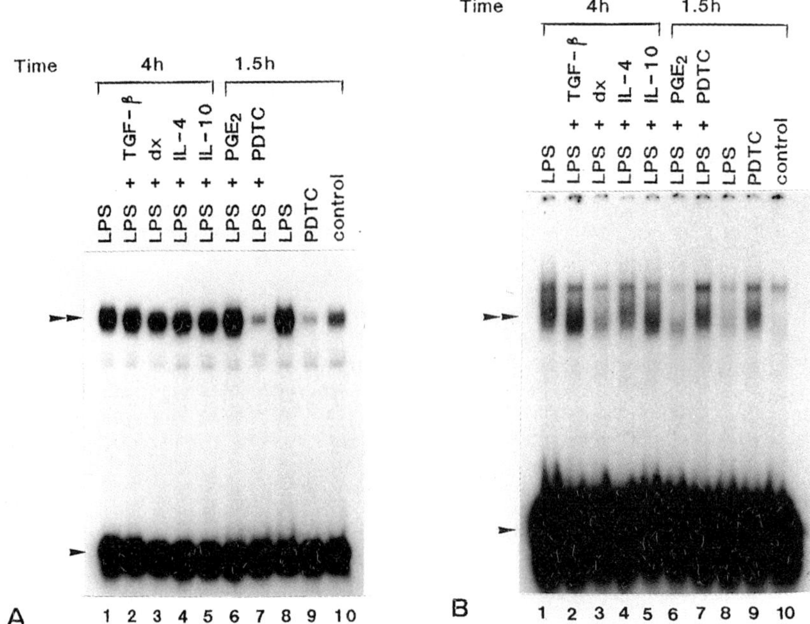

Fig. 2 Modulation of activation of NF-κB and AP-1 elicited by LPS. The conditions used were the same as described in the legend of Table 1. Activation of NF-κB (**A**) and AP-1 (**B**) was assayed as described in Materials and methods. dx: dexamethasone

colony stimulating factor (M-CSF) activated NF-κB. All other cytokines tested (IL-1β, IL-4, IL-6, IL-8, IL-10, interferon-γ and granulocyte-macrophage colony stimulating factor) had no effect on either NF-κB or on AP-1 (Fig. 3A,B).

Since reactive oxygen intermediates (ROI) have been proposed to activate NF-κB[17,18] and since phorbol 12-myristate 13-acetate (PMA) and zymosan stimulated the production of superoxide in Kupffer cells[19–21], we tested whether these two agents can activate NF-κB. However, none of them was active (Fig. 3A). While PMA activated AP-1, zymosan strongly induced the activation of a modified form of AP-1 (Fig. 3B). These results indicate that superoxide generated by NADPH oxidase in Kupffer cells does not activate NF-κB. As reported by Meyer et al.[22] not all reactive oxygen intermediates are able to activate NF-κB. For instance in the Jurkat T cell line, H_2O_2 was the best activator, while O_2^- generated by paraquat and doxorubicin, and $NO^\bullet$ delivered by sodium nitroprusside failed to activate NF-κB.

In this study, we have shown that LPS and TNF-α largely activate NF-κB in primary cultures of Kupffer cells. The activated transcription factor then induces transcription and biosynthesis of TNF-α, a proinflammatory cytokine. The TNF-α gene has been reported to be under transcriptional control of NF-κB. Direct evidence that this is also the case in Kupffer cells comes from our finding that the antioxidant inhibitor of NF-κB, PDTC, was a very potent inhibitor of TNF-α production. This indicates that reactive oxygen intermediates played a role as messengers in LPS-induced NF-κB activation. The responsible

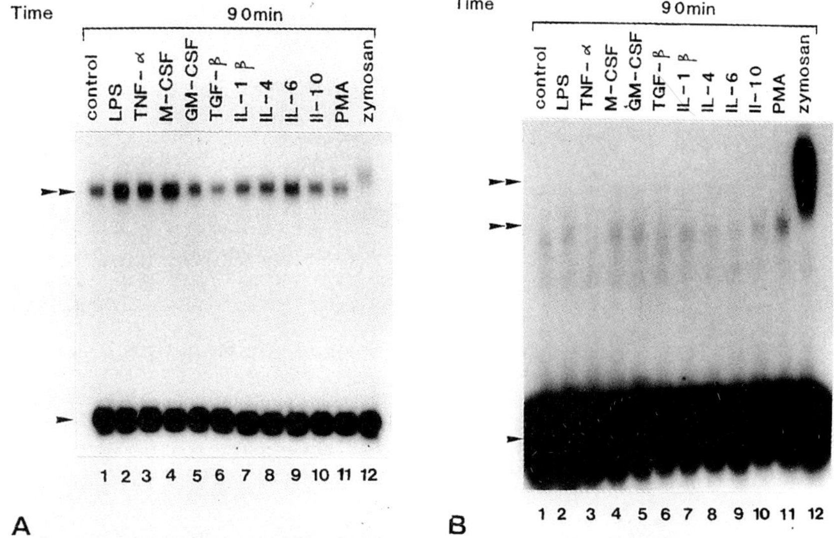

Fig. 3 Activation of NF-κB and AP-1 in response to LPS, cytokines, zymosan and PMA. Lane 1: control, 2: LPS 500 ng/ml; 3: TNF-α 4000 U/ml; 4: M-CSF 2000 U/ml, 5: GM-CSF, 100 ng/ml, 6: TGF-β, 10 ng/ml, 7: IL-1β 170 ng/ml, 8: IL-4 10 U/ml, 9: IL-6, 470 U/ml, 10: IL-10, 70 ng/ml, 11: 1 μM PMA, 12: zymosan 0.5 mg/ml. Activation of NF-κB (**A**) and AP-1 (**B**) was assayed as described in Materials and methods

intermediate was not superoxide because stimuli known to induce superoxide production in Kupffer cells, such as zymosan, had no effect. In conclusion, the behaviour of Kupffer cells with respect to NF-κB inducing and inhibiting conditions is very similar to that of monocytes[23].

The behaviour of transcription factor AP-1 was quite distinct from that of NF-κB. As reported for HeLa cells[10], PDTC directly induced AP-1. The effect of LPS on AP-1 seemed very indirect since it took hours before strong DNA binding activity appeared. Of particular interest was the strong induction of an AP-1-like activity by zymosan. Although the activity requires further analysis using antibodies, it appears that AP-1 underwent a covalent modification. This was also apparent after a 24 h LPS treatment (see Fig. 1B). Future studies have to determine the nature and function of this modification.

ACKNOWLEDGEMENTS

This work was supported by the Deutsche Forschungsgemeinschaft, Bonn through SFB 154 and the Fonds der Chemischen Industrie, Frankfurt-M, Germany.

REFERENCES

1. Baeuerle PA. The inducible transcription activator NF-κB: regulation by distinct protein subunits. Biochem Biophys Acta. 1991;1072:63–80.

2. Mathison JC, Ulevitch RJ. The clearance, tissue distribution and cellular localization of intravenously injected lipopolysaccharide in rabbits. J Immunol. 1979;123:2133–44.

3. Freudenberg MA, Freudenberg N, Galanos C. Time course of cellular distribution of endotoxin in liver, lungs and kidney of rats. Br J Exp Pathol. 1982;63:55–65.

4. Karck U, Peters T, Decker K. The release of tumor necrosis factor from endotoxin-stimulated rat Kupffer cells is regulated by PGE_2 and dexamethasone. J Hepatol. 1988;7:352–61.

5. Shirahama M, Hishibashi H, Tsuchiya Y, Kurokawa S, Okumura Y, Niho Y. Kinetics and parameters of interleukin 1 secretion by rat Kupffer cells. J Clin Lab Immunol. 1988;27:127–32.

6. Busam KJ, Bauer TM, Bauer J, Gerok W, Decker K. Interleukin-6 release by rat liver macrophages. J Hepatol. 1990;11:367–73.

7. Angel P, Karin M. The role of Jun, Fos and the AP-1 complex in cell proliferation and transformation. Biochim Biophys Acta. 1991;1072:129–57.

8. Brouwer A, Barelds R, Knook DL. Centrifugal separations of mammalian cells. In: Rickwood D, editor. Centrifugation, a practical approach. Oxford: IRL, Press 1984:183–218.

9. Eyhorn S, Schlayer HJ, Dieter P et al. Rat hepatic sinusoidal endothelial cells in monolayer cultures. Biochemical and ultrastructural characteristics. J Hepatol. 1988;6:23–35.

10. Meyer M, Schreck R, Baeuerle P. H_2O_2 and antioxidants have opposite effects on activation of NF-κB and AP-1 in intact cells: AP-1 as secondary antioxidant-responsive factor. EMBO J. 1993;12:2005–15.

11. Flick DA, Gifford GE. Comparison of in vitro cell cytotoxic assays for tumor-necrosis factor. J Immunol Methods. 1984;68:167–75.

12. Bradford MM. A rapid and sensitive method for the quantitation of microgram quantities of protein utilizing the principle of protein-dye binding. Anal Biochem. 1976;72:248–54.

13. Tran-Thi A, Weinhold L, Weinstock C et al. Production of tumor necrosis factor-α, interleukin-1 and interleukin-6 in the perfused rat liver. Eur Cytokine Netw. 1993;4:363–70.

14. Hart PH, Vitti PF, Burgess DR, Whitty GA, Piccoli DS, Hamilton JA. Potential antiinflammatory effects of interleukin-4: Suppression of human monocyte tumor necrosis factor α, interleukin 1 and prostaglandin E_2. Proc Natl Acad Sci USA. 1989;86:3803–7.

15. Bogdan C, Paik J, Vodovotz Y, Nathan C. Contrasting mechanism for suppression of macrophage cytokine release by transforming growth factor-β and interleukin-10. J Biol Chem. 1992;267:23301–8.

16. Grewe M, Gausling R, Gyufko K, Decker K. Regulation of the mRNA for tumor necrosis factor α in rat liver macrophages. In: Knook DL, Wisse E, eds. Cells of the hepatic sinusoid, vol. 4. Leiden: The Kupffer cell foundation; 1993:13–16.

17. Schreck R, Rieber P, Baeuerle PA. Reactive oxygen intermediates as apparently widely used messengers in the activation of the NF-κB transcription factor and HIV-1. EMBO J. 1991;10:2247–58.

18. Schreck R, Baeuerle PA. A role for oxygen radicals as second messenger. Trends Cell Biol. 1991;1:39–42.

19. Bhatnagar R, Schirmer R, Ernst M, Decker K. Superoxide release by zymosan-stimulated rat Kupffer cells in vitro. Eur J Biochem. 1981;119:171–5.

20. Birmelin M, Decker K. Synthesis of prostanoids and cyclic nucleotides by phagocytosing rat Kupffer cells. Eur J Biochem. 1984;142:219-25.

21. Dieter P, Schulze-Specking A, Decker K. Differential inhibition of prostaglandin and superoxide production by dexamethasone in primary cultures of rat Kupffer cells. Eur J Biochem. 1986;159:451-7.

22. Meyer M, Schreck R, Müller JM, Baeuerle PA. Redox control of gene expression by eukaryotic transcription factors NF-κB, AP-1 and SRF/TCF. In: Pasquier C, et al, eds. Oxidative stress, cell activation and viral infection. Basel: Birkhäuser Verlag; 1994:217–35.

23. Ziegler Heitbrock HWL, Sterndorf T, Liese J et al. Pyrrolidine dithiocarbamate inhibits NF-κB mobilization and TNF production in human monocytes. J Immunol. 1993;151:6986–93.

4
Cytokines and adhesion molecules in the liver

K. TANIKAWA

INTRODUCTION

Cytokines have been widely studied in investigations of diseases in various organs. Recently they have been found to be important in the pathogenesis of liver injuries[1–5] and our studies have focused on how the cytokines are involved with adhesion molecules in various liver injuries. Four main studies carried out recently in our department are presented here.

The first study concerns the need to consider the spleen when discussing cytokines in the liver. The next study found that tumour necrosis factor-α (TNF-α) or interleukin-1 (IL-1) stimulated the expression of the adhesion molecule ICAM-1 on the surface of cultured hepatic sinusoidal endothelial cells (SEC). The third study found an interaction between polymorphoneutrophils (PMN) and hepatic SEC induced by cytokines in experimental liver injuries, while the fourth was a clinical study on the usefulness of serum sICAM-1 and IL-8 measurement in alcoholic hepatitis.

SOURCES OF CYTOKINES INDUCING THE EXPRESSION OF ADHESION MOLECULES IN THE LIVER

When considering the sources of cytokines affecting the liver, it is important to include the spleen, which contains about one-third of the lymphoid tissue of the body. In addition, all the blood that flows through the spleen, including a large amount of cytokines produced there, flows next into the liver[6].

TNF-α is one of the most potent cytokines inducing ICAM-1 expression and is produced mainly in macrophages. We compared the productivity of TNF-α in Kupffer cells and splenic macrophages. Isolated Kupffer cells or splenic macrophages were incubated and after addition of lipopolysaccharide (LPS) the culture medium of splenic macrophages contained much higher levels of TNF-α than did medium from Kupffer cells (Fig. 1)[7]. TNF-α levels after LPS treatment, measured by reverse transcription-polymerase chain reaction also showed

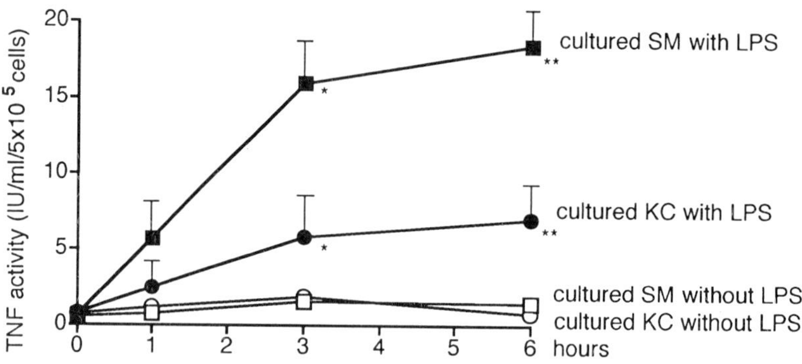

Isolated rat SM and KC were stimulated with and without 1 μ g/ml of LPS for various hours(0,1,3 and 6 hours), and the activities of TNF in the culture medium were determined on the bioassay. *vs*, **vs**: p<0.01(Student's t-test)

Fig. 1 TNF-α levels in the culture medium of splenic macrophages are significantly higher than in those of Kupffer cells after addition of LPS

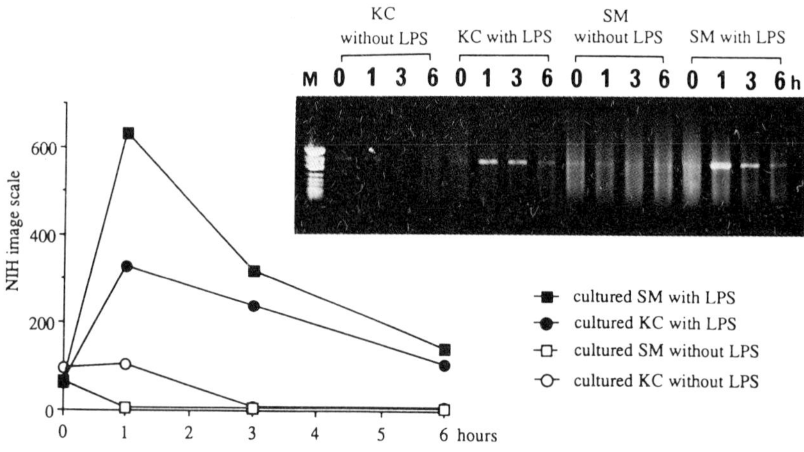

KC and SM were incubated for various periods in 1 ml RPMI1640/10% FBS with and without 1 µg/ml of LPS, and isolated total RNA was used for PCR.

Fig. 2 TNF-α mRNA expression in cultured splenic macrophages is higher than that in cultured Kupffer cells after addition of LPS

significantly higher levels in the splenic macrophages than in the Kupffer cells (Fig. 2). Splenectomized rats or mice showed remarkably low levels of serum TNF-α after i.v. administration of LPS (Fig. 3).

These data indicate that splenic macrophages are important sources of TNF-α in the liver and we must consider the role of the spleen in the pathogenesis of various hepatic injuries.

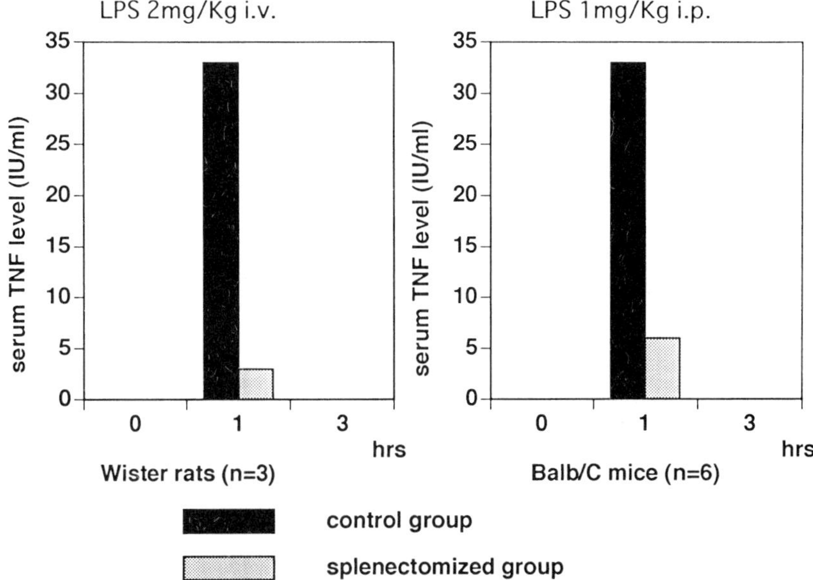

Fig. 3 Serum TNF-α levels are significantly lower in splenectomized rats or mice after i.v. administration of LPS

EXPRESSION OF ICAM-1 ON HEPATIC SEC INDUCED BY TNF-α OR IL-1 IN VITRO

It is well known that various adhesion molecules of vascular endothelial cells such as ICAM-1 are involved in the infiltration of inflammatory cells into tissue from vessels[8]. ICAM-1, for instance, is up-regulated by inflammatory cytokines such as TNF-α or IL-1[9–11] and closely related to the interaction between vascular endothelial cells and leukocytes[12–14]. Various studies have shown an increased expression of adhesion molecules on the sinusoidal lining cells and hepatocytes in liver diseases, especially around areas which appear damaged by light microscopy.

We examined the expression of ICAM-1 on hepatic SEC induced by TNF-α and IL-1 in vitro by electron microscopy[15]. As shown in Figure 4, electron microscopy showed immunoreactive gold particles directed against mouse anti-rat ICAM-1 on the surface of a cultured hepatic SEC. More gold particles were present on the surface of cells treated with TNF-α or IL-1 than on the surface of untreated cells. Cultured hepatic SEC treated with TNF-α or IL-1α were incubated with mouse anti-rat ICAM-1 for cell surface labelling, and semi-quantitative analysis of ICAM-1 on these cells was carried out by cytofluorometry. The fluorescence intensity of ICAM-1 on these cells was significantly increased in a dose-dependent manner (Fig. 5).

These studies indicated that stimulation by cytokines such as TNF-α and IL-1α enhances the ICAM-1 expression on hepatic SEC. This enhanced ICAM-1 expression appeared to be related to an increase in the number of leukocytes which adhered to the hepatic SEC and then migrated into the Disse space to

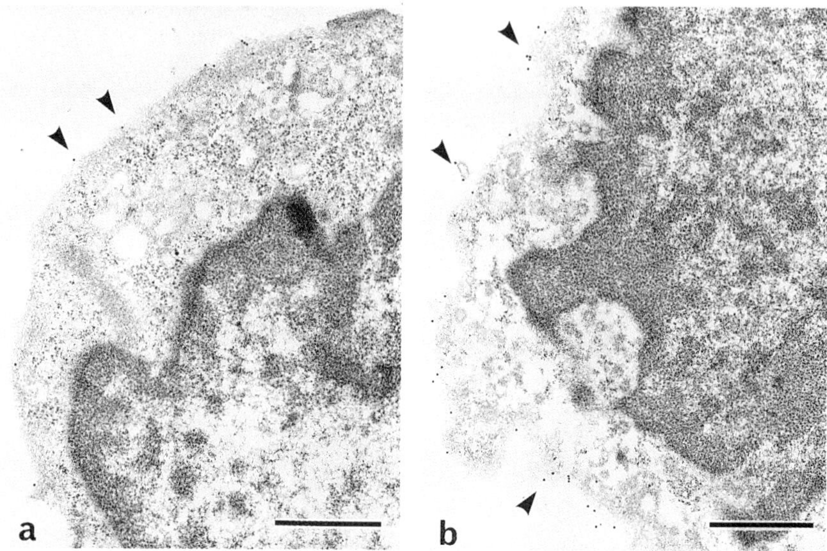

Fig. 4   Electron micrographs of the immunoreactive gold particles against mouse anti-rat ICAM-1 on the surface of the cultured hepatic SEC. More gold particles are seen on the surface of cells treated with TNF-α or IL-1 (**a**) than on the surface of untreated cells (**b**)

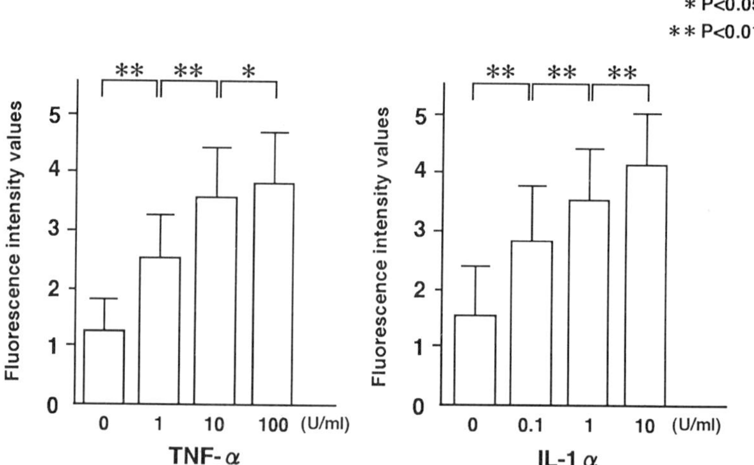

Fig. 5   Fluorescence intensity of ICAM-1 expression on cultured hepatic SECs treated with TNF-α or IL-1 is remarkably increased in a dose-dependent manner

interact with the hepatocytes. The effect of TNF-α on adhesion of PMN to the cultured hepatic SEC was dose dependent (Fig. 6).

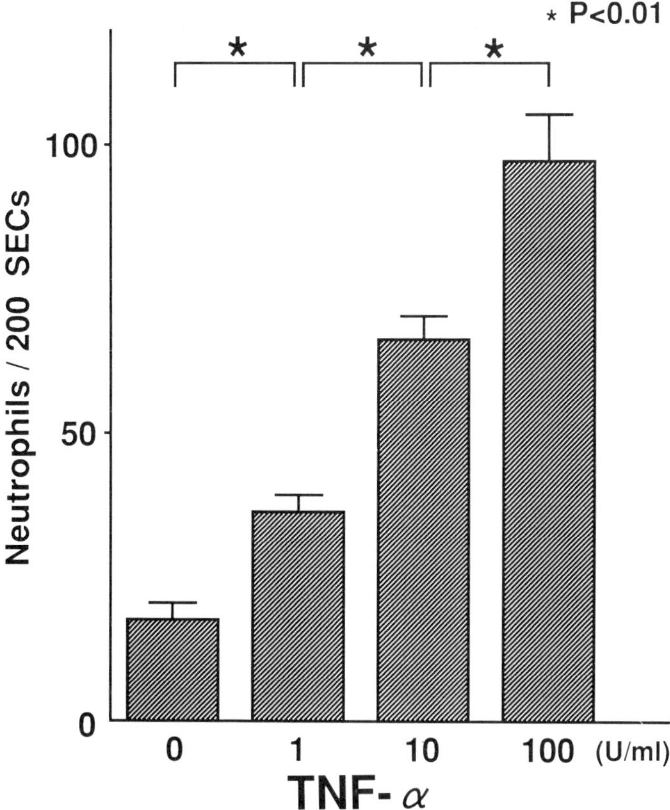

Fig. 6 Neutrophil adhesion to cultured hepatic SEC treated with TNF-α is increased in a dose-dependent manner

CYTOKINES AND ADHESION MOLECULES IN EXPERIMENTAL LIVER INJURIES

The interaction between PMN and hepatic SEC is probably involved in the pathogenesis of acute liver injuries, including alcoholic hepatitis and various experimental liver injuries[16–18]. In LPS-induced liver injury in the rat, TNF-α levels peak at 1 h, and the IL-8 level at 3 h, after LPS treatment. An increase in the number of PMN in the liver is seen as early as 1 h and continues until 12 h after the LPS exposure. ICAM-1 was strongly expressed on SEC (Fig. 7), and PMN adhering to the SEC expressed both LFA-1α and Mac-1 (Fig. 8) under light and electron immunomicroscopy. ICAM-1 was also observed on the hepatocytes[19]. From these data it was concluded that increased interactions between PMN and hepatic SEC and between PMN and hepatocytes occurred via the leukocyte adhesion molecules, regulated by the inflammatory cytokines such as TNF-α and IL-8. These interactions may be deeply involved in LPS-induced acute liver injury.

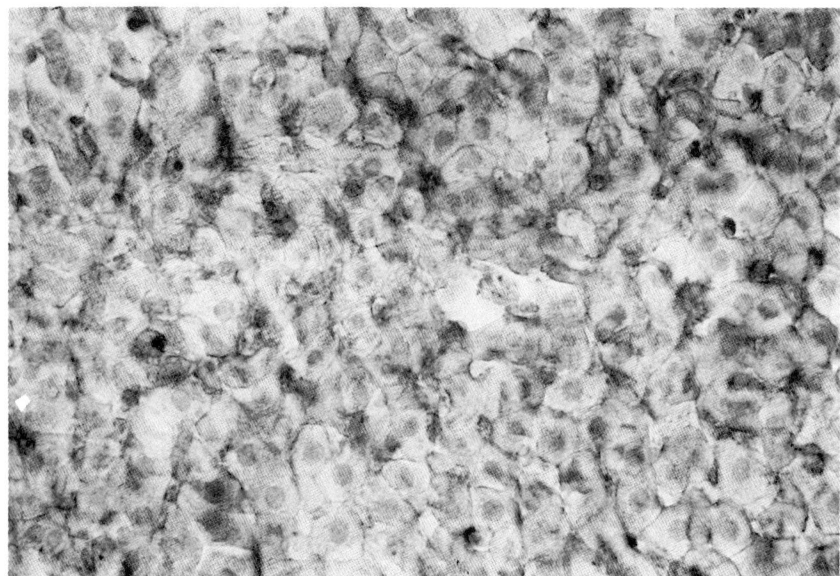

Fig. 7   Light micrograph showing the expression of ICAM-1 along the hepatic SEC in endotoxin-induced rat liver injury

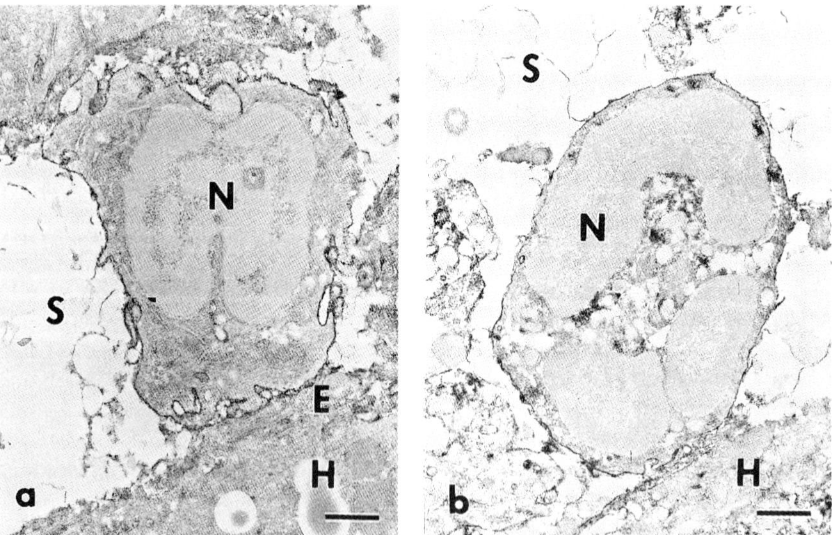

Fig. 8   Electron micrographs showing the expression of LFA-1α (**a**) and Mac-1 (**b**) on the surface of a PMN in endotoxin-induced rat liver injury

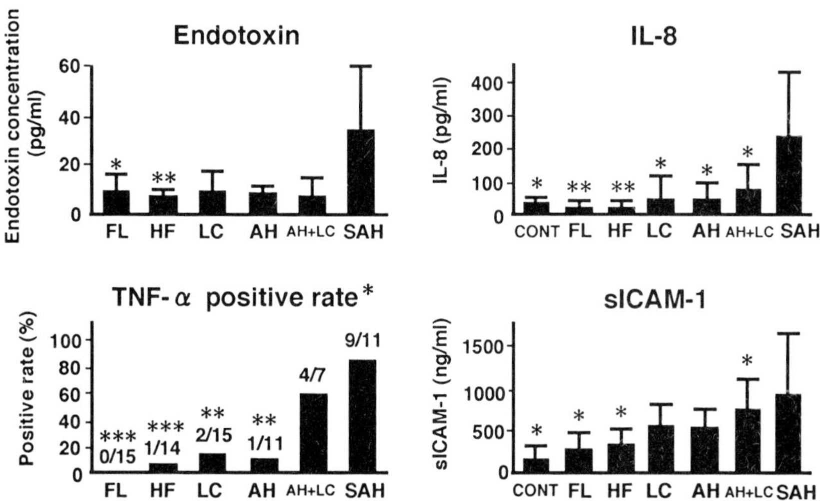

Fig. 9 Serum endotoxin, TNF-α, IL-8 and sICAM-1 are elevated with progression of various types of alcoholic liver diseases

SERUM sICAM-1 AND IL-8 IN HUMAN ALCOHOLIC HEPATITIS

In alcoholic hepatitis, significant numbers of PMN infiltrate the liver and are considered to play a primary role in the pathogenesis. Endotoxaemia is often associated with alcoholic liver injuries because of depressed Kupffer cell function and an increased permeability to endotoxin at the intestinal barrier[20]. Levels of cytokines such as TNF-α or IL-1 are high in the sera of alcoholic hepatitis patients; these are probably generated by macrophages or lymphocytes stimulated by endotoxin. As described earlier, the spleen appears to be a main source of cytokines in the serum. On the other hand, IL-8, a chemoattractant for PMN and also the rapid activator CD11/CD18 integrin of PMN[21], is generated in the liver tissue in response to TNF-α and by other cytokines. The whole process of the pathogenesis of alcoholic hepatitis is thus well understood; TNF-α and other cytokines, initially generated mainly from the spleen by endotoxin, induce the expression of adhesion molecules on the hepatic SEC and the generation of IL-8 in liver tissue. These result in an accumulation of the PMN in the liver, which then attach to hepatic SEC, leading finally to hepatic injury.

As shown in Figure 9, levels of endotoxin, TNF-α, IL-8 and sICAM-1 are elevated as alcoholic liver injuries progress. Serum IL-8 levels are closely correlated with the number of PMN in liver biopsy specimens (Fig. 10) and IL-8 tends to remain high in the clinical course of severe alcoholic hepatitis. Serum IL-8 or sICAM-1 levels appear to be correlated with liver function such as T. Bil, albumin, AST or prothrombin time in alcoholic hepatitis and are good indicators of prognosis[22].

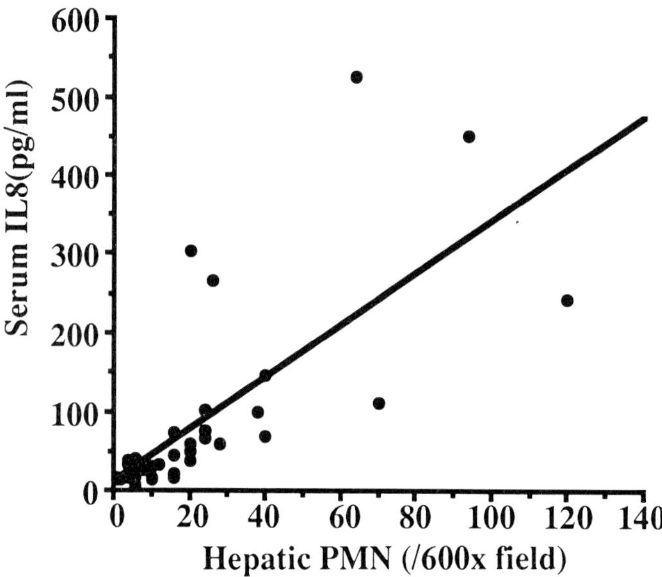

Fig. 10 Correlation of serum IL-8 and hepatic neutrophils in alcoholic liver diseases. Serum IL-8 levels and the number of neutrophils in biopsy specimens are well correlated

References

1. Volpes R, Oord JJ, Desmet VJ. Vascular adhesion molecules in acute and chronic liver inflammation. Hepatology. 1992;15:269–75.
2. Volpes R, Oord JJ, Desmet VJ. Hepatic expression of intercellular adhesion molecule-1 (ICMA-1) in viral hepatitis B. Hepatology. 1990;12:148–54.
3. Volpes R, Oord JJ, Desmet VJ. Adhesive molecules in liver disease. Immunohistochemical distribution of thrombospondin receptors in chronic HBV infection. J Hepatol. 1990;10: 297–304.
4. Volpes R, Oord JJ, Desmet VJ. Immunohistochemical study of adhesion molecules in liver inflammation. Hepatology. 1990;12:59–65.
5. Adams DH, Hubscher SG, Shaw J et al. Increased expression of intercellular adhesion molecule 1 on bile ducts in primary biliary cirrhosis and primary sclerosing cholangitis. Hepatology. 1991;14:426–31.
6. Tanaka S, Kumashiro R, Tanikawa K. Role of the spleen in endotoxin-induced hepatic injury in chronic alcohol-fed rats. Liver. 1992;12:306–10.
7. Shimauchi Y. Functional differences between rat Kupffer cells and splenic macrophages. Acta Hepatol Jap. 1992;33:779–86.
8. Rothlein R, Dustin ML, Marlin SD, Springer TA. A human intercellular adhesion molecule (ICAM-1) distinct from LFA-1. J Immunol. 1986;137:1270–4.
9. Pober JS, Gimbrone MA Jr, Lagierre LA et al. Overlapping patterns of activation of human endothelial cells by interleukin 1, tumor necrosis factor and immune interferon. J Immunol. 1986;137:1893–6.
10. Dustin ML, Singer KH, Tuck DT, Springer TA. Adhesion of T lymphoblasts to epidermal karatinocytes is up regulated by interferon gamma and is mediated by intercellular adhesion

molecule-1 (ICAM-1). J Exp Med. 1988;167:1323–40.

11. Dustin ML, Rothlein R, Bhan AK, Dinarello CA, Springer TA. Induction by IL-1 and interferon-α: tissue distribution, biochemistry, and function of a natural adherence molecule (ICAM-1). J Immunol. 1986;137:245–54.

12. Springer TA. Adhesion receptor of the immune system. Nature. 1990;346:425–34.

13. Munro JM, Pober JS, Cotran RS. Tumor necrosis factor and interferon-α induce distinct patterns of endothelial activation and associated leukocyte accumulation in skin of Papio ancebis. Am J Pathol. 1989;135:121–33.

14. Butcher EC. Leukocyte-endothelial cell recognition: three (or more) steps to specificity and diversity. Cell. 1991;67:1033–6.

15. Ohira H, Ueno T, Shakado S et al. Cultured rat hepatic sinusoidal endothelial cells express intercellular adhesion molecule-1 (ICAM-1) by tumor necrosis factor-α or interleukin-1α stimulation. J Hepatol. 1994;20:729–34.

16. Doi F, Goya T, Torisu M. Potential role of hepatic macrophages in neutrophil-mediated liver injury in rats with sepsis. Hepatology. 1993;17:1086–95.

17. Burra P, Hubscher SG, Shaw J, Elias E, Adams D. Is the intercellular adhesion molecule-1/leukocyte function associated antigen-1 pathway of leukocyte adhesion involved in the tissue damage of alcoholic hepatitis? Gut. 1992;33:268–71.

18. Furudera S, Kumashiro R, Tanaka S et al. Roles of the splenic cytokines and arachidonic acid metabolites in severe hepatic injury after lipopolysaccharide injection in chronically alcohol-fed rats. Alcohol Alcoholism. 1993;28(S1):91–5.

19. Ohira H, Ueno T, Torimura T, Tanikawa K, Kasukawa R. Leukocyte adhesion molecules in the liver and plasma cytokine levels in endotoxin-induced rat liver injury. (Submitted).

20. Nolan JP, Camara DS. Endotoxin, sinusoidal cells, and liver injury. In: Popper H, Schaffner F, editors. Progress in liver disease. Vol. VII. New York: Grune and Stratton, 1982:361–76.

21. Lo SK, Detmers PA, Levin SM, Wright SD. Transient adhesion of neutrophils to endothelium. J Exp Med. 1989;169:1779-93.

22. Seo J, Kumashiro R, Ishii K, Sata M, Tanikawa K. Significance of interleukin-8 and intercellular adhesion molecule-1 in alcoholic hepatitis. (Submitted).

Part B
Cell biological aspects

Section III
Inflammation and fibrogenesis

5
Role of sinusoidal endothelial cells in liver fibrosis

G. RAMADORI and K. NEUBAUER

INTRODUCTION

Liver sinusoidal endothelial cells differ from endothelial cells of other sites in various morphological and functional characteristics[1,2]. A main morphological characteristic of sinusoidal endothelial cells is the numerous fenestrae that are arranged as sieve plates along the sinusoidal lining[3]. Sinusoidal endothelial cells regulate the number and size of the fenestrae by means of cytoskeletal components such as actin and myosin[4]. This allows control of molecular exchange at the sinusoidal surface of hepatocytes.

Although sinusoids of the normal liver are devoid of basement membrane, a delicate reticular network of matrix proteins is present beneath sinusoidal endothelial liver cells, such as in the space of Disse[5]. Under normal circumstances this matrix contains collagen types I, III, and IV, glycoproteins such as fibronectin and small amounts of undulin[6], thrombospondin[7], laminin[8], entactin[9], and proteoglycans such as heparan sulphate[10].

Liver fibrogenesis is a result of response of the liver to toxic, infectious or metabolic agents and is characterized by an increase and altered deposition of newly formed extracellular matrix components. Fibrogenesis is initiated by hepatocyte damage leading to recruitment of inflammatory blood cells and activation of Kupffer cells with subsequent release of cytokines and growth factors. Ito cells seem to be the primary target cells for inflammatory stimuli: these proliferate, transform into myofibroblast-like cells ('activated Ito cells') and synthesize large amounts of connective tissue components.

The composition of extracellular matrix proteins in expanded portal areas, in septa and in cirrhotic nodules is similar to that of the normal portal tracts and consists of collagen I, III, IV, V and VI and various members of the structural glycoprotein family and the major subclasses of glycosaminoglycans. Deposition of large amounts of collagen type IV, perlecan, laminin, and entactin in the perisinusoidal space results in the formation of a complete basement membrane, a process called collagenization or capillarization of the sinusoids. Capillarization of the sinusoids is an early event in liver fibrogenesis and seems to be of crucial importance for the liver function, since the exchange of macromolecules between the sinusoidal blood and hepatocytes is fundamentally affected.

In vitro, activated Ito cells produce large amounts of these extracellular matrix proteins, and because these cells are situated in the space of Disse they were considered the most important cell type in this respect. In situ hybridization studies showed that during fibrogenesis sinusoidal or parasinusoidal cells contain mRNA for collagen type I, III, and IV[11-13], laminin[14] and cellular fibronectin[15]. The endothelial cell also seems to be involved in the process of capillarization. During developing liver fibrogenesis morphological changes have been demonstrated in an animal model of thioacetamide-induced rat liver cirrhosis[16]. Using ultrastructural immunochemistry, collagen type I, III, IV, and fibronectin were identified in endothelial cells[17,18]. However, as sinusoidal endothelial cells endocytose matrix proteins, synthesis had to be proven.

In order to study synthetic activities of sinusoidal endothelial cells, these cells had to be isolated free of contaminants in a functionally intact state. Guinea pig sinusoidal liver cells were prepared by pronase and collagenase digestion of the perfused liver, followed by density gradient centrifugation and centrifugal elutriation[19]. After 5 days in culture these cells formed a confluent monolayer (Fig. 1a). Recently, in our laboratory rat sinusoidal endothelial cells were cultured on collagen type I coated surfaces and formed a confluent monolayer after 4 days of culture. Cells prepared in this way are >85% pure. It is still a matter of debate whether von Willebrand factor is a useful marker for sinusoidal endothelial liver cells: it is well established that the endothelium of the large hepatic vessel contains abundant amounts of von Willebrand factor. It is not clear, however, whether von Willebrand factor-related positivity along the sinusoids reflects staining of sinusoidal cells or extracellular von Willebrand factor deposits. There seem to be species-related differences, since cultured guinea pig sinusoidal endothelial cells express von Willebrand factor (Fig. 1b)[20], whereas only a small proportion of cultured rat sinusoidal endothelial cell show von Willebrand factor positivity[21] (unpublished personal results), which may be related to contaminating endothelial cells of the large vessels. As von Willebrand factor seems not to be an appropriate marker for rat sinusoidal endothelial cells, the purity of rat cultures has to be checked by electron microscopy and the uptake of dil-Ac-LDL[22].

CELL–MATRIX ADHESION PROTEINS EXPRESSED BY SINUSOIDAL ENDOTHELIAL CELLS

Since it is now well established that most interactions between endothelial cells and matrix are mediated through specialized membrane proteins, it is likely that sinusoidal endothelial cells express distinct sets of adhesion molecules, concurrent with the structural and microenvironmental characteristics of the sinusoidal wall. Cell–matrix interactions operating in the endothelial lining of the sinusoids differ from those in other capillary vessels. Capillary endothelial cells adhere to the constituents of their basement membrane through the expression of specialized proteins, including the integrin family[23,24], the

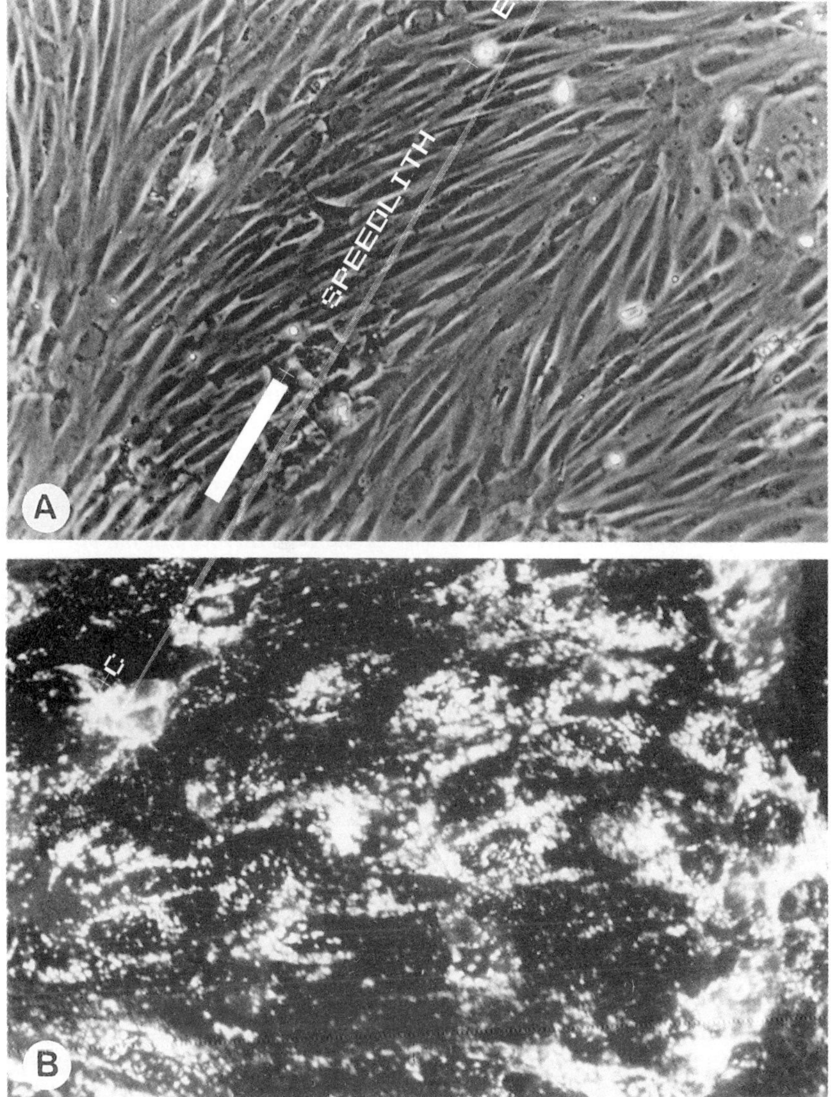

Fig. 1 (a) Phase contrast microscopy of guinea pig sinusoidal endothelial cells 7 days after isolation, with permission from Mosby-Year Book, Inc. (×86). (b) Indirect immunofluorescence staining of guinea pig endothelial cells fixed at day 7 after isolation with a polyclonal antibody against human von Willebrand factor, with permission from W.B. Saunders Company. (Original magnification×172)

thrombospondin receptor (CD36 molecule) and the hyaluronate receptor (CD44 molecule). On the contrary sinusoidal endothelial cells display significant levels of CD36[25] and hyaluronate receptor[26] but express a very restricted set of integrins, which parallels the composition of the perisinusoidal matrix. Only $\alpha_1\beta_1$

Table 1   Extracellular matrix protein expression in liver sinusoidal endothelial cells

Protein	Reference
Cellular fibronectin (guinea pig)	20
Laminin (rat)	31
Collagen type IV (guinea pig)	30
Thrombospondin (guinea pig)	7
Entactin (rat)	9
von Willebrand factor (guinea pig)	17

and $\alpha_5\beta_1$ integrins are expressed in high levels on the sinusoidal endothelium[27]. Both integrins are receptors for collagen and fibronectin. Collagen as well as fibronectin are present in large amounts in the perisinusoidal space.

β_3 integrins are strongly expressed by microvascular endothelial cells, but are only faintly detectable along the sinusoidal wall[28]. Some of their ligands, such as von Willebrand factor and thrombospondin, are present in small amounts in the extracellular matrix along the sinusoids; others such as vitronectin are undetectable. Integrin chains characteristic of the laminin receptor including α_2, α_3, α_6, and β_4 are undetectable on sinusoidal endothelial cells[28]. This lack of expression is correlated with the near absence of laminin in the perisinusoidal space[29].

The restrictive set of integrins expressed by sinusoidal cells is therefore adapted to the specific microenvironment of this endothelial subset. Recent evidence shows that sinusoidal endothelial cells may express an expanded repertoire of adhesion molecules in response to microenvironmental changes as they occur during liver fibrogenesis.

CONTRIBUTION OF LIVER SINUSOIDAL CELLS TO THE SYNTHESIS OF EXTRACELLULAR MATRIX PROTEINS

Isolated and cultivated guinea pig sinusoidal endothelial cells synthesize fibronectin[20], collagen type IV[30] and other glycoproteins of the sinusoidal space such as thrombospondin[7,30], entactin[9] and probably laminin[24] (Table 1). Maher and McGuire found that freshly isolated rat endothelial cells contain more mRNA specific for collagen type III, IV and laminin than Ito cells[31]. The authors also found that endothelial cells isolated from fibrotic liver contain an increased amount of transcripts specific for collagen type I[31]. The increased deposition of von Willebrand factor (Fig. 2) and thrombospondin in developing fibrotic septa could be demonstrated in an animal model of fibrosing liver damage[7,32].

MODULATION OF PROTEIN SYNTHESIS BY TRANSFORMING GROWTH FACTOR-β1

In liver fibrosis, transforming growth factor-β1 (TGF-β1) seems to play a central role. In an experimental model[33] and in human liver fibrosis due to viral

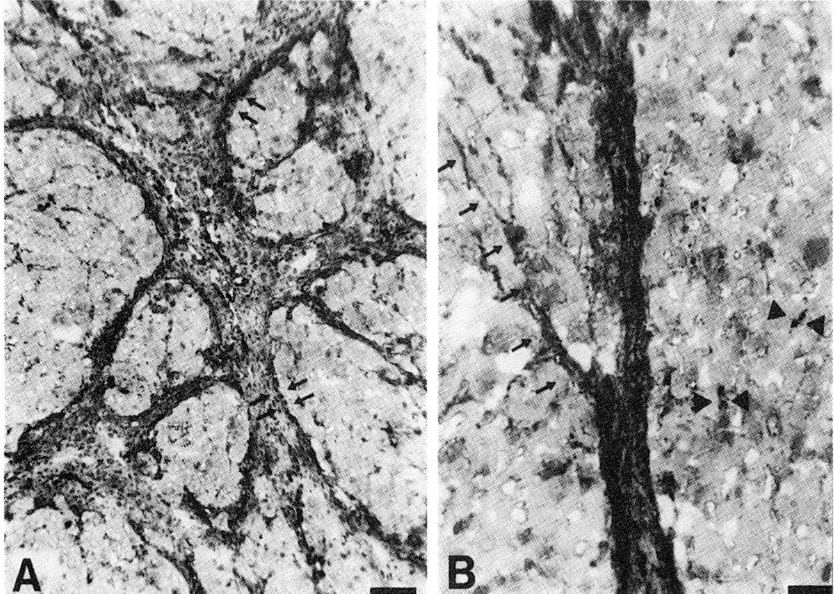

Fig. 2 Immunohistochemical detection of von Willebrand factor in chronically damaged rat liver tissue (cirrhosis). Cryostat sections of rat liver tissue were immunostained with an antibody directed against von Willebrand factor followed by the incubation with peroxidase-conjugated anti rabbit immunoglobulins, with permission from W.B. Saunders Company. [bars represent $30\,\mu$m (a), $15\,\mu$m (b)]

hepatitis[34], the expression of TGF-β1 mRNA in the liver is correlated with ongoing deposition of collagenous proteins.

Guinea pig sinusoidal endothelial liver cells have been shown to express TGF-β1 receptors[35]. The synthesis of extracellular matrix proteins in cultured guinea pig sinusoidal endothelial cells is stimulated in vitro by TGF-β[30]. TGF-β regulates fibrotic processes not only by stimulation of matrix proteins but also at the level of proteinase activity[36]. The most important protease degrading glycoprotein of extracellular matrix seems to be plasmin[37]. Endothelial cells use the plasmin system for intravascular fibrinolysis[38] and vascular remodelling[39]. Sinusoidal endothelial cells contribute to liver fibrosis by the synthesis and release of matrix degradation inhibition proteins such as plasminogen activator inhibitor type I[35]. TGF-β1 stimulated the production of plasminogen activator inhibitor type I[35]. Furthermore, TGF-β responsiveness of endothelin synthesis in sinusoidal endothelial cells could be demonstrated[40]. The main target of endothelin seems to be Ito cells expressing the endothelin A and B receptor, which respond upon endothelin stimulation by contraction and mitogenesis[41].

In conclusion, sinusoidal endothelial cells are not mere innocent bystanders, but seem to contribute to liver fibrogenesis by different pathways. Preliminary data obtained in CCl_4-induced rat liver cirrhosis might indicate that fibrous septa develop inside liver sinusoids crucially involving sinusoidal endothelial cells.

REFERENCES

1. Brouwer A, Wisse E, Knook DL. Sinusoidal endothelial cells and perisinusoidal fat storing cells. In: Arias IM, Jacoby WB, Popper H, Schachter D, Shafritz DA, editors. The liver: biology and pathobiology, 2nd Edn. New York: Raven Press; 1988:665–82.
2. Smedsröd B, Bertoft H, Gustafson S, Laurent TC. Scavenger function of liver endothelial cell. Biochem J. 1990;266:313–27.
3. Wisse E. An electron microscopic study of the fenestrated endothelial lining of rat liver sinusoids. J Ultrastruct Res. 1970;31:125–50.
4. Arias IM. The biology of hepatic endothelial cell fenestrae. In: Schaffer F, Popper H, editors. Progress in liver disease. Vol IX. Philadelphia: WB Saunders; 1990:11–26.
5. Martinez-Hernandez A. The hepatic extracellular matrix. I. Electron immunohistochemical studies in normal rat liver. Lab Invest. 1984;51:57–74.
6. Knittel T, Odenthal M, Schuppan D et al. Synthesis of undulin by rat liver fat-storing cells: Comparison with fibronectin and tenascin. Exp Cell Res. 1992;203:312–20.
7. Rieder H, Ramadori G, Schwögler S, Meyer zum Büschenfelde KH. Thrombospondin, a matrix protein of the Disse space, is mainly produced by sinusoidal endothelial liver cells. In: Gressner AM, Ramadori G, editors. Molecular and cell biology of liver fibrogenesis. Kluwer Academic Publishers; 1992:172–5.
8. Friedman SL. Cellular sources of collagen and regulation of collagen production in liver. Semin Liver Dis. 1990;10:20–9.
9. Schwoegler S, Neubauer K, Knittel T. Chung AE, Ramadori G. Entactin expression in normal and in fibrotic rat liver and in rat liver cells. Lab Invest. 1994;70:525–36.
10. Gressner AM. Hepatic proteoglycans: a brief review of their pathobiochemical implications. Hepatogastroenterology. 1983;20:225–9.
11. Milani S, Herbst H, Schuppan D, Hahn EG, Stein H. In situ hybridization for procollagen type I, III and IV messenger RNA in normal and fibrotic rat liver. Evidence for prodominant expression in non-parenchymal liver cells. Hepatology. 1989;10:84–92.
12. Milani S, Herbst H, Schuppan D, Kim KY, Riecken EO, Stein H. Procollagen expression by nonparenchymal rat liver cells in biliary fibrosis. Gastroenterology. 1990;98:175–84.
13. Milani S, Herbst H, Schuppan D, Surrenti C, Riecken EO, Stein H. Cellular localization of type I, III, and procollagen gene transcripts in normal and fibrotic human liver. Am J Pathol. 1990;137:59–70.
14. Milani S, Herbst H, Schuppan D, Surrenti C, Riecken EO, Stein H. Cellular localization of laminin gene transcripts in normal and fibrotic human liver. Am J Pathol. 1989;143:1175–82.
15. Odenthal M, Neubauer K, Meyer zum Büschenfelde KH, Ramadori G. Localization and mRNA steady-state level of cellular fibronectin in rat liver undergoing a CCl_4-induced acute damage or fibrosis. Biochem Biophys Acta. 1993;1181:266–72.
16. Mori T, Okanoue T, Sawa Y, Hori N, Ohta M, Kagawa K. Defenestration of the sinusoidal endothelial cell in a rat model of cirrhosis. Hepatology. 1993;17:891–97.
17. Clement B, Emonhrad H, Rissel M et al. Cellular origin of collagen and fibronectin in the liver. Cell Mol Biol. 1984;30:489–96.
18. Clement B, Grimaud JA, Campion JP, Deugnier Y, Guillouzo A. Cell types involved in collagen and fibronectin production in normal and fibrotic human liver. Hepatology. 1986;6:225–34.
19. Knook DL, Sleyster ECH. Separation of Kupffer and endothelial cells of the rat liver by centrifugal elutriation. Exp Cell Res. 1976;99:444–9.
20. Rieder H, Ramadori G, Dienes HP, Meyer zum Büschenfelde KH. Sinusoidal endothelial cells from guinea pig liver synthesize and secrete cellular fibronectin in vitro. Hepatology. 1987;7:856–61.
21. Lenzi R, Alpini G, Lin MH, Rand JH, Tavoloni N. Von Willebrand factor related antigen is not an accurate marker of rat and guinea pig liver endothelial cells. Liver. 1990;10:372–9.
22. Gustafson S, Ostlund-Lindquists AM. Uptake and degradation of human very low density lipoproteins by rat liver endothelial cells in culture. Biochem Biophys Acta. 1985;834:308–15.
23. Hynes RO. Integrins: a family of surface receptors. Cell. 1987;48:549–54.
24. Ruoshlati E. Integrins. J Clin Invest. 1981;87:1–5.
25. Greenwalt DE, Lipsky RH, Ockenhouse CF, Ikeda H, Tandon NN, Jamieson GA. Membrane glycoprotein CD36: a review of its role in adherence, signal transduction and transfusion medicine. Blood. 1992;80:1105–15.

26. Volpes R, van den Oord JJ, Desmet CJ. Vascular adhesion molecules in acute and chronic liver inflammation. Hepatology. 1992;16:169–75.
27. Scoazec JY, Feldmann G. The cell adhesion molecules of hepatic sinusoidal endothelial cells. J Hepatology. 1994;20:296–300.
28. Coulevard A, Scoazec JY, Feldmann G. Expression of cell–cell and cell–matrix adhesion molecules by sinusoidal endothelial cells in the normal and cirrhotic human liver. Am J Pathol. 1993;143:738–52.
29. Griffith MR, Keir S, Burt AD. Basement membrane proteins in the space of Disse: a reappraisal. J Pathol. 1991;44:646–8.
30. Rieder H, Ramadori G, Meyer zum Büschenfelde KH. Liver sinusoidal cells are activated by transforming growth factor β and Kupffer cell supernatants to an increased biosynthesis of matrix proteins. In: Wisse E, Knook DL, McCuskey R, editors. Cells of the hepatic sinusoids. Leiden: The Kupffer Cell Foundation; 1991;Vol. 3:171–6.
31. Maher JJ, McGuire RF. Extracellular matrix protein expression increases preferentially in rat lipocytes and sinusoidal endothelial cells during hepatic fibrosis in vivo. J Clin Invest. 1990;86:1641–48.
32. Knittel T, Neubauer K, Armbrust T, Ramadori G. Expression of von Willebrand factor in normal and diseased rat liver and in activated rat liver cells. Hepatology. 1995;in press.
33. Nakatsukasa H, Nagy P, Evarts RP, Hsia LC, Marsden E, Thorgeirsson SS. Cellular distribution of transforming growth factor $\beta 1$ and procollagen types I, III, and IV transcripts in carbon tetrachloride induced rat liver fibrosis. J Clin Invest. 1990;85:1833–43.
34. Castilla A, Prieto J, Fausto N. Transforming growth factor $\beta 1$ and α in chronic liver disease: effects of interferon α therapy. N Engl J Med. 1991;324:933–40.
35. Rieder H, Armbrust T, Meyer zum Büschenfelde KH, Ramadori G. Contribution of sinusoidal liver cells to liver fibrosis: Expression of transforming growth factor $\beta 1$ receptors and modulation of plasmin generating enzymes by transforming growth factor $\beta 1$. Hepatology. 1993;18:938–44.
36. Roberts AB, Sporn MB. The transforming growth factor β. In: Sporn MB, Roberts AB, editors. Peptide growth factors and their receptors. Berlin: Springer; 1990:419–71.
37. Keski-Oja J, Raghow R, Sawdey M et al. Regulation of mRNAs for type-1 plasminogen activator inhibitor, fibronectin and type I procollagen by transforming growth factor β. J Biol Chem. 1988;263:3111–15.
38. Erickson LA, Schleef RR, Ny T, Loskutoff DJ. The fibronolytic system of the vascular wall. Clin Haematol. 1985;14:513–30.
39. Yasunaga C, Nakashima Y, Suliski K. A role of fibronolytic system in angiogenesis. Lab Invest. 1989;61:698–704.
40. Rieder H, Ramadori G, Meyer zum Büschenfelde KH. Sinusoidal endothelial cells in vitro release endothelin – augmentation by transforming growth factor β and Kupffer cell conditioned media. Klin Wochenschr. 1991;69:387–91.
41. Housset C, Rockey DC, Bissell DM. Endothelin receptors in rat liver: lipocyte as contractile target for endothelin 1. Proc Natl Acad Sci USA. 1993;15:9266–70.

6
The contribution of hepatocytes to cytokine-directed activation of fat-storing cells – a pathogenetic key mechanism in liver fibrogenesis

A. M. GRESSNER, C. HOFFMANN, M. G. BACHEM, G. SCHÜFTAN, B. LAHME and A. BRENZEL

INTRODUCTION

Chronic acute liver diseases of diverse aetiologies are complicated by the development of liver fibrosis, i.e. the accumulation, histological redistribution, and molecular rearrangement of virtually all components of the extracellular matrix (ECM). Collagens (types I, III, IV, V, VI), proteoglycans (proteoheparan sulphate, and dermatan and chondroitin sulphate isomers), hyaluronan, and structural glycoproteins (fibronectin isotypes, laminin, nidogen, tenascin, undulin) constitute the main fractions of ECM[1–3]. The fibrotic accumulation of liver ECM is brought about mainly by increased synthesis of matrix molecules (i.e. fibrogenesis), but histological and molecular rearrangement of the various ECM components leading to preferential perisinusoidal and early perivenular deposition of ECM and increases of predominantly dermatan and chondroitin sulphates and of types I and IV collagens is thought to be mainly the result of preferential degradation (i.e. fibrolysis) of some ECM components by the activity of various substrate-specific matrix metalloproteinases (MMPs)[4] and their respective tissue inhibitors (TIMPs)[5,6].

Recent analyses point clearly to fat-storing cells (FSC) (perisinusoidal lipocytes, vitamin A-storing cells, stellate cells)[7] as the main (precursor) cell type responsible for fibrogenesis[8,9] and partially also for fibrolysis[8,10]. Before full competency for fibrogenesis is reached, FSC have to be activated[8,9,11]. Activation includes (i) stimulation of cellular proliferation[12], (ii) phenotypic transition (transformation) from the retinoid storing to ECM secreting cell type (termed myofibroblast), (iii) enhanced expression of almost all matrix genes, and (iv) the acquisition of contractility mediated by endothelin-1, angiotensin II, and other agonists[9]. The fully transformed counterpart of FSC, i.e. the myofibroblast,

Table 1 Principal pathways of fat storing cell activation

'traditional' pathway (!)	complementary pathway (?)
paracrine by inflammatory cells	paracrine by (damaged) hepatocytes (PC)
• cells increase in number • activated macrophages • generation of FSC activating factors in culture (e.g. TGF-β_1, TGF-α)	• PC closely associated with FSC in situ • PC damage precedes (always?) fibrogenesis • alcoholic fibrosis is initiated in centrilobular zone where PC injury is most prominent • p-oncogene expression in FSC follows directly CCl_4-damage of PC • fibrogenesis proceeds in the absence of conspicuous inflammation, e.g. in haemochromatosis

characteristically expresses smooth muscle α-actin filament[13] and a broad spectrum of growth factors, (proinflammatory) cytokines and chemokines, including transforming growth factors (TGF) α and β, insulin-like growth factor (IGF), and monocyte chemotactic peptide (MCP)-1[9].

Lipocyte activation in situ is the result of interactions between FSC and activated macrophages/Kupffer cells (KC)[14,15], platelets[16], and endothelial cells[17]. These produce cytokines and some non-peptide molecular mediators that stimulate one or several partial reactions of FSC activation in vitro. TGF-β, TGF-α, tumour necrosis factor (TNF) α and platelet-derived growth factor (PDGF) have been identified as main 'fibrogenic' mediators discharged from these cells upon stimulation. The present study was focused on the role which hepatocytes (PC) might play in the activation process of FSC. We hypothesized on the basis of histological, recent cell biological and clinical findings and observations (Table 1) that PC, the cell type which is located in situ nearest to FSC, could play a prominent, permissive or additive role in the pathogenetically most relevant process of FSC activation.

MATERIALS AND METHODS

Isolation and culture of cells

Isolation and culture of rat liver FSC have been described in detail previously[18]. In brief, non-parenchymal liver cells were isolated by the pronase–collagenase method. FSC were purified by a single step density gradient centrifugation with Nycodenz and identified by their typical light microscopic appearance, transmission electron microscopy, immunofluorescent stainings for desmin and vimentin, vitamin A-specific autofluorescence and, negatively, by the inability to phagocytose latex beads, to stain for peroxidase, and to express Fc receptors. The mean purity of freshly isolated cells was $90 \pm 5\%$, cell viability was $>95\%$. FSC were seeded normally with a density of 0.2×10^6 cells/10 cm^2/2 ml medium and were maintained as monolayers in 6-well culture plates with DMEM containing 4 mmol/l L-glutamine, penicillin (100 IU/ml), streptomycin (100 μg/ml), and 0.5% (v/v) fetal calf serum (FCS). The cells were cultured in a humidified atmosphere of 5% CO_2–95% air. The first change of the medium was made about 16h after seeding, after which the purity of FSC was >97%. The medium was changed from 10% FSC at seeding to 0.5%.

PC were isolated from rats (250-320 g body weight, fasted overnight) by the collagenase method of Seglen[19], modified as described previously[20]. The viability of the final parenchymal cell suspension was between 80 and 90%. Contamination with non-parenchymal cells was <1%. Cells were seeded at a density of 4.5×10^6 cells/75 cm^2 flask and cultured at 37°C in a humidified atmosphere of 5% CO_2 and 95% air in 15 ml DMEM supplemented with 4 mmol/l L-glutamine, 10% FCS, 2 mg/ml insulin (from bovine pancreas), penicillin (100 IU/ml), and streptomycin (100 μg/l). The first change of the medium was 2h after plating. Cells were cultured for another 16h in DMEM with 10% FCS. Thereafter, medium was aspirated, the cell layer was washed with HBSS to remove traces of FCS, and cultured further in DMEM without FCS and insulin. The conditioned medium (PCcM) was then harvested and the DNA content of the cell layer measured.

KC were isolated separately from FSC and purified by elutriation as described[21]. Kupffer cells recovered from eluates were collected by centrifugation and resuspended in culture medium identical with that described above for FSC. The cells were seeded at a density of 30×10^6 cells/75 cm^2 culture flask in 15 ml of the above medium containing 10% FCS. About 40 min after seeding the cells were washed with HBSS to remove FCS. KC were then cultured in DMEM without FCS for a period of 24h after which time conditioned medium (KCcM) was collected. Viability was >90%. Assessment of the purity of KC (>95%) was performed by electron microscopy, peroxidase staining, by phagocytosis of latex beads, and by demonstration of positive immunofluorescence staining for vimentin as described[21].

Treatment of hepatocytes

Before and during collection of hepatocyte-conditioned media, the cells were exposed to various chemical toxins: carbonyl-cyanide m-chlorophenylhydrazone (CCCP), t-butylhydroperoxide (TBHP), and calcium ionophore A23187, respectively[22]. In other experiments PC were exposed either continuously up to 96h or only temporarily for 1h and 3h, respectively, to human recombinant TGF-β_1 (0.25 – 3 ng/ml).

Preparation of cell-conditioned media

Media harvested from cultures of PC and KC, respectively, were centrifuged and dialysed for 24h against 3 changes of each 20 vol of DMEM at 4°C in tubing with a molecular weight cutoff of 3500 Da. Thereafter, the medium was gassed with CO_2, sterilized by filtration and aliquots were frozen at −40°C until use. The concentration of total protein was determined in the medium.

Determination of proliferation of fat-storing cells

One day after seeding the medium of nonconfluent monolayers of FSC was changed from 10% to 0.5% FCS. After 24h various dilutions of conditioned media of hepatocytes (PCcM) and Kupffer cells (KCcM), separately or in combination, were added. Other agonists were added similarly and 24h thereafter the cells were exposed to [³H]thymidine for 24h. Control cultures received an equivalent amount (up to 100 μg/ml) of protein (bovine albumin, fraction V, cell culture tested) instead of PCcM or KCcM. Radioactivity incorporated into DNA was measured as described previously[21]. Modifications of this regimen are described in the legends of the appropriate figures and tables.

For standardization, stimulation of [³H]thymidine incorporation into DNA of FSC by PCcM was related to that provoked by addition of 10% FCS in relation to 0.5% FCS. A stimulation index (SI) was defined to be the following ratio of incorporation:

$$SI = \frac{PCcM - 0.5\% \text{ FCS}}{10\% \text{ FCS} - 0.5\% \text{ FCS}}$$

Measurement of bromodeoxyuridine incorporation

Cells were labelled for 24h with 5-bromo-2′-deoxyuridine (BrdUrd, final concentration 5×10^{-5} mol/l, Sigma Chemical Co.) and thereafter carefully washed with cold PBS. Fixation was performed with ethanol/acetic acid (95:5, v/v) for at least 20min at 4°C. BrdUrd was detected with an anti-BrdUrd IgG antibody followed by incubation with peroxidase-conjugated antimouse IgG. Nuclei which had taken up BrdUrd were stained with DAB. The percentage of BrdUrd positive nuclei was calculated. Details of the method have been described elsewhere[23,24].

Determination of total and specific proteoglycan synthesis

The synthesis of sulphated proteoglycans (PG) was measured by the incorporation of [³⁵S]sulphate into glycosaminoglycans (GAG) during a labelling period of 24h. Labelled PG were assayed only in the medium, because FSC were shown previously to secrete nearly 80% of newly synthesized PG into the culture medium[18]. Specific types of GAG were analysed by subjecting total PG to consecutive degradations with nitrous acid to yield the incorporation of [³⁵S]sulphate into heparan sulphate and to enzymatic digestions with chondroitin AC- and -ABC-lyases, to obtain chondroitin-4,6-sulphate and dermatan sulphate fractions, respectively. Details have been reported previously[18].

Determination of the catalytic activity of arginase (L-arginine amidinohydrolase, EC 3.5.3.1)

Arginase was determined in PCcM by hydrolysis of L-arginine to L-ornithine and urea at 37°C in 0.1 mol/l carbonate buffer, pH 9.5. Ornithine was measured after stopping the reaction with glacial acetic acid which results in the presence of ninhydrin in a red colour with a maximal absorbance at 515 nm[25].

Inhibition of paracrine stimulation of FSC by α_2-macroglobulin (α_2M)

α_2M was added at concentrations of 50, 200, 500, and 2000 μg/ml to transiently acidified (pH 2.0, 30 min) media conditioned by myofibroblasts and KC and to transiently acidified platelet lysate. Thereafter, these media were added in the absence of FCS to primary cultured FSC three days after seeding. Twelve hours later the cells were labelled with [³H]thymidine and [³⁵S]sulphate for 24 h. Thereafter, cultures were stopped and [³H]thymidine incorporation, DNA and proteoglycan synthesis were determined.

Inhibition of autocrine stimulation of myofibroblasts by α_2-macroglobulin

α_2M was added in concentrations of 50, 500, and 2000 μg/ml to secondary cultured myofibroblasts on the 6th day after passage in the absence of FCS. Twelve hours later cells were labelled with [³H]thymidine and [³⁵S]sulphate. Cultures were stopped 24 h later and cell proliferation, proteoglycan synthesis, DNA and cellular fibronectin were determined.

Determination of cellular fibronectin

Cellular fibronectin was measured in medium using MAB-anti-c-fn clone DH1 (ICN, Costa Mesa, USA) with time-resolved fluorescence[26].

Determination of active TGF-β

TGF-β was activated by transient acidification (pH 2.0, 30 min) of the conditioned media using HCl. Thereafter, the medium was neutralized and dialysed. Active TGF-β was measured by a slightly modified method described by Danielpour[27] using a proliferation inhibition assay of MV1-Lu cells.

Western ligand blotting

PCcM and its chromatographic fractions were dialysed, concentrated and subjected to electrophoresis and ligand blot analysis, essentially as described by Hossenlopp et al.[28]. The separated proteins were transferred to nitrocellulose membranes by electroblotting. The membranes were incubated overnight at 4°C with [¹²⁵I]IGF-1, washed, air-dried and exposed for 6 days at −80°C to Hyperfilm MP using an intensifying screen.

Immunofluorescent stainings of cytoskeletal and extracellular matrix proteins

Cells were washed with PBS and fixed with ethanol/acetic acid. After repeated washings they were incubated with appropriate dilutions of monoclonal mouse antibodies directed against human desmin, vimentin and the α-actin isoform of smooth muscle cells. Extracellular matrix proteins were identified similarly with rabbit polyclonal antibodies to rat fibronectin, rat laminin and rat type I and type III collagen. They were made visible by incubation with biotinylated rabbit anti-mouse immunoglobulin and swine antirabbit antibodies, respectively, followed by FITC- or rhodamine-conjugated streptavidine.

General analytical procedures

Cells were quantitated by fluorometric determination of DNA[29]. Viability was assayed by estimation of the percentage of unstained cells when incubated with 0.25% trypan blue (trypan blue exclusion test), by measurement of LDH and AST activity in the medium using standard clinical chemical procedures, and by fluorochromasia[30], respectively. Total protein in the medium was determined with Coomassie brilliant blue G-250[31].

RESULTS AND DISCUSSION

Growth promoting activity for FSC in the medium conditioned by hepatocytes

The addition of hepatocyte-conditioned medium (PCcM) reproducibly stimulated the incorporation of [³H]thymidine and BrdUrd (not shown) into DNA of FSC 4- to 6-fold compared with untreated control cultures (Fig. 1). The DNA content per culture well increased by about 40% during an exposure time of 48h of FSC with PCcM relative to control cultures kept in 0.5% FCS. The stimulatory effect of PCcM on proliferation of FSC was dose dependent and the magnitude was almost similar to that of 10% FCS. Dilutions of PCcM of 1:8 still enhanced the incorporation of [³H]thymidine about 4-fold (Fig. 1). The mitogenic effect of PCcM on FSC resulted in clear morphological alterations: cells exhibited high density and the shape was more compact than that of control cultures. Perinuclear arrangements of lipid droplets were clearly visible and appeared to be more prominent than in untreated cultures. Immunostaining of ECM components in PCcM-treated FSC cultures showed more intense deposition of both type I and type III collagen and also of fibronectin and laminin than in control cultures. However, the expression of matrix components per cell seemed to be almost unaffected by PCcM, indicating that the increase in matrix deposition per culture is mainly due to the enhancement of FSC number[32]. The exposure of FSC for 5 days with PCcM greatly reduced the spontaneous expression of smooth muscle α-actin. The intensity and arrangement of cytochemically stained lipid droplets in FSC were not affected by treatment of cultures with PCcM. The data support the notion that PCcM does not promote the phenotypic transition of FSC to myofibroblasts and the level of matrix protein expression.

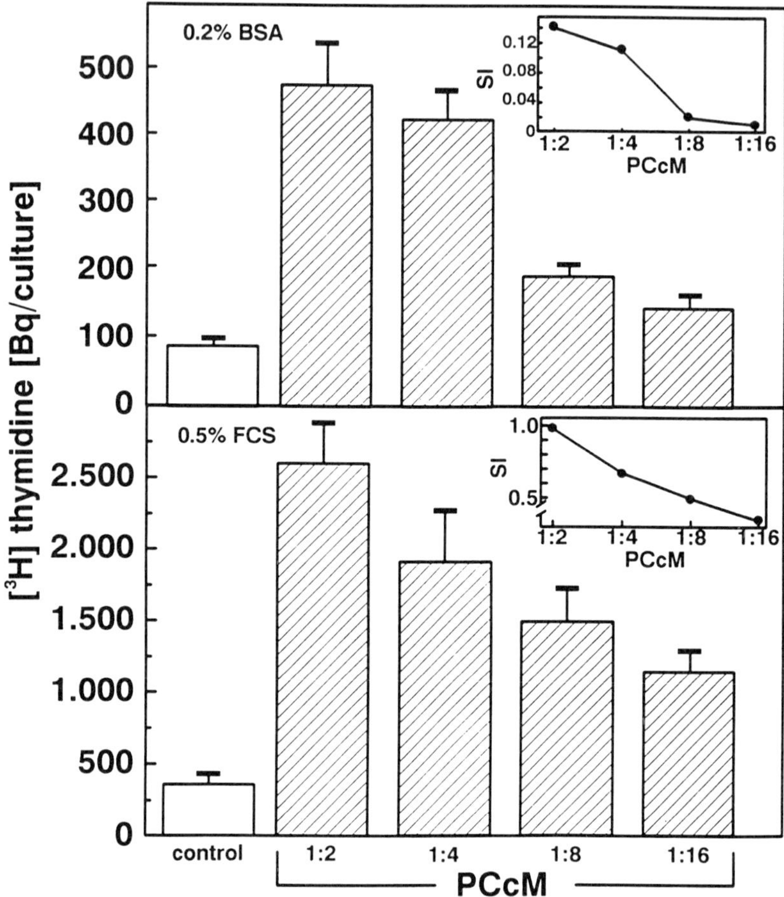

Fig. 1 The stimulatory effects of various dilutions of hepatocyte-conditioned medium (PCcM) on the proliferation of FSC cultured in 0.5% fetal calf serum (FCS) and 0.2% bovine serum albumin (BSA), respectively[32]. The stimulation index (SI) is given in the inset

Synergistic action of hepatocyte-derived mitogenic activity with media conditioned by Kupffer cells

Media conditioned by PC and KC, respectively, stimulated FSC proliferation in a dose-dependent manner (Fig. 2). Combinations of PC- and KC-conditioned media were most potent and increased the incorporation of [³H]thymidine up to 4 times above control values. The multiplication stimulatory effects of PC and KC visualized by labelling cell nuclei with BrdUrd and the increase of cell number per culture well were additive. Whereas KCcM stimulated transformation of FSC, as indicated by more elongated cells with spindle-like cellular extensions and reduction of retinoid droplets, PCcM did not stimulate the transformation to myofibroblasts as described above. Both media act synergistically on the deposition of fibronectin and laminin in FSC cultures[33].

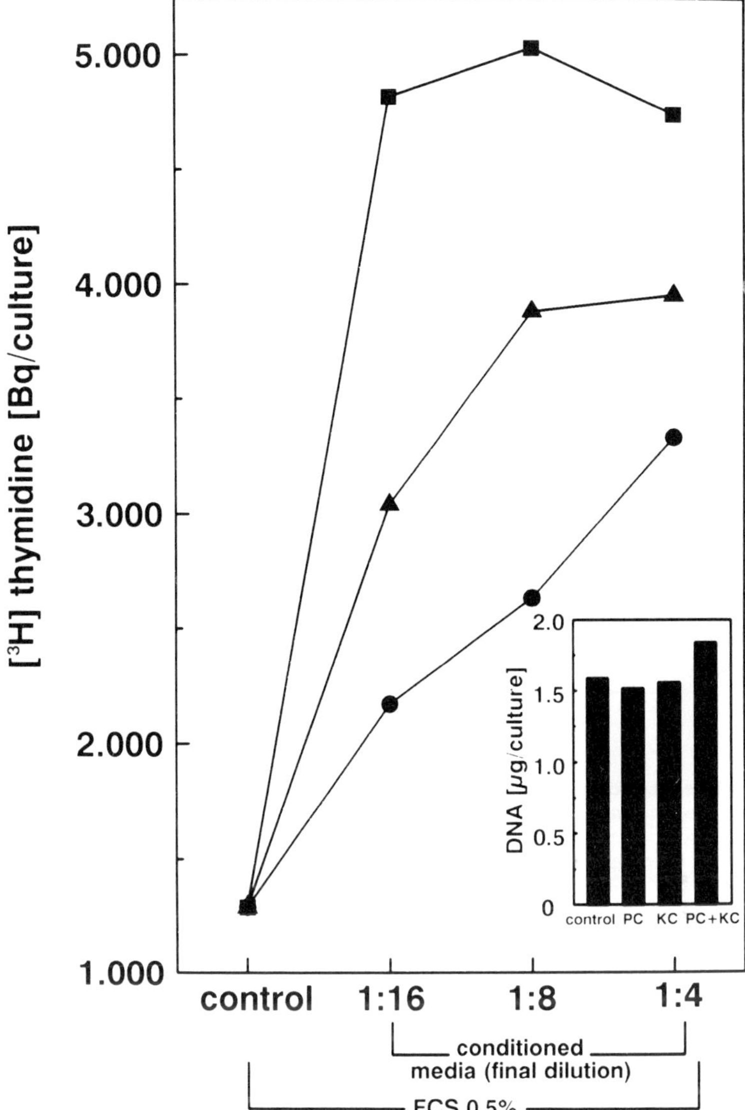

Fig. 2 The effects of hepatocyte-conditioned medium (PCcM, ●—●), Kupffer cell-conditioned medium (KCcM, ▲—▲) and of the combined PCcM/KCcM (■—■) on proliferation of cultured FSC[33]

Similarly, proteoglycan synthesis was maximally enhanced if FSC were exposed to PC and KC media simultaneously[33]. These data suggest that PC and KC might act synergistically, perhaps in a spatial and time-dependent manner, on the activation of FSC in situ. Whereas PCcM represents essentially a non-inflammatory mechanism, KCcM is a prototype inflammatory mechanism of activation of FSC.

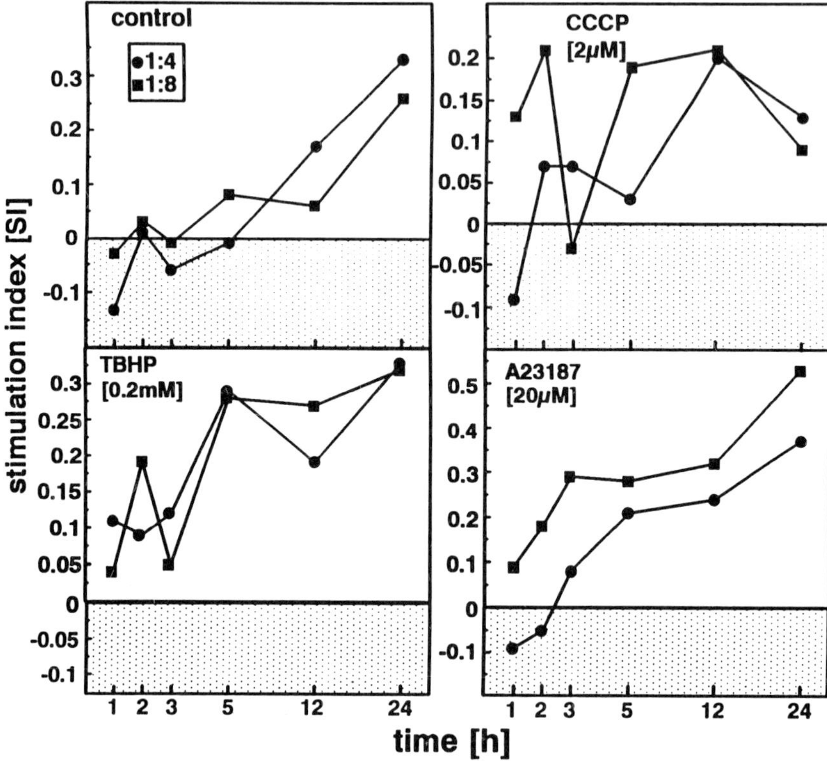

Fig. 3 Time course of the occurrence of mitogenic activity in the medium of untreated PC (control) and PC exposed for up to 24 h to m-chlorophenylhydrazone (CCCP), t-butylhydroperoxide (TBHP), and the calcium ionophore A23187. Control cultures received an equivalent amount of solvent. Dilutions of the conditioned media harvested at the times indicated were added for 48 h to FSC monolayers in 0.5% FCS. The dotted area indicates the inhibitory range. Mean values of triplicate determinations of two independent experiments are shown[22]

Enhancement of hepatocyte-derived mitogenic activity by toxic damage and TGF-β_1-induced apoptosis of cultured parenchymal cells

PC damage frequently (if not always) precedes the activation of FSC in situ and, hence, the development of liver fibrosis. It is not yet known what role damaged PC might play in the process of FSC activation. Defined PC injury was therefore initiated by several toxic chemicals before PCcM was collected and assayed for mitogenic activity in FSC cultures as described above. Data summarized in Figure 3 clearly show that there is a time-dependent increase of mitogenic activity in the conditioned media of control PC; this is more pronounced in PC damaged by various chemicals. The increase of the growth promoting activity in the conditioned media was paralleled by the elevation of LDH and AST activities in these media (Fig. 4) and by the decrease of cell viability. Under these conditions the growth promoting activity of PCcM was correlated highly

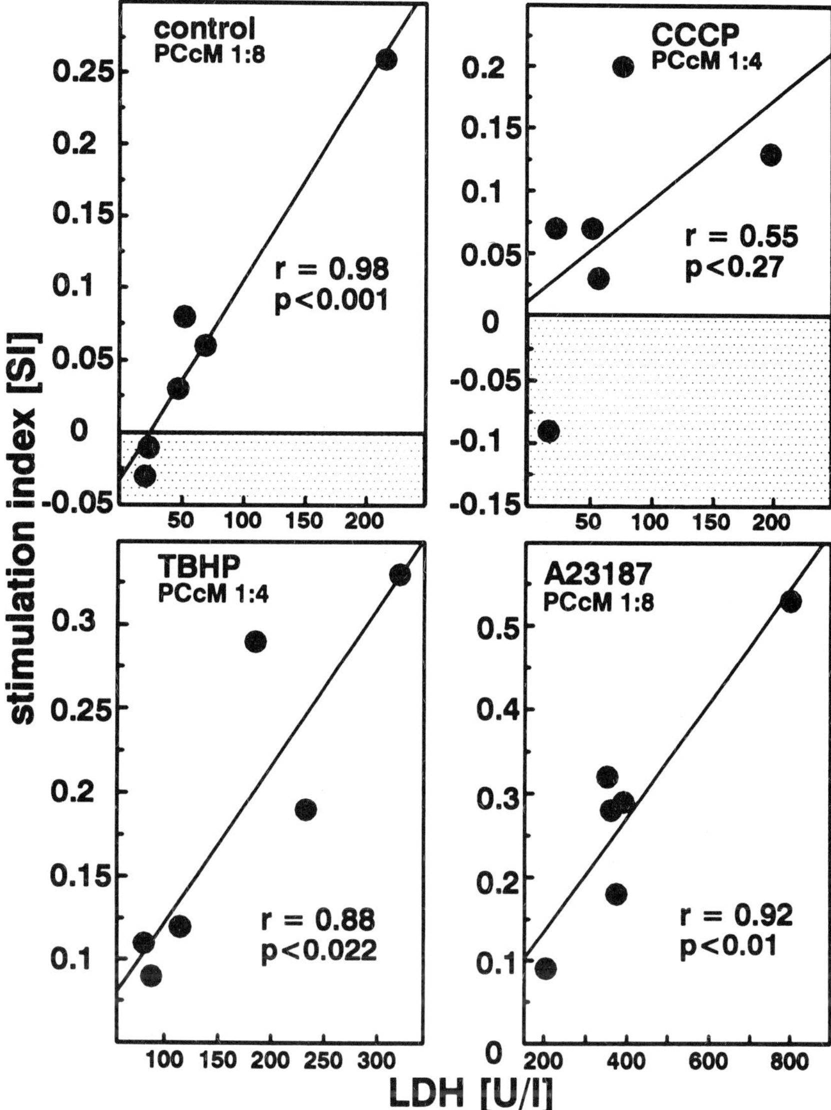

Fig. 4 Correlation between the mitogenic activities for FSC and the catalytic activities of LDH in medium (PCcM) conditioned by untreated PC (control) and PC exposed for various times to cytotoxic agents described in Fig. 3. The dilution of the medium (PCcM), the coefficient of the correlation (r) and the level of statistical significance (p) are given. Mean values of triplicate determinations of two independent experiments are presented[22]

positively and significantly with LDH (Fig. 4) and total protein concentration ($r=0.82$, $p<0.05$). In previous experiments we demonstrated that PC cultured under hypoxic or anoxic conditions released similar or even higher mitogenic activity into the medium than PC cultured under adequate conditions[32]. Thus, PC damage does not abolish but rather augments the mitogenic activity for FSC, which suggests the release of a 'wound hormone' in damaged liver tissue. The chemical characterization and molecular mechanism of action of this mitogen are only incompletely known[32]. The data point to a trypsin-, heat-, and pH-sensitive protein, which is resistant to reducing agents. It does not bind to heparin and wheat germ lectin but is partially fixed to Con-A-lectin. Leupeptin did not reduce its biological activity.

As well as accidental cell death (necrosis), programmed cell death (apoptosis) has been shown to occur in experimental liver diseases[34]. Apoptosis of PC can be induced by some cytokines including TNF-α[35] and TGF-β[36]. Since fully transformed myofibroblasts, activated Kupffer cells/macrophages and disintegrated platelets express and release TGF-β_1 (see Chapter 7), PC in diseased liver may be primed to undergo apoptosis, which in turn may discharge a mitogenic mediator for untransformed FSC similar to that reported above for damaged PC. In fact, myofibroblast-conditioned media in which latent TGF-β had been activated by transient acidification measured in the mink lung epithelial cell bioassay[27] was able to induce apoptosis of primary cultured PC, similar to the action of authentic human recombinant TGF-β_1. Apoptosis was proven by increased activity of endonuclease, electrophoretic DNA ladder, detachment of PC from the plastic support, decrease of mitochondrial dehydrogenase activity measured by reduced formazane dye generation, and by enzyme release (LDH, AST, ALT) into the medium. It was found that PCcM recovered from TGF-β apoptotic PC stimulated mitogenesis of FSC significantly more potently than control PCcM (Fig. 5). Even short exposures to low concentrations of TGF-β_1 produced significant fractions of apoptotic PC. These results suggest a pathogenetic vicious circle based on TGF-β_1 primed parenchymal cell apoptosis, which in turn stimulates FSC to proliferate. Beside of its pleiotropic action on FSC transformation, matrix gene expression, and modulation of matrix degradation, TGF-β_1 might have additional profibrogenic activity via its attack (maybe together with TNF-α) on the integrity of PC.

Scavenging of TGF-β by α_2-macroglobulin (α_2M) produced by hepatocytes and myofibroblasts

α_2M which is synthesized by hepatocytes[37] and myofibroblasts[38,39] was shown to be able to bind and inactivate several growth factors including TGF-β[40–42]. α_2M is also known by its function in binding and scavenging of proteases[43]. The complex binds to specific receptors on hepatocytes[44], fibroblasts[45], myofibroblasts[39] and macrophages[46] and is rapidly eliminated from circulation by endocytosis.

As shown in Figure 6 activated α_2M binds radiolabelled TGF-β very avidly: binding can be demonstrated within 30 s. We evaluated whether α_2M is able to reduce paracrine and autocrine stimulatory loops in FSC and myofibroblasts, respectively. Addition of 500 and 2000 μg/ml α_2M to transiently acidified KCcM, MFBcM and platelet lysate reduced proteoglyan synthesis per DNA significantly and dose-dependently (Fig. 7). This inhibition was comparable to that obtained by adding 12.5 μg/ml TGF-β neutralizing antibodies to the

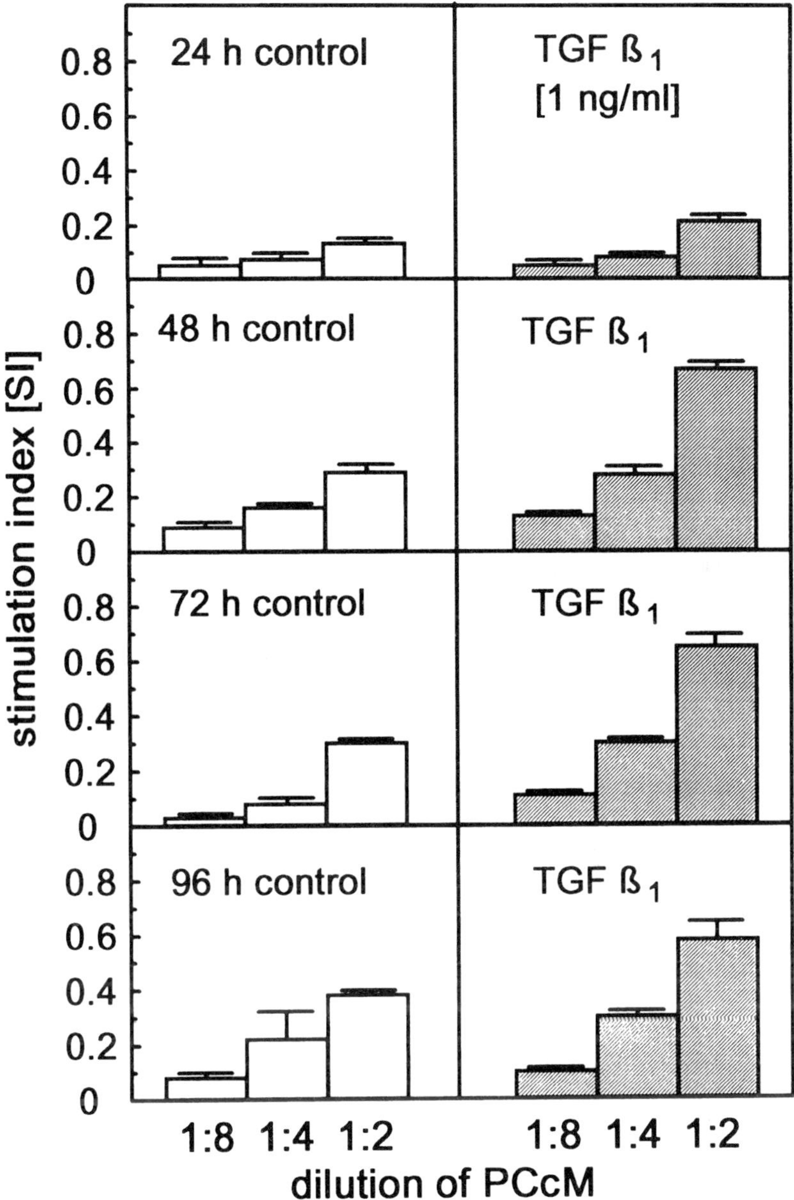

Fig. 5 Comparison of the mitogenic effects on FSC in primary culture of various dilutions of PCcM harvested at different times from control and TGF-β_1-treated PC cultures. TGF-β_1 has been neutralized with anti-TGF-β antibodies before PCcM was added to FSC cultures

conditioned media (data not shown). To inhibit autocrine stimulation α_2M was added at concentrations between 50 and 2000 μg/ml to highly active

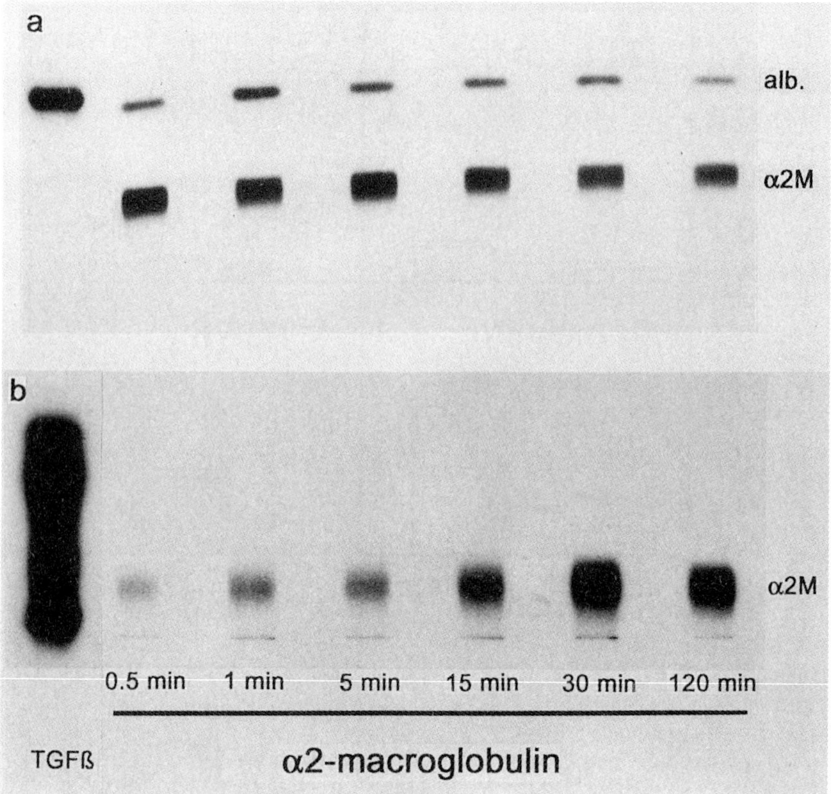

Fig. 6 Binding of [^{125}I]TGF-β to α_2M. [^{125}I]TGF-β was incubated with active α_2M for 30 s, 1, 5, 15, 30 and 120 min, respectively. Thereafter, native agarose electrophoresis followed by autoradiography was performed. (a) Coomassie staining showing α_2M and albumin. (b) Autoradiographic signals demonstrating binding of [^{125}I]TGF-β to α_2M. First line, left side, TGF-β alone; alb, albumin band; α_2M, α_2-macroglobulin

myofibroblasts in secondary culture. Proteoglycan synthesis and cellular fibronectin synthesis were reduced by 50% at a α_2M concentration of 200 μg/ml (Fig. 8). Interestingly, low concentrations of α_2M (50–500 μg/ml) stimulated cell proliferation but high concentrations (2000 μg/ml) reduced mitogenesis. These results suggest that low concentrations of α_2M predominantly bind active TGF-β, which acts as a growth inhibitor[23], but high concentrations neutralize mitogens resulting in growth inhibition.

Determination of active TGF-β in native and acidified conditioned media and in platelet lysate demonstrates that native media contain predominantly latent TGF-β. Transient acidification activated latent TGF-β: this reached concentrations of 1.76±0.45 ng/ml in MFBcM, 2.47±0.56 ng/ml in KCcM, and 9.77 ±1.68 ng/ml in platelet lysate (10^9 platelets/ml), respectively. Addition of 200 μg/ml α_2M for 30 min to these media reduced active TGF-β significantly resulting in a fraction of latent TGF-β >90% in MFBcM and >70% in KCcM and platelet lysate, respectively (Fig. 9).

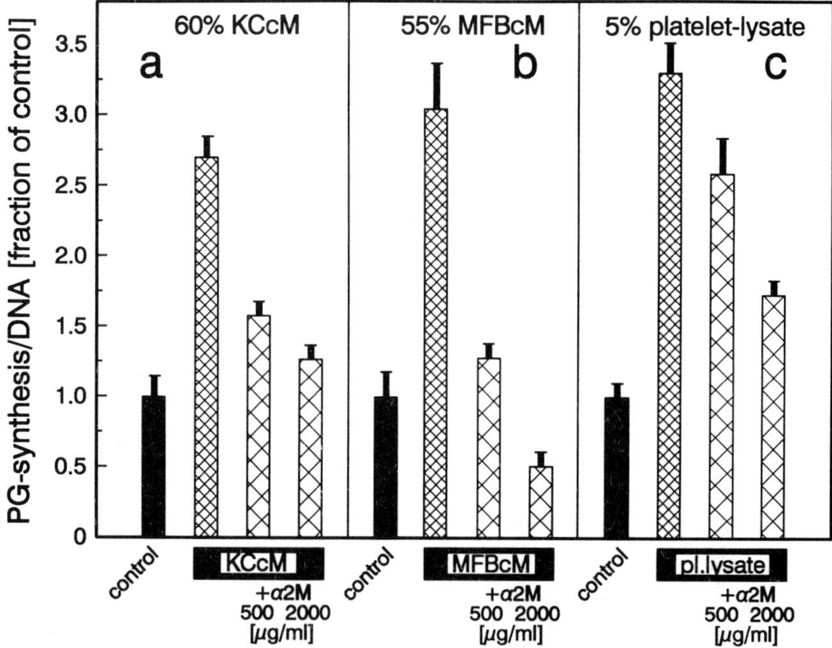

Fig. 7 Inhibition of paracrine stimulation of FSC by α_2M. KCcM, MFBcM, and platelet lysate were transiently acidified to activate latent TGF-β. Thereafter, these media were incubated with α_2M at concentrations of 500 and 2000 μg/ml for 30 min at room temperature. 12 h after adding the media to primary cultured FSC the cells were labelled for 24 h with [^{35}S]sulphate. DNA and proteoglycan synthesis were measured. Results represent mean $\pm$ SD of two experiments (each $n=3$)

Hepatocytes modulate the action of insulin-like growth factors (IGF) on FSC by secretion of IGF-binding proteins (IGFBPs)

The proliferation of FSC in culture was stimulated dose-dependently by IGF-I and IGF-II[47]. PCcM also stimulated FSC proliferation in a dose-dependent manner (see above). If applied in combination a distinct enhancement (more than additive) of both proliferative effects was observed[47].

Native PCcM contains about 100 ng IGF-I/3×10^5 cells per 48 h as determined by radioreceptor assay. Its IGFBP content appears to be heterogeneous as detected by Western ligand blot analysis. A major binding fraction is found in a range of M_r 28–34 kDa, possibly including IGFBPs -1, -2, -5 and -6, and a smaller binding protein fraction is identified at M_r 24 kDa, pointing to IGFBP-4 (Fig. 10).

For identification of the IGFBPs with modulatory effects on IGF activity, concentrated PCcM was subjected to different chromatographic steps which resulted in depletion of growth inhibitory arginase[48] and in enrichment of IGFBP-containing fractions. Maximum proliferation potency, with and without IGF supplementation, was demonstrated by two different final purification procedures: FPLC gel filtration fraction M_r 40–20 kDa and the low salt elution

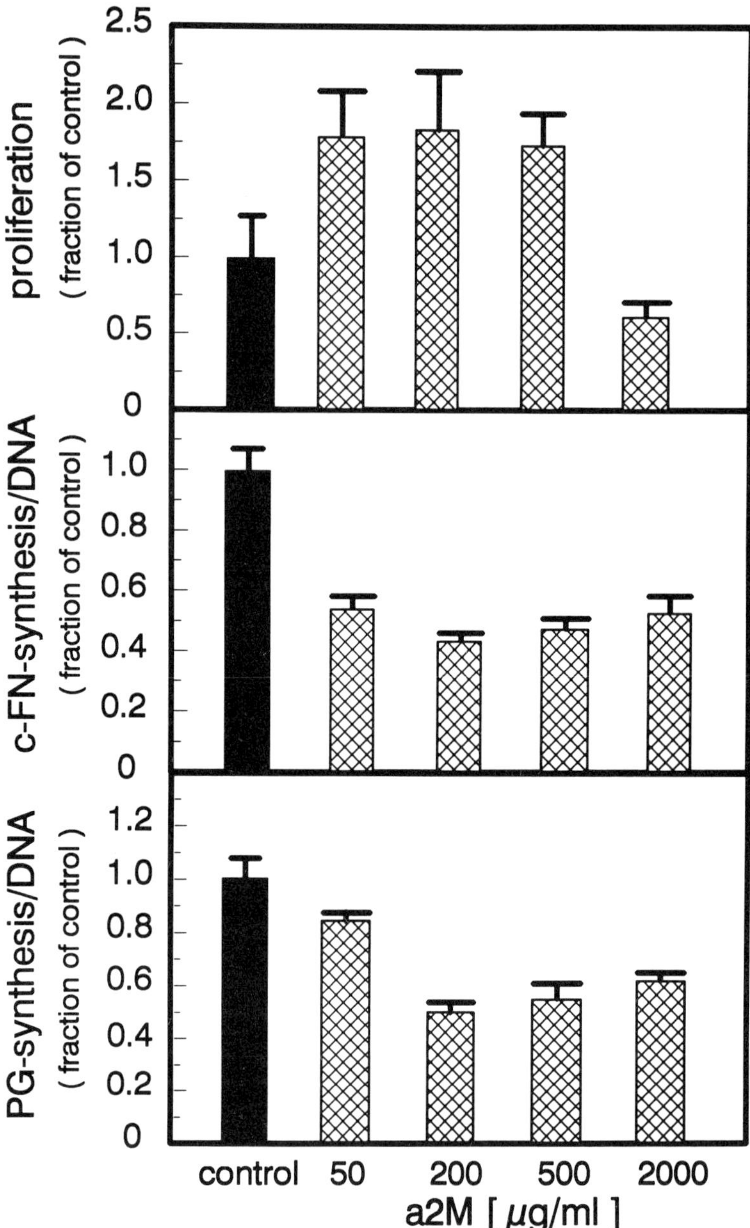

Fig. 8   Inhibition of autocrine stimulation of proteoglycan and cellular fibronectin synthesis, and proliferation of myofibroblasts by α_2-macroglobulin (α_2M). α_2M (50–2000 μg/ml) was added to secondary cultured myofibroblasts at the 5th day after passage. 12h later the cells were labelled for 24h with [^{35}S]sulphate. Proteoglycan synthesis and cellular fibronectin were measured in the medium; proliferation was measured by DNA

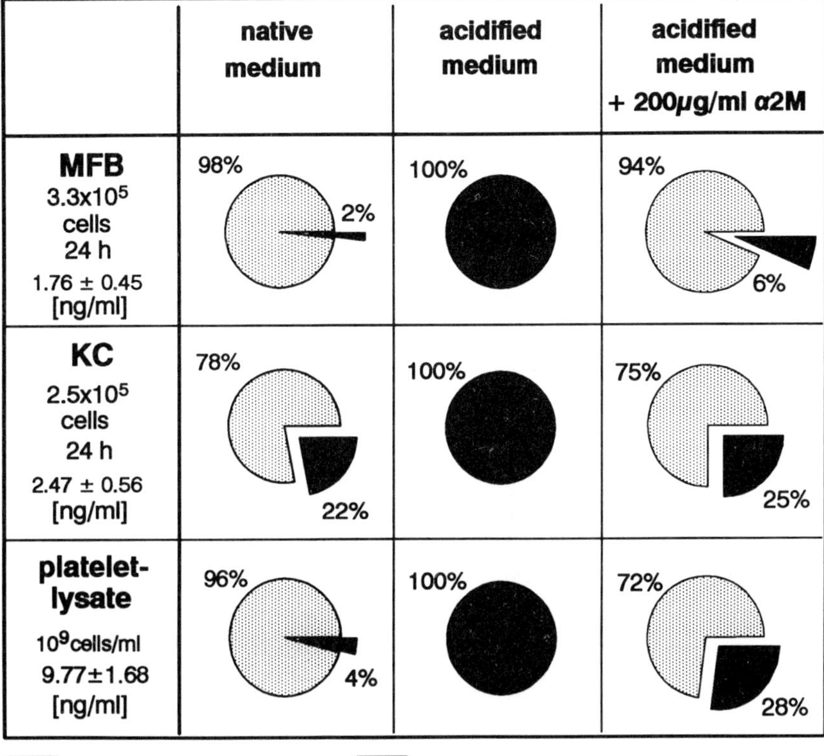

Fig. 9 Determination of active TGF-β in conditioned media and platelet lysate before and after addition of α_2M. TGF-β-concentration was measured with the proliferation inhibition assay using Mv1-LU cells in native and acidified media conditioned by myofibroblasts and Kupffer cells and in platelet lysate before and after incubation with 200 μg/ml α_2M for 30 min. The first row gives the absolute concentrations of active TGF-β in conditioned media, the circle segments indicate the fraction of latent and active TGF-β, respectively

fraction 1 of anion-exchange chromatography (Fig. 10a). Western ligand blot analysis revealed one strong band of M_r 24 kDa, possibly IGFBP-4; the faint band at M_r 29 kDa might be IGFBP-5 (Fig. 10b, lane 1).

Fractions eluting at elevated salt concentrations contained high amounts of IGFBP-1 together with minor portions of IGFBPs -4 and -5 (Fig. 10b, lanes 2 and 3). As shown in the FSC proliferation assay IGFBP-1 may cause a significant reduction in the stimulatory activity of IGFBP-4 and -5 on IGF (Fig. 10a, fractions 2 and 3). Corresponding observations concerning inhibitory effects of IGFBP-1 on IGF action have been reported[49,50].

From these data we conclude that PCcM contains IGF as well as IGFBP, probably associated in complex binding. Though proliferation of FSC is moderately stimulated by IGFs alone it is distinctly enhanced in combination with PCcM. Enhancement obviously occurs when IGFs, mainly derived from IGF-producing PC[51,52] are combined with the specific binding proteins such as

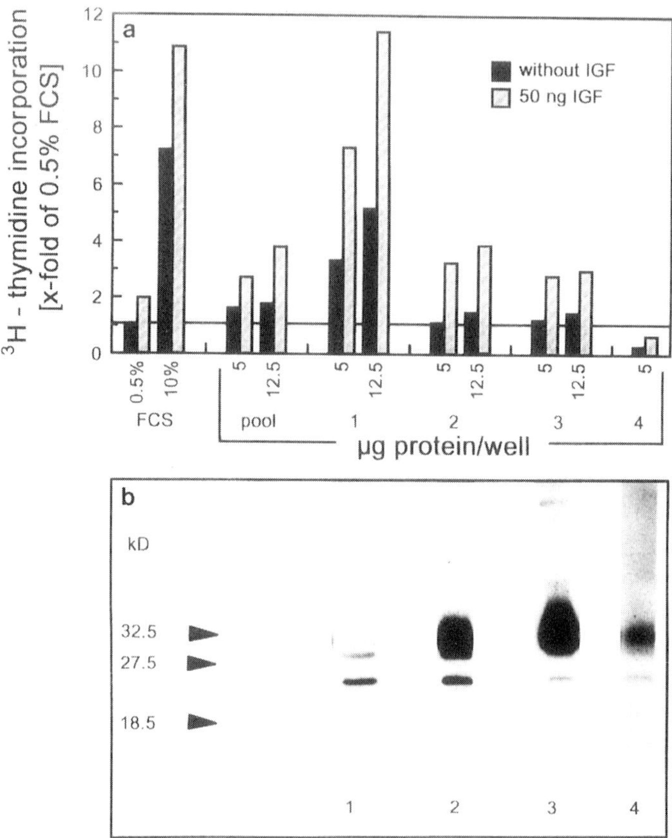

Fig. 10 (a) [³H]thymidine incorporation of cultured FSC displaying the original (■) and IGF-enhanced (□) stimulation caused by IGFBP-containing fractions (fraction 1–4) of chromatographically prepurified pools of concentrated PCcM processed on an anion-exchange FPLC-column correlated with (b) the respective Western ligand blot autoradiographies using [¹²⁵I]IGF-I as detecting ligand (arrows indicate positions of mol. wt markers)

IGFBP-4 and -5, which might be secreted by (damaged) hepatocytes predominantly in case of liver injury. This release may serve as a paracrine stimulus for adjacent FSC to proliferate and transform into myofibroblasts.

Membrane-bound arginase of hepatocytes suppresses proliferation, transformation, and matrix gene expression of cultured FSC

The loss of topographical relationship (cell–cell contact) between FSC and hepatocytes in consequence of hepatocellular damage might play an important role in the initiation of DNA synthesis, mitosis, and transformation of FSC. Therefore, the effect of isolated liver cell membranes and its subfractions on

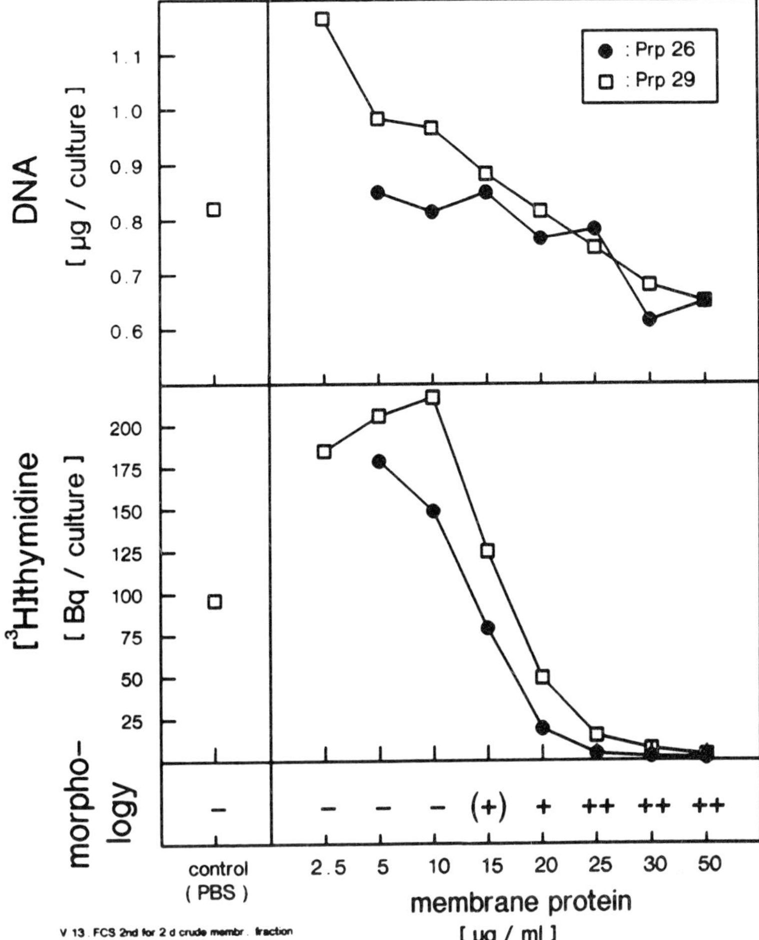

Fig. 11 Dose-dependent inhibition of FSC growth by ultrasonicated liver cell membranes. FSC were incubated at day 2 of primary culture for a further 2 days with increasing amounts of hepatocyte membranes. Labelling with [³H]thymidine was performed during the last 24h. Morphological changes were viewed by phase contrast microscopy. Two independent experiments (prp 26, 29) are shown[48]

some basic functions of FSC was studied in vitro[48]. Crude liver cell membranes and isolated subfractions are able to inhibit the growth, proteoglycan synthesis, and general protein synthesis of FSC in vitro (Fig. 11). Treated cells show characteristic morphological changes characterized by thin cytoplasmic extensions. For crude membranes the ID_{50} was about 17.5 μg protein/ml; for the partially purified inhibitor ID_{50} was 1.5 μg protein/ml[48]. The inhibitor was identified by several criteria to be arginase (EC 3.5.3.1), which acts by depletion of arginine in the medium on the growth activity of FSC[48]. Arginase is present both in the cytosol and, as an ectoenzyme, at the outer surface of hepatocellular membranes. A functional role in situ of the hepatocellular membrane-located arginase for growth regulation of adjacent FSC has not been established. It is possible that the enzyme reduces the concentration of arginine in the immediate microenvironment of FSC, which in turn could suppress some key mechanisms related to DNA replication and mitosis. Our results add support to arginase as an inhibitor of activity in hepatocellular membranes capable of arresting growth of FSC and other cell types in vitro. The possibility that loss of membrane-bound arginase during damage of PC might play a role in the activation of FSC exists. By this mechanism PC might be sensitized to the various 'fibrogenic' cytokines elaborated by inflammatory cells and damaged hepatocytes (see above).

SUMMARY AND CONCLUSIONS

In an attempt to compile present knowledge on the molecular and cellular interactions of FSC in a hypothetical model of cell activation, we propose a three-step cascade mechanism of FSC activation, which implies the sequential cross-talk between FSC, hepatocytes, KC, thrombocytes, endothelial cells and myofibroblasts (transformed FSC) (Fig. 12). In the preinflammatory phase complete or only subtle hepatocellular damage leading to membrane leakage facilitates the release of paracrine acting mitogen(s), which acts like a 'wound hormone'[53] to initiate proliferation of FSC (Fig. 12). In addition, ethanol-metabolizing PC produce acetaldehyde and lipid peroxides, which stimulate matrix gene expression in nearby FSC before inflammatory mediators (second phase) become effective[54].

Proliferation of FSC adjacent to PC might also be initiated by the decrease of membrane arginase as a consequence of hepatocellular damage. In the subsequent inflammatory phase cytokines of activated Kupffer cells/macrophages (e.g. TGF-β_1, TGF-α, TNF-α) and of disintegrated platelets (e.g. TGF-β_1, EGF-like factors, PDGF) stimulate FSC to proliferate and to transform into myofibroblasts (Fig. 12). Activation of resident KC and invaded monocytes is initiated partially by phagocytosis of cell debris at the locus of necrosis. These activated cells might induce hepatocellular damage and/or apoptosis via release of proteases, toxic cytokines (TNF-α) and oxygen radicals. Toxic oxygen metabolites generated by polymorphonuclear leukocytes attracted and activated by IL-8-producing ethanol-metabolizing hepatocytes[55] might contribute to a pathogenetic vicious circle, at least in alcoholic liver injury. In the inflammatory phase TGF-β, the prototype of a fibrogenic cytokine[56] promotes the transformation of FSC to myofibroblasts. The latter cell type is stimulated during the post-inflammatory phase via an autocrine loop generated by TGF-α, TGF-β_1 and FGF, which are expressed and secreted by myofibroblasts (Fig. 12). In combination with further paracrine stimulation of still untransformed FSC by myofibroblasts, the post-inflammatory phase potentially contributes to self-perpetuation of fibrogenesis even after cessation of the initiating event[57]. The matrix formed by the myofibroblast might modulate the activity of secreted cytokines and growth factors (e.g. TGF-β) by forming a sink or sponge of cytokines providing the possibility of their sustained release. In addition, α_2-macroglobulin, produced by hepatocytes and also by myofibroblasts[38], might act

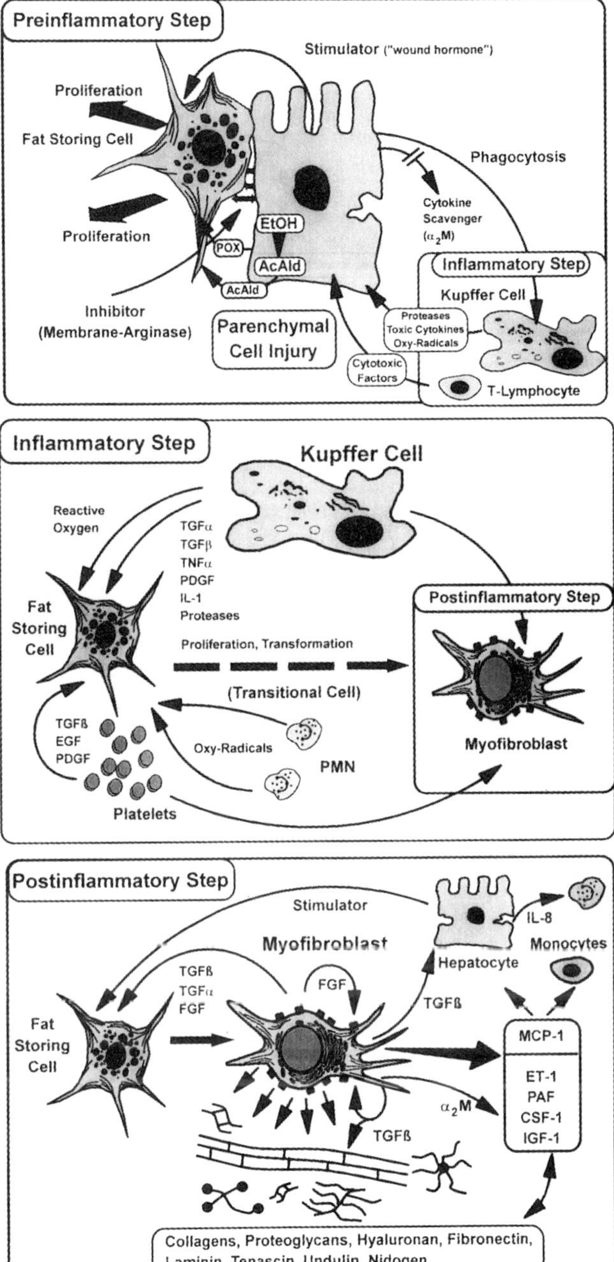

Fig. 12 The three step cascade model of fat-storing cell activation. The **preinflammatory** stage is initiated by damage of hepatocytes, which releases stimulators of fat-storing cell proliferation and decreases membrane-associated inhibitors like membrane arginase. In addition, metabolism of

(continued)

as a pleiotropic scavenger of cytokines (e.g. TGF-β_1, TNF-α, PDGF)[58]. The concept proposed ascribes direct roles for (damaged) hepatocytes and myofibroblasts in the sequential activation of FSC, and may provide an explanation for the clinical finding that inflammation is not necessarily required for developing fibrosis[59].

Acknowledgements

The excellent technical assistance of Brigitte Heitmann, Marcus Fischer, and Lothar Scheckel are gratefully acknowledged. The studies are supported by grants from the Duetsche Forschungsgemeinschaft (Gr 463/9-1 and 9-2) and the Kempkes Stiftung.

References

1. Martinez-Hernandez A, Amenta PS. The hepatic extracellular matrix I. Components and distribution in normal liver. Virchows Arch A Pathol Anat Histol. 1993;423:1–11.
2. Martinez-Hernandez A. The hepatic extracellular matrix. Electron immunohistochemical studies in rats with CC14-induced cirrhosis. Lab Invest. 1985;53:166–86.
3. Schuppan D. Structure of the extracellular matrix in normal and fibrotic liver: collagens and glycoproteins. Semin Liver Dis. 1990;10:1–10.
4. Milani S, Herbst H, Schuppan D et al. Differential expression of matrix-metalloproteinase-1 and -2 genes in normal and fibrotic human liver. Am J Pathol. 1994;144:528–37.
5. Arthur MJP. Matrix degradation in the liver. Semin Liver Dis. 1990;10:47–55.
6. Woessner JF. Matrix metalloproteinases and their inhibitors in connective tissue remodeling. Faseb J. 1991;5:2145–54.
7. Ramadori G. The stellate cell (Ito-cell, fat-storing cell, lipocyte, perisinusoidal cell) of the liver. Virchows Arch B Cell Pathol. 1991;61:147–58.
8. Friedman SL. The cellular basis of hepatic fibrosis. New Engl J Med. 1993;328:1828–35.
9. Gressner AM. Hepatic fibrogenesis: the puzzle of interacting cells, fibrogenic cytokines, regulatory loops, and extracellular matrix molecules. Z Gastroenterol. 1992;30(Suppl. 1):5–16.
10. Arthur MJP, Friedman SL, Roll FJ, Bissell DM. Lipocytes from normal rat liver release a neutral metalloproteinase that degrades basement membrane (type IV) collagen. J Clin Invest. 1989;84:1076–85.
11. Bissell DM. Lipocyte activation and hepatic fibrosis. Gastroenterology. 1992;102:1803–5.
12. Geerts A, Lazou JM, De Bleser P, Wisse E. Tissue distribution, quantitation and proliferation kinetics of fat-storing cells in carbon tetrachloride-injured rat liver. Hepatology. 1991;13:1193–202.
13. Rockey DC, Boyles JK, Gabbiani G, Friedman SL. Rat hepatic lipocytes express smooth muscle actin upon activation in vivo and in culture. J Submicrosc Cytol Pathol. 1992;24:193–203.

Fig. 12 (*continued*) ethanol (EtOH) to acetaldehyde (AcAld) and the generation of lipid peroxides initiate matrix gene expression before inflammatory stimuli (2nd step) become effective. In the **inflammatory** step mitogens from activated Kupffer cells (macrophages) and disintegrated platelets are most potent stimulators of fat-storing cell proliferation and transformation into myofibroblasts. Activated Kupffer cells in turn can cause, via the release of proteases, toxic cytokines (e.g. TNF-α) and oxygen radicals, membrane damage of hepatocytes. In the **post-inflammatory** step the fully transformed fat-storing cells (myofibroblast) release various cytokines and growth factors, which stimulate in a paracrine way non-transformed fat-storing cells and in an autocrine loop the myofibroblast itself. The cytokines interact with extracellular matrix components secreted by the myofibroblast. Abbreviations: MCP-1, monocyte chemotactic peptide; ET-1, endothelin-1; PAF, platelet activating factor; CSF-1, colony stimulating factor; IGF-1, insulin-like growth factor 1; FGF, fibroblast growth factor; TGF-β, transforming growth factor β; TGF-α, transforming growth factor α; α_2M, α_2-macroglobulin; PMN, polymorphonuclear leukocytes

14. Friedman ASL, Arthur JP. Activation of cultured rat hepatic lipocytes by Kupffer cell conditioned medium. J Clin Invest. 1989;84:1780–5.
15. Matsuoka M, Zhang MY, Tsukamoto H. Sensitization of hepatic lipocytes by high-fat diet to stimulatory effects of Kupffer cell-derived factors: implication in alcoholic liver fibrogenesis. Hepatology. 1990;11:173–82.
16. Bachem MG, Melchior R, Gressner AM. The role of thrombocytes in liver fibrogenesis: Effects of platelet lysate and thrombocyte-derived growth factors on the mitogenic activity and glycosaminoglycan synthesis of cultured rat liver fat storing cells. J Clin Chem Clin Biochem. 1989;27:555–65.
17. Rieder H, Armbrust T, Meyer-zum-Büschenfelde KH, Ramadori G. Contribution of sinusoidal endothelial liver cells to liver fibrosis: Expression of transforming growth factor-b1 receptors and modulation of plasmin-generating enzymes by transforming growth factor-b1. Hepatology. 1993;18:937–44.
18. Schäfter S, Zerbe O, Gressner AM. The synthesis of proteoglycans in fat-storing cell of rat liver. Hepatology. 1987;7:680–7.
19. Seglen PO. Preparation of isolated rat liver cells. In: Prescott DM, editor. Methods in cell biology. New York: Academic Press; 1987:Vol. 8:29–83.
20. Gressner AM, Pfeiffer T. Preventive effects of acute inflammation on liver cell necrosis and inhibition of heparan sulfate synthesis in hepatocytes. J Clin Chem Clin Biochem. 1986;24:821–9.
21. Zerbe O, Gressner AM. Proliferation of fat storing cells is stimulated by secretions of Kupffer cells from normal and injured liver. Exp Mol Pathol. 1988;49:87–101.
22. Hoffmann C, Lahme B, Brenzel A, Gressner AM. The relation between hepatocellular damage and activation of fat-storing cell proliferation in vitro. Inter Hepatol Commun. 1994;2:29–36.
23. Bachem MG, Riess U, Gressner AM. Liver fat storing cell proliferation is stimulated by epidermal growth factor/transforming growth factor alpha and inhibited by transforming growth factor beta. Biochem Biophys Res Commun. 1989;162:708–14.
24. Gressner AM. Proliferation and transformation of cultured liver fat storing cells (perisinusoidal lipocytes) under conditions of β-D-xyloside induced abrogation of proteoglycan synthesis. Exp Mol Pathol. 1991;55:143–69.
25. Colombo JP, Konarska L. Arginase. In: Bergmeyer HU, editor. Methods in enzymatic analysis. Weinheim, Germany: Verlag Chemie, 1983:285–92.
26. Kropf J, Quitte E, Gressner AM. Time-resolved immunofluorometric assays with measurement of a europium chelate in solution. Application for sensitive determination of fibronectin. Anal Biochem. 1991;197:258–65.
27. Danielpour D, Dart LL, Flanders KC, Roberts AB, Sporn MB. Immunodetection and quantitation of the two forms of transforming growth factor-beta (TGF-beta1 and TGF-beta2) secreted by cells in culture. J Cell Physiol. 1989;138:79–86.
28. Hossenlopp P, Seurin D, Segovia-Quinson B, Hardouin S, Binoux M. Analysis of serum insulin-like growth factor binding proteins using Western blotting: Use of the method for titration of the binding proteins and competitive bindng studies. Anal Biochem. 1986;154:138–43.
29. Labarca C, Paigen K. A simple, rapid, and sensitive DNA assay procedure. Anal Biochem. 1980;102:344–52.
30. Rotman B, Papermaster BW. Membrane properties of living mammalian cells as studied by enzymatic hydrolysis of fluorogenic esters. Proc Natl Acad Sci USA. 1966;55:134–41.
31. Bradford MM. A rapid and sensitive method for the quantitation of microgram quantities of protein utilizing the principle of protein-dye binding. Anal Biochem. 1976;72:248–54.
32. Gressner AM, Lotfi S, Gressner G, Lahme B. Identification and partial characterization of a hepatocyte-derived factor promoting proliferation of cultured fat storing cells (parasinusoidal lipocytes). Hepatology. 1992;16:1250–66.
33. Gressner AM, Lotfi S, Gressner G, Haltner E, Kropf J. Synergism between hepatocytes and Kupffer cells in the activation of fat-storing cells (perisinusoidal lipocytes). J Hepatol. 1993;19:117–32.
34. Baroni GS, Marucci L, Benedetti A, Mancini R, Jezequel AM, Orlandi F. Chronic ethanol feeding increases apoptosis and cell proliferation in rat liver. J Hepatol. 1994;20:508–13.
35. Leist M, Gantner F, Bohlinger I, Germann PG, Tiegs G, Wendel A. Murine hepatocytes apoptosis induced in vitro and in vivo by TNF-alpha requires transcriptional arrest. J Immunol. 1994; in press.

36. Oberhammer FA, Pavelka M, Sharma S, et al. Induction of apoptosis in cultured hepatocytes and in regressing liver by transforming growth factor beta-1. Proc Natl Acad Sci USA. 1992;89: 5408–12.

37. Okuba H, Miyanaga O, Nagano M et al. Purification and immunological determination of alpha2-macroglobulin in serum from injured rats. Biochim Biophys Acta. 1981;668:257–67.

38. Andus T, Ramadori G, Heinrich PC, Knittel T, Meyer-zum-Büschenfelde KH. Cultured Ito cells of rat liver express the alpha2-macroglobulin gene. Eur J Biochem. 1987;168:641–6.

39. Bachem MG, Burschel G, Boers W et al. Feedback regulation between alpha2-macroglobulin and TGF-b1. Its putative role in liver fibrogenesis. In: Knook DL, Wisse E, editors. Cells of the hepatic sinusoid. Leiden: The Kupffer Cell Foundation, Vol. 4, 1993:218–21.

40. LaMarre J, Hayes MA, Wolleberg GK, Hussaini I, Hall SW, Gonias SL. An alpha2-macroglobulin receptor-dependent mechanism for the plasma clearance of TGF-beta1 in mice. J Clin Invest. 1991;87:39–44.

41. McCaffrey TA, Falcone DJ, Brayton CF, Agarwal LA, Welt GFP, Weksler BB. Transforming growth factor-beta activity is potentiated by heparin via dissociation of the transforming growth factor-beta/alpha-macroglobulin inactive complex. J Cell Biol. 1989;109:441–8.

42. O'Connor-McCourt MD, Wakefield LM. Latent transforming growth factor beta in serum. A specific complex with alpha 2-macroglobulin. J Biol Chem. 1987;262:14090–9.

43. Sottrup-Jensen L, Stepanik TM, Kristensen T. Primary structure of human alpha2-macroglobulin. J Biol Chem. 1984;259:8318–27.

44. Feldman RS, Rosenberg MR, Ney KA, Michalopoulos G, Pizzo SV. Binding alpha2-macroglobulin to hepatocytes: mechanism of in vivo clearance. Biochem Biophys Res Commun. 1985;28:795–802.

45. Hanover JA, Cheng S, Willingham MC, Pastan I. Alpha2-macroglobulin binding to cultured fibroblasts. J Biol Chem. 1983;258:370–7.

46. Kaplan J, Nielsen ML. Analysis of macrophage surface receptors. J Biol Chem. 1979;254: 7323–8.

47. Gressner AM, Brenzel A, Vossmeyer T. Hepatocyte-conditioned medium potentiates insulin-like growth factor (IGF) 1 and 2 stimulated DNA synthesis of cultured fat-storing cells. Liver. 1993;13:86–94.

48. Gressner AM, Lahme B. Inhibitory actions of hepatocyte plasma membranes on proliferation, protein- and proteoglycan synthesis of cultured rat fat storing cells. In: Wisse E, Knook DL, McCuskey RS, editors. Cells of the hepatic sinusoid. Vol. 3, 1991:237–41.

49. Rechler MM, Brown AL. Insulin-like growth factor binding proteins: gene structure and expression. Growth Reg. 1992;2:55–68.

50. Clemmons DR. IGFBPs-regulation of cellular action. Growth Reg. 1992;2:80–7.

51. Scott CD, Martin JL, Baxter RC. Production of insulin-like growth factor I and its binding protein by adult rat hepatocytes in primary culture. Endocrinology. 1985;116:1094–101.

52. Lamas E, Zindy F, Seurin D, Guguen-Guillouzo C, Brechot C. Expression of insulin-like growth factor II and receptors for insulin-like growth factor II, insulin-like growth factor I and insulin in isolated and cultured rat hepatocytes. Hepatology. 1991;13:36–40.

53. Muthukrishnan L, Warder E, McNeil PL. Basic fibroblast growth factor is efficiently released from a cytosolic storage site through plasma membrane disruptions of endothelial cells. J Cell Physiol. 1991;148:1–16.

54. Bedossa P, Houglum K, Trautwein C, Holstege A, Chojkier M. Stimulation of collagen alpha1 (I) gene expression is associated with lipid peroxidation in hepatocellular injury: A link to tissue fibrosis? Hepatology. 1994;19:1262–71.

55. Shiratori Y, Takada H, Hikiba Y et al. Production of chemotactic factor interleukin-8, from hepatocytes exposed to ethanol. Hepatology. 1993;18:1477–82.

56. Border WA, Ruoslahti E. Transforming growth factor-beta in disease – the dark side of tissue repair. J Clin Invest. 1992;90:1–7.

57. Bachem MG, Meyer DM, Melchior R, Sell KM, Gressner AM. Activation of rat liver perisinusoidal lipocytes by transforming growth factors derived from myofibroblast-like cells – a potential mechanism of self perpetuation in liver fibrogenesis. J Clin Invest. 1992;89:19–27.

58. LaMarre J, Wollenberg GK, Gonias SL, Hayes MA. Biology of disease: cytokine binding and clearance properties of proteinase-activated alpha2-macroglobulins. Lab Invest. 1991;65:3–14.

59. Friedman SL. Acetaldehyde and alcoholic fibrogenesis: fuel to the fire, but not the spark. Hepatology. 1990;12:609–12.

Section IV
Function of stellate cells and growth regulation

7
On the contraction and relaxation of stellate cells induced by Kupffer cell-derived vasoactive substances

N. KAWADA and K. DECKER

INTRODUCTION

Using the isolated perfused rat liver model, some bioactive substances have been shown to influence the fluid dynamics of the liver. A thromboxane A_2 (TXA_2) analogue, U46619, prostaglandin $F_{2\alpha}$ ($PGF_{2\alpha}$), leukotriene D_4 and nucleotides increase the perfusion pressure of isolated rat liver[1,2]. An endothelium-derived peptide mediator, endothelin (ET), was also shown to increase the portal pressure[3,4]. A gaseous and radical mediator, nitric oxide, produced by both Kupffer cells and hepatocytes is speculated to take part in regulating the sinusoidal microcirculation[5]. However, neither a cellular target of these vasoactive substances in the liver nor the molecular mechanism that regulates sinusoidal tonus has been fully defined.

Hepatic stellate cells reside in the space of Disse and encompass the external surface of endothelial cells. Because of this anatomical location and their similarity to vascular smooth muscle cells, the cells have been postulated to be involved in regulating the luminal size of hepatic sinusoid and the local microcirculation[6]. The present study provides a direct evidence of the reversible contractility of stellate cells after exposure to various vasoactive substances. Stellate cells grown on inert silicone rubber films were found to form wrinkles in the substrate which are indicative of tension development[7,8]. The data presented here also show the movement of intracellular signal molecules after receptor–ligand couplings on the surface of stellate cells.

MATERIALS AND METHODS

Isolation and culture of stellate cells

Livers of male Wistar rats were perfused with a Ca^{2+}/Mg^{2+}-free medium for 5 min at 37°C at a flow rate of 10 ml/min. The liver was then perfused with a solution containing 3.8 mM $CaCl_2$ and 300 mg/l collagenase. After perfusion, the liver was excised and incubated with gentle stirring in a solution containing pronase and DNAase at 37°C. The digested liver was filtered through a nylon mesh. Residual liver cells were centrifuged. The stellate cell-enriched fraction was obtained by centrifugation with an 8.2% Nycodenz cushion at 1400*g* for 20 min. Cells in the upper layer were washed by centrifugation, resuspended in DMEM supplemented with 10% fetal bovine serum and antibiotics, and cultured at 37°C in a CO_2 incubator. After 2 days, stellate cells revealed a typical star-like structure, possessed a lot of lipid droplets and immunoreactive desmin.

Measurement of cell contraction

A rapid response of stellate cells to test ligands was detected by a silicone-rubber-membrane method[9,10]. Changes in cell shape and wrinkle number were constantly monitored by phase-contrast microscopy connected with a video camera system.

Long-lasting contraction of stellate cells was observed by a collagen gel method. Hydrated collagen gels were prepared using collagen type 1 solution[11,12]. In brief, 2 ml of collagen solution were added to each well and incubated for 2 h at 37°C to allow gelation. Stellate cells were kept in primary culture for 5–7 days and they detached from culture plates with 0.025% trypsin-EDTA solution, suspended in DMEM (1×10^6 cells/ml) and plated on collagen gels for 2 h at 37°C (1 ml/well). After detaching the cell-associated gels (35 mm in diameter) from the plate, they were incubated in 2 ml DMEM in the presence of various ligands. At the indicated times after incubation, contraction of adherent cells was monitored by measuring diameter of the gel.

Staining of F-actin

Cells were fixed with 3.7% formaldehyde in the presence of 0.1% Triton X-100 for 15 min at room temperature. Cells were further permeabilized in a buffer containing 0.1% saponin for 10 min at room temperature. After washing three times with the saponin-containing buffer, cell-associated F-actin was stained by 0.5 μg/ml TRITC-phalloidin for 1 h at room temperature. After washing and fixation with glycerol, the specimens were observed under the fluorescence microscope.

Measurement of [³H]inositol phosphate

Stellate cells cultured on 6-well plates were radiolabelled with myo-[2-³H]-inositol and incubated for 15 min at 37°C in a buffer supplemented with 10 mM LiCl and 0.1% bovine serum albumin. Reaction was started by adding various ligands. After incubation for various intervals the reaction was stopped by removing the medium and adding of 1 ml of 5% trichloroacetic acid. Trichloroacetic acid extracts were then washed four times with 5 ml each of water-saturated diethylether. After adjusting the pH to 7.2, the washed samples were subjected to column chromatography on a 0.5 ml Bio-Rad AG1-X8 resin. Ins$P$ was eluted from the column with 10 ml of 0.1 M formic acid/0.4 M ammonium formate[13]. Radioactivity of the eluted fractions was determined in a liquid scintillation spectrophotometer.

Measurement of cellular cAMP and cGMP

Stellate cells grown on 6-well culture plates were washed twice with 1 ml buffer. After incubating cells in 1 ml buffer containing 0.5 mM 3-isobutyl-1-methylxanthine at 37°C for 10 min, various concentrations of stimulants were added. The reaction was terminated by adding 5% trichloroacetic acid. cAMP and cGMP contents in the extract were measured by radioimmunoassay.

Measurement of cytosolic free Ca²⁺ using indo-1

Cells were grown in primary culture as subconfluent monolayers on quartz coverslips. They were loaded with indo-1 (indo-1/AM). After incubation, the coverslips with the cells were washed three times and put into a quartz cuvette filled with Hepes buffer (pH 7.35). Fluorescence was measured in a thermostatted fluorometer. The cytosolic free Ca²⁺ concentration was measured and calculated.

RESULTS

Contraction and relaxation of hepatic stellate cells

Contraction of stellate cells cultured for 3–5 days on a silicone rubber membrane was detected by the increasing number of wrinkles around individual cells. A TXA$_2$ analogue, U46619, PGF$_{2\alpha}$ and ETs triggered stellate cell contraction as early as 0.5 min after addition of these ligands. Figure 1 shows typical wrinkles produced by stellate cells stimulated with 10 nM ET-1; after addition of 10 nM ET-1, 78, 87, 59 and 56% of stellate cells were contracted at 2.5, 5, 10 and 20 min, respectively. The increase in number of wrinkles around cells was usually accompanied with an apparent diminution of cell body size. ET-1 was the strongest elicitor of the cell contraction; U46619 and PGF$_{2\alpha}$ induced a transient movement of stellate cells while ETs triggered a long-lasting contraction of the cells.

The collagen gel method was also useful to detect a long-lasting contraction of stellate cells. Serum and ETs but not U46619 and PGF$_{2\alpha}$ were able to stimulate the contraction of stellate cells on the gel (Fig. 2).

On the other hand, a prostacyclin analogue, Iloprost, PGE$_2$ and nitric oxide relaxed contracted stellate cells; the number of wrinkles in the silicone membrane that were produced by contracted stellate cells decreased in a time-dependent manner after addition of these substances. Iloprost was strongest in relaxing stellate cells; 47, 75 and 82% of contracted stellate cells had relaxed within 5, 10 and 20 min, respectively, after addition of 2 μM Iloprost.

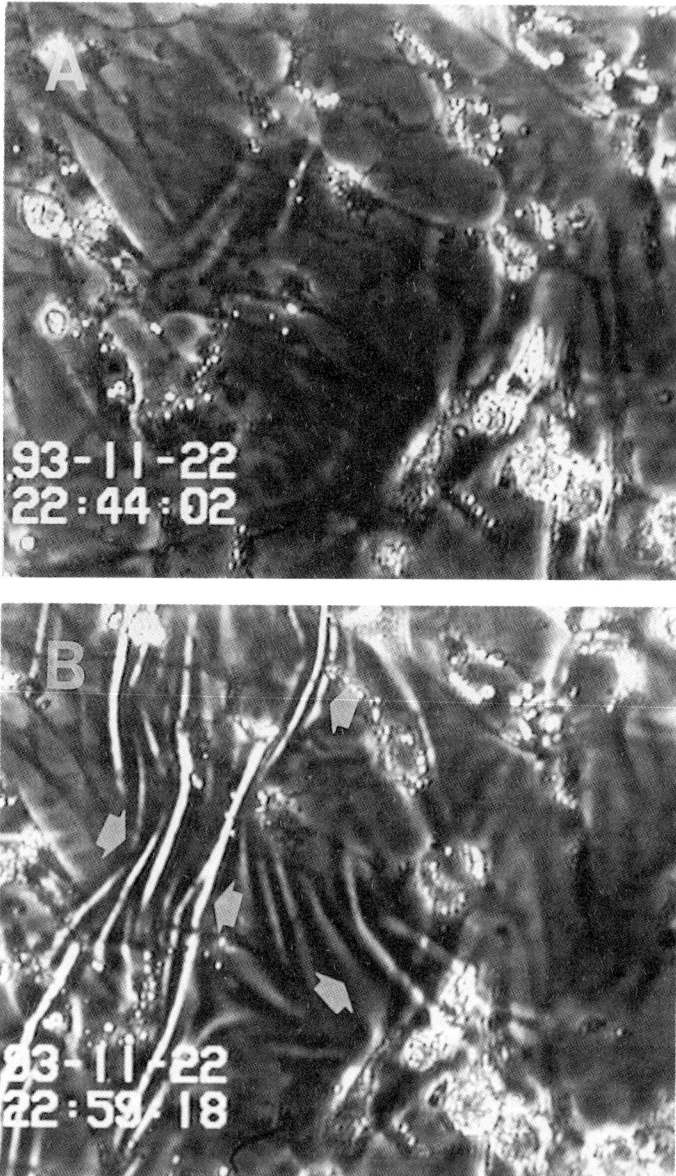

Fig. 1 Effect of endothelin-1 on stellate cell contraction. Stellate cells cultured for 3 days on silicone rubber membrane were stimulated with 1 nM endothelin-1. Changes in the appearance of wrinkles were constantly monitored under microscope equipped with a video-camera system. Cell contraction was judged by increase in the number of wrinkles of silicone membrane around stellate cells. (**A**) Basal tonic state; (**B**) 8 min after addition of endothelin-1. Many wrinkles of silicone membrane are seen (×200)

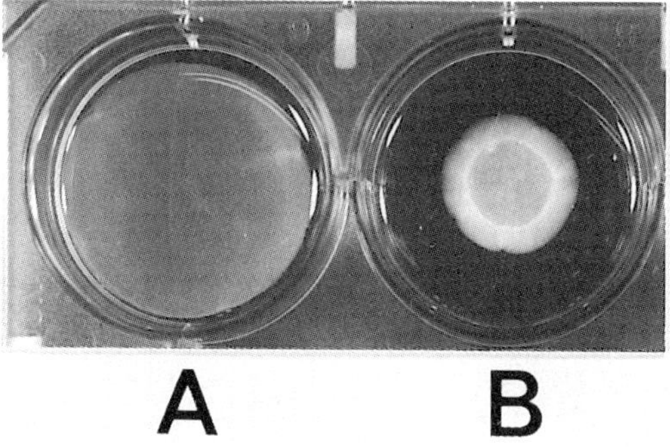

Fig. 2   The contraction of hydrated collagen gels by endothelin-1-stimulated stellate cells. Primary cultures of stellate cells were transferred to collagen gels (diameter, 35 mm). After the cells attached to the gels, reactions were started by adding 10 nM endothelin-1 to the culture medium (Dulbecco's MEM). The diameter of the gels was determined at various time. (**A**) Dulbecco's MEM only. (**B**) Dulbecco's MEM + 10 nM endothelin-1. Diminution of gel size is apparent

Interestingly, addition of Iloprost (10 μM) induced de-aggregation of actin stress fibres, accompanied by transformation of the cell shape. Stellate cells cultured for 7 days displayed stress fibres of F-actin filaments. However, stellate cells exposed to Iloprost lost viable fibres 30 min after addition of the ligands. PGE_2 and sodium nitroprusside mimicked the effect of Iloprost on actin stress fibres.

Inositol-phosphate formation in stellate cells

The formation of Ins$P$, InsP_2 and InsP_3 by stellate cells previously radiolabelled with [^{3}H]inositol was analysed after addition of eicosanoids, ETs and NO donors. A significant accumulation of Ins$P$ in stellate cells was induced by ET-1, 2, 3 and $PGF_{2\alpha}$, while PGE_2, PGD_2, Iloprost, U46619, sodium nitroprusside or sin-1 had negligible effects on Ins$P$ production (Fig. 3). ETs were much more potent in stimulating inositol-phosphate metabolism than $PGF_{2\alpha}$. A time course study also showed that ETs had a long-lasting effect on InsP_3 formation. Additionally we found that ET-dependent Ins$P$ formation was regulated by pertussis toxin-sensitive G protein; treatment of stellate cells with pertussis toxin (100 μg/ml) restrained the Ins$P$ production in ET-stimulated stellate cells. Thus, some pertussis-toxin sensitive G protein might control cellular metabolism evoked by coupling of receptor and ligand on stellate cells.

Measurement of the intracellular Ca²⁺ level

To analyse second messenger systems operating in stimulated stellate cells. $[Ca^{2+}]_i$ was measured in indo-1-loaded stellate cells. $[Ca^{2+}]_i$ of non-stimulated stellate cells on quartz cover slips was 121 ± 9 nM. ET-1 (10 nM) and $PGF_{2\alpha}$ (5 μM) increased this to 1015 ± 86 and 711 ± 85 nM, respectively. U46619 was a weaker elicitor than ET-1 and $PGF_{2\alpha}$. Neither PGE_2, PGD_2 and Iloprost, nor sodium nitroprusside increased the intracellular Ca^{2+} level (Table 1).

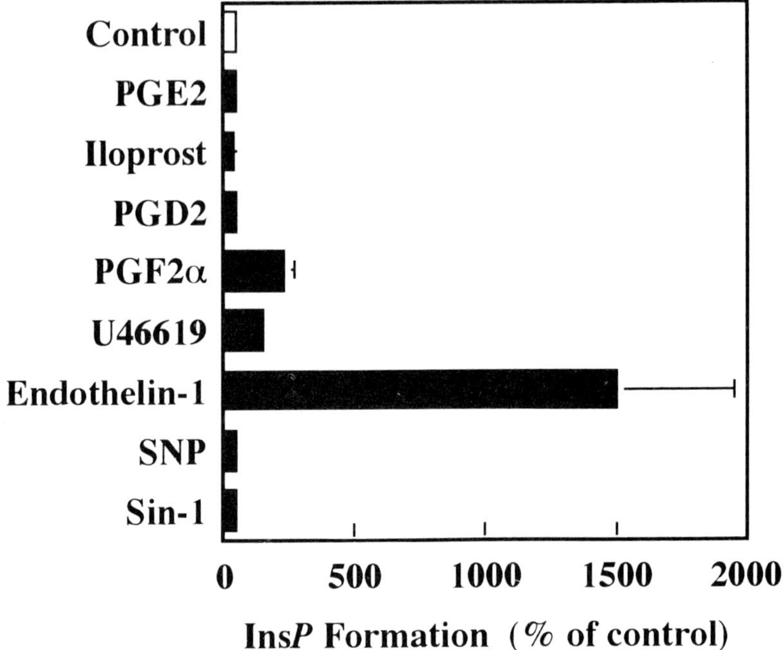

Ins*P* Formation (% of control)

Fig. 3 Ins*P* accumulation in stimulated stellate cells. Stellate cells in primary culture were radiolabelled with [2-³H]inositol. Reactions were started by adding various ligands to the incubation medium supplemented with 10 mM LiCl. Accumulated Ins*P* species were extracted from the cells and analysed using Dowex AG1 X8 column chromatography

Table 1 Change of intracellular Ca^{2+} level in stellate cells

Stimulants	$[Ca^{2+}]_i$ level (nM)
Basal	121 ± 9
ET-1 (10 nM)	1015 ± 86
$PGF_{2\alpha}$ (5 μM)	711 ± 85
U46619 5 μM)	205 ± 37
PGE_2 (5 μM)	142 ± 12
SNP (100 μM)	125 ± 32

Stellate cells were cultured on quartz cover slips for 5–7 days. Cells were then labelled with indo-1 using 10 μM indo-1/AM. After washing, the stellate cells were challenged with test substances. Indo-1-derived fluorescence was monitored by fluorometer and the cytosolic free Ca^{2+} concentration was calculated

Measurement of the intracellular level of cAMP and cGMP

Intracellular accumulation of cAMP and cGMP in stimulated stellate cells was determined in the presence of 3-isobutyl-1-methylxanthine, an inhibitor of 3′,5′-

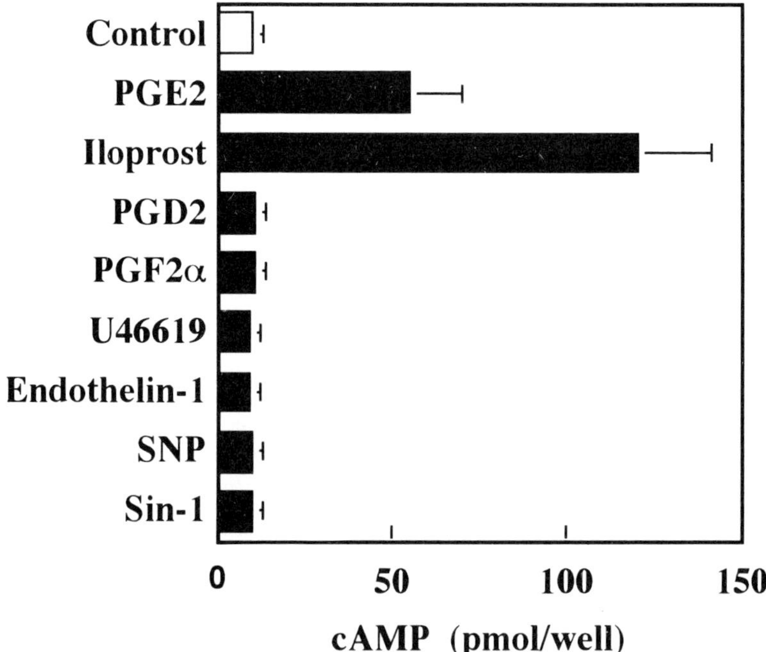

Fig. 4 cAMP accumulation in stimulated stellate cells. Stellate cells in primary culture were incubated with various substances for 20 min in the presence of 3-isobuthylmethylxanthine. Accumulated cAMP was extracted from the cells and quantified by using radioimmunoassay

cyclic nucleotide phosphodiesterase. Iloprost ($5\,\mu$M) and PGE_2 ($5\,\mu$M) increased the level of cAMP from 9.2 ± 0.8 to 122 ± 12 and 55.1 ± 8.0 pmol/well, respectively. On the other hand, sodium nitroprusside and sin-1 induced the accumulation of cGMP in stellate cells; cGMP increased from a basal level of 0.91 ± 0.07 to 3.1 ± 0.6 and 1.2 ± 0.4 pmol/well, respectively, when stimulated with $100\,\mu$M sodium nitroprusside and $10\,\mu$M sin-1. By contrast, ETs, $PGF_{2\alpha}$ and U46619, that elicited the contraction of stellate cells, hardly affected the cellular level of cAMP and cGMP (Figs 4 and 5).

DISCUSSION

The effect of PGs on the resistance of the porto-hepatic vasculature has been demonstrated using perfusion experiments in isolated rat liver; TXA_2 and PGF_{2a} increased the perfusion pressure[1]. More recently, endothelins, endothelial cell-derived vasocontracting factors, have been reported to act as agonists to the liver[3,4]. Despite these findings, cellular target for prostaglandins and endothelins in the liver has not been fully elucidated. Anatomical observations by Wake indicated clearly that stellate cells encompass the external surface of sinusoidal endothelial cells with their well-branching cytoplasmic processes[6]. Therefore, it has been assumed that stellate cells undergo contraction and function as pericytes. The present study shows directly that stellate cells undergo reversible

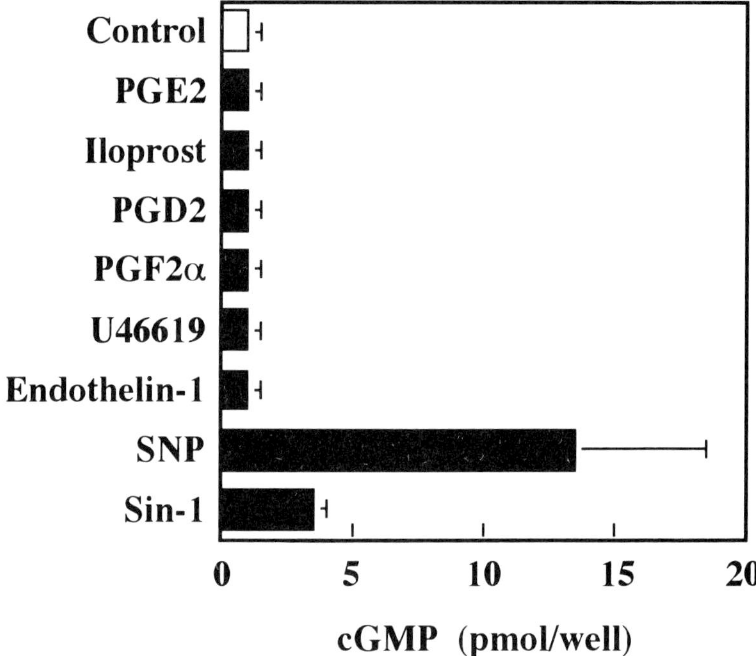

Fig. 5 cGMP accumulation in stimulated stellate cells. Stellate cells in primary culture were incubated with various substances for 20 min in the presence of 3-isobuthylmethylxanthine. Accumulated cGMP was extracted from the cells and quantified by using radioimmunoassay

contraction in response to substances derived from Kupffer cells and sinusoidal endothelial cells, and also reveals that stellate cells have binding sites for prostaglandins and endothelins that are closely coupling to cellular metabolism of inositol phospholipid, Ca^{2+} and cAMP.

Endothelin is the most potent agent known to induce stellate cell contraction and to achieve a long-lasting increase of perfusion pressure. Stellate cells have B type endothelin receptors because they respond equally to every isotype of endothelins. They also express mRNA for the ET_B receptor as well as the ET_A receptor[14]. An activation of phospholipase C and an increase in $[Ca^{2+}]_i$ are possible signal transductions caused by receptor–endothelin coupling in stellate cells. Protein kinase C may be also involved in the long-lasting action of endothelins as staurosporin and H-7 (a protein kinase C inhibitor) antagonizes the effect. Clinical investigations have also revealed an increased concentration of endothelin-1 in portal blood of patients with chronic liver inflammation[15]. Thus, endothelin may be one of important mediators that modify the function of stellate cells and the circulatory status in the liver.

Nitric oxide is a radical mediator produced in the liver by Kupffer cells and hepatocytes[5,16,17]. Using inhibitors of nitric oxide synthase, it has also been demonstrated that nitric oxide takes part in the regulation of sinusoidal tonus[18]. The present study indicates that stellate cells respond to nitric oxide donors, sodium nitroprusside and sin-1, and relax by some cGMP-dependent mechanism.

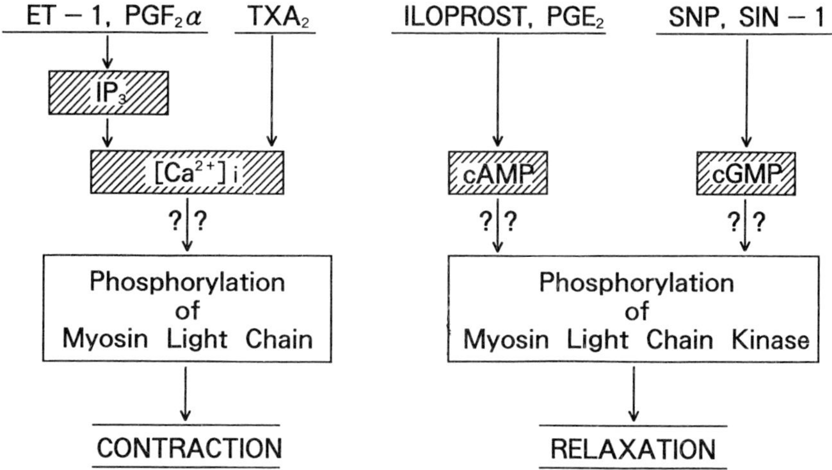

Fig. 6 Possible mechanism of stellate cell contraction

As stellate cells reside in the space of Disse, nitric oxide derived from both hepatocytes and Kupffer cells might affect the contractility of stellate cells *in vivo*.

Thus, stellate cells undergo reversible contraction in response to various mediators derived from Kupffer cells in vitro. Various signal transductions seem to be employed in the activation of phospholipase C and/or the elevation of the intracellular Ca^{2+} level and, finally, in the contraction of the stellate cells. However, cAMP and cGMP appear to promote relaxation (Fig. 6). As the contractile response of stellate cells is concomitant with the rise in portal vein pressure during the perfusion experiment, the motility of stellate cells and the resulting diminution of sinusoidal diameter may account for part of the increase in hepatic resistance *in vivo*.

ACKNOWLEDGEMENTS

Thanks are due to Prof. Masayasu Inoue, Department of Biochemistry, Osaka City University Medical School for his valuable suggestions. The authors also thank Dr Thuy-Anh Tran-Thi, Biochemisches Institut der Albert-Ludwigs-Universität Freiburg, Dr Kazuo Ikeda and Dr Shigekazu Takemura, Department of Surgery, Osaka City University Medical School, for their co-working in this project. This work was supported by grants-in-aid for scientific research from the Ministry of Education, Science and Culture of Japan and by the Osaka Foundation for Promotion of Clinical Immunology.

REFERENCES

1. Häussinger D, Stehle T, Gerok W. Effect of leukotrienes and the thromboxane A2 analogue U-46619 in isolated perfused rat liver. Metabolic, hemodynamic and ion-flux responses. Biol Chem Hoppe-Seyler. 1988;369:97 – 107.

2. Häussinger D, Busshardt E, Stehle T, Stoll B, Wettstein M, Gerok W. Stimulation of thromboxane release by extracellular UTP and ATP from perfused rat liver. Role of eicosanoids in mediating the nucleotide responses. Eur J Biochem. 1988;178:249–56.

3. Gandhi CR, Behal RH, Harvey SAK, Nouchi TA, Olson MS. Hepatic effects of endothelin. Receptor characterization and endothelin-induced signal transduction in hepatocytes. Biochem J. 1992;287:897–904.

4. Tran-Thi TA, Kawada N, Decker K. Regulation of endothelin-1 action on the perfused rat liver. FEBS Lett. 1993;318:353–7.

5. Billiar TR, Curran RD, Harbrecht BG, Stuehr DJ, Demetris AJ, Simmons RL. Modulation of nitrogen oxide synthesis in vivo: Ng-monomethyl-L-arginine inhibits endotoxin-induced nitrite/nitrate biosynthesis while promoting hepatic damage. J Leuk Biol. 1990;48:565–9.

6. Wake K. Perisinusoidal stellate cells (fat-storing cells, interstitial cells, lipocytes), their related structure in and around the liver sinusoids, and vitamin A-storing cells in extrahepatic organs. Int Rev Cytol. 1980;66:303–53.

7. Kawada N, Tran-Thi TA, Klein H, Decker K. The contraction of hepatic stellate (Ito) cells stimulated with vasoactive substances. Possible involvement of endothelin 1 and nitric oxide in the regulation of the sinusoidal tonus. Eur J Biochem. 1993;213:815–23.

8. Kawada N, Klein H, Decker K. Eicosanoid-mediated contractility of hepatic stellate cells. Biochem J. 1992;285:367–71.

9. Kelley C, D'Amore P, Hechtman HB, Shepro D. Microvascular pericyte contractility in vitro: comparison with other cells of the vascular wall. J Cell Biol. 1987;104:483–90.

10. Murray TR, Marshall BE, Macarak EJ. Contraction of vascular smooth muscle in cell culture. J Cell Physiol. 1990;143:26–38.

11. Guidry C, Grinnell F. Heparin modulate the organization of hydrated collagen gels and inhibits gel contraction by fibroblast. J Cell Biol. 1987;104:103–9.

12. Montesano R, Orci L. Transforming growth factor β stimulates collagen-matrix contraction by fibroblasts: implication for wound healing. Proc Natl Acad Sci USA. 1988;85:4894–7.

13. Berridge MJ, Dawson RMC, Downes CP, Heslop JP, Irvine RF. Changes in the levels of inositol phosphates after agonist-dependent hydrolysis of membrane phosphoinositide. Biochem J. 1983;212:473–82.

14. Housset C, Rockey DC, Bissell DM. Endothelin receptor in rat liver: Lipocytes as a contractile target for endothelin 1. Proc Natl Acad Sci USA. 1993;90:9266–70.

15. Schrader J, Tabbe U, Borries M et al. Plasma-endothelin bei Normalpersonen und Patienten mit nehrologisch-rhematologischen und kardiovaskularen Erkrankungen. Klin Wochenschr. 1990;68:774–9.

16. Nussler AK, Di Silvio M, Billiar T et al. Stimulation of the nitric oxide synthase pathway in human hepatocytes by cytokines and endotoxin. J Exp Med. 1992;176:261–4.

17. Gaillard T, Mulsch A, Busse R, Klein H, Decker K. Regulation of nitric oxide production by stimulated rat Kupffer cells. Pathobiology. 1991;59:280–3.

18. Harbrecht BG, Stadler J, Demetris AJ, Simmons RL, Billiar TR. Nitric oxide and prostaglandins interact to prevent hepatic damage during murine endotoxemia. Am J Physiol. 1994;266:G1004–G1010.

8
The initiation of liver regeneration and the regulation of liver growth by transforming growth factor alpha (TGF-α)

N. FAUSTO

INTRODUCTION

The liver can regulate its growth and size, and in adult animals and humans, the functional hepatic mass maintains a close relationship with body mass[1]. Disruption of the optimal hepatic functional mass, either by tissue deficit or by the addition of extra capacity is rapidly corrected by tissue growth or cellular death. Decreased functional capacity can be caused by surgical removal of portions of the liver (partial hepatectomy) or by hepatocyte cell death caused by toxic agents and viruses. Regardless of the inducing agent, through mechanisms that may involve metabolic signals or growth factor/receptor activation, hepatocytes sense the functional deficit and undergo a series of sequential changes in gene expression that culminate in DNA replication of the normally quiescent cell. Despite the fact that the process of liver growth in these situations is referred to as 'regeneration' it is important to understand what the term means when applied to hepatic growth. It is also useful for understanding the basic mechanisms of liver growth to establish general distinctions between hepatic regeneration induced by partial hepatectomy and that which develops as a response to cell death.

The standard partial hepatectomy performed in rats or mice involves the excision of 2/3 of liver by removing intact, complete liver lobes without cutting through liver tissue[2]. The remaining lobes are undisturbed and constitute an intact miniature liver, the cells of which begin to grow to compensate for the loss of tissue mass. However, there is no regrowth or 'regeneration' of the lost lobes. It is also to be noted that in this procedure no wound surface is produced and the inflammatory and vascular events normally associated with the healing of wounds do not occur because the tissue is intact. Nevertheless the operation involves the severing of blood vessels, and causes an immediate increase in flow of blood and metabolites to the hepatic tissue as well as rapid changes in ion fluxes, redox potential and membrane polarization in hepatocytes[1,3]. All of these factors may alter gene expression and transcription factor binding and may also trigger the release of cytokines in liver and other tissues. Partial hepatectomy in humans is actually a segmentectomy and requires different techniques from those used to remove liver lobes of rodents. It does not result in true 'regeneration', that is, the regrowth of tissue which is removed[4]. Instead, hepatocytes in the liver remnant proliferate, leading to an expansion in size of the acinar units in the remnant which eventually compensates for the tissue loss[5]. The situation referred to as 'small-for-size' transplants in humans, in which the transplanted liver is small relative to the optimal liver mass appropriate for the host, is in many respects very similar to a partial hepatectomy in man or rodents[6,7]. It is remarkable that a small-for-size transplant grows until it reaches the optimal size for the host, at which time the growth process terminates[7].

In contrast to the situation described above for liver regeneration after partial hepatectomy in humans and laboratory animals, hepatocyte proliferation induced by toxic chemicals and viruses is preceded by cell death. In this type of regeneration, cytokines and other chemotactic and inflammatory mediators may be released as a result of tissue necrosis[8]. Whether the release of these mediators constitutes the stimulus which triggers hepatocyte proliferation is an issue of major significance which has not yet been studied in detail. Normal restitution of tissue after toxic injury occurs only if the liver scaffolding, that is, the extracellular components that constitute the tissue framework, remains intact[5,9]. Otherwise the normal architecture of the organ is not restored and fibrosis and nodular regeneration occur despite hepatocyte proliferation. This type of outcome commonly occurs in cases of repeated, relatively mild injury alternating with periods of healing[10].

This brief introduction provides a background for the discussion of two aspects of liver regeneration after partial hepatectomy which are essential for understanding the growth response: the mechanisms involved in making hepatocytes enter the cell cycle and the role played by growth factors in hepatic regeneration.

TRANSCRIPTION FACTOR ACTIVATION AND THE INITIATION OF LIVER REGENERATION

During the first hour after partial hepatectomy expression of a number of genes, including the protooncogenes c-*fos*, c-*jun* and c-*myc* among many others, is increased[11,12]. This class of genes show rapid protein synthesis-independent activation after the application of a mitogenic stimulus. Activation of these genes, known as immediate early genes, occurs in hepatocytes and cells of other tissues, both in vivo and in culture. Because many of these genes code for proteins which are transcription factors, their activation is considered to be a very early step in mitogenic gene activation[13]. The primary response of immediate early genes is further expanded by induction of the transcription of secondary genes which may be essential for DNA replication.

Given the importance of immediate early genes as the intermediate step between the triggering signals for liver regeneration and the activation of secondary response genes, it is essential to understand how the expression of immediate early genes is regulated. One likely possibility that we have examined is that the initiation of liver regeneration involves the rapid post-translational modification of transcription factors which bind to DNA and trigger the primary gene response. Based on the findings of Tewari et al.[14] we studied in detail the activation of the transcription factor NFkB and other related members of the same family. As indicated by its name, nuclear factor for the kappa enhancer in B cells, NFkB was originally isolated from B cells but has since been found to be active in many different cell types[15]. We have found that NFkB, which is composed of two subunits, p65 and p50, shows a dramatic increase in its binding to DNA in the first 30 min after partial hepatectomy[16]. In addition, binding of a homodimer composed of p50 subunits as well as binding of another dimeric product referred to as post-hepatectomy factor (PHF) is also increased[14]. The increase in NFkB binding to DNA also occurs after one-third hepatectomy, but this occurs more slowly than after 2/3 hepatectomy. The importance of this finding is two-fold: first, because 1/3 hepatectomy is not a sufficient stimulus to induce hepatocyte DNA synthesis[17], we conclude that NFkB binding might be needed for DNA synthesis but it is not sufficient by itself to cause it. Second, because 1/3 hepatectomy makes hepatocytes become competent to enter the cell cycle ('primed'), we suggest that the enhanced NFkB binding to DNA observed shortly after partial hepatectomy is a component of the priming process by which hepatocytes move from their quiescent state and enter the cell cycle[18,19].

It is clearly important to determine whether the NFkB response which we have described occurs in hepatocytes and/or non-parenchymal cells (NPC) after 2/3 partial hepatectomy. We have found, using isolated cells fractions, that NPC display a significant amount of NFkB binding in the normal liver. However, after partial hepatectomy the binding activity in NPC remains approximately constant while that in hepatocytes it increases significantly. These results have been further substantiated by the demonstration that NFkB binding occurs in hepatocytes and liver epithelial cells in culture and can be modulated by mitogenic stimuli[16]. Taken together, these results suggest that enhanced NFkB binding to DNA is a very early response of hepatocytes to partial hepatectomy and may precede the activation of immediate early genes.

The results on NFkB binding reviewed above have led us to propose that hepatocytes go through a series of steps as they enter the cell cycle and eventually replicate during liver regeneration (Fig. 1). We suggest that binding of transcription factor to DNA may be one of the initial steps of the process. Subsequent steps are regulated by various growth factors and, as cells reach the G1/S junction, cyclins and cyclin-dependent kinase come into play as important regulatory elements[1]. As all of these events unfold the effect of inhibitory factors needs to be overcome. Although one would expect that the expression of inhibitory proteins such as transforming growth factor (TGF) β1 and activin to decrease during liver regeneration, the levels of mRNAs for these proteins actually increase in the regenerating liver. Thus a critical question in liver regeneration is to understand how positive and negative growth factors act to enhance or repress hepatocyte replication. To analyse the role of stimulatory

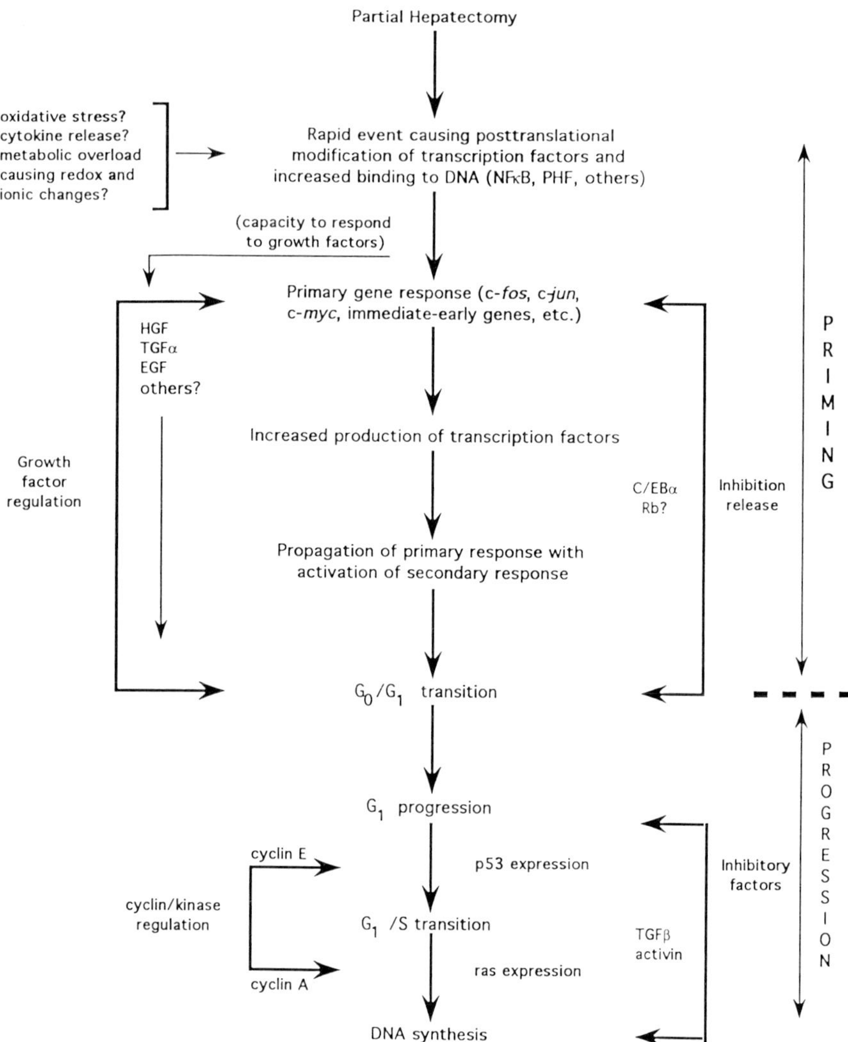

Fig. 1 Proposed sequence of events during liver regeneration after partial hepatectomy. The events are divided into two phases indicated in the figure as priming and progression. Priming involves the passage of quiescent hepatocytes into the cell cycle; progression involves the transit of hepatocytes through G1 and S. The priming phase may be initiated by post-translational modification and DNA binding of transcription factors, particularly of NFkB and derivatives. These alterations occur immediately after partial hepatectomy and may be caused by oxidative changes, cytokine release or other events. DNA binding of transcription factors induces a secondary gene response that propagates the initial events. The figure indicates the likely phases of growth factor control and cyclin/kinase activation. It also indicates that the effect of inhibitory factors has to be overcome during the growth process

growth factors in hepatocyte replication, we have studied in detail the expression of TGF-α in liver development, regeneration and carcinogenesis. In these studies we have used various animal models and technologies, including transgenic

Table 1 Relationship between hepatocyte proliferation and TGF-α production

Growth stage	TGF-α production	Consequence
Neonatal hepatocytes	High	Cell proliferation
Adult hepatocytes	Low	Quiescence
Hepatocytes in regenerating liver	High, transient	DNA replication (transient)
Hepatocytes in TGF-α transgenic mice	High, persistent	Hepatocyte proliferation eventually leading to transformation

mouse lines that overexpress TGFα and cultured cells in which the expression of the factor is inhibited by an antisense gene.

HEPATIC HYERPLASIA, ALTERATIONS IN PLOIDY AND NEOPLASIA CAUSED BY TGF-α OVEREXPRESSION

Expression of TGF-α by hepatocytes correlates well with the proliferative state of the cell (Table 1). It is high until approximately 1 week after birth and drops to low levels in adult quiescent hepatocytes. Transient expression of TGF-α is detected during liver regeneration after partial hepatectomy or toxic injury in vivo and in cultured hepatocytes stimulated to undergo DNA replication by growth factors[20–23]. Constitutive overexpression in transgenic mice causes liver hyperplasia and increased hepatocyte proliferation[24]. This increased proliferative capacity remains a regulated process that is compensated by increased cell turnover. After several months, the proliferative state becomes constitutive in some hepatocytes, at an age in which hepatocyte replication is negligible in non-transgenic mice. The cells that continuously replicate appear to be mostly diploid hepatocytes which overexpress TGF-α, and these cells are considered to be the progenitors of the hepatocellular tumours that develop in more than 80% of the animals at 12–15 months of age[25–27]. Proliferative indices (labelling after [^{3}H]thymidine infusion for 3 and 7 days, PCNA staining and mitotic index) for non-transgenic and TGF-α transgenic mice at 4 weeks and 8 months of age[24] are shown in Table 2. In TGF-α mice with enhanced hepatocyte proliferation in the first 4 weeks of life, the development of polyploidy in hepatocytes is delayed[24]. As shown in Figure 2, at 1 month of age, the majority of the hepatocytes in most transgenic mice are either diploid or tetraploid. In contrast, in non-transgenic mice there is only a small proportion of diploid hepatocytes while the percentage of octoploid cells is high.

It is clear from the available data that increased TGF-α expression causes hepatocyte hyperplasia, that the hyperplastic state can persist for many months and that neoplastic transformation eventually develops in hepatocytes which have become constitutively proliferative. What mechanisms may account for the change from regulated hyperproliferation to neoplastic development? The tumours that develop in the liver of these mice show no alterations in c-*ras* genes and no p53 mutations[26,27]. However, almost invariably, tumour development is associated with increased expression of insulin-like growth factor (IGF)-II[25]. The association between hepatocarcinogenesis and overexpression of IGF-II (and often also that of c-*myc*) has now been observed in many different animal models of liver carcinogenesis and in human hepatocellular carcinomas[28]. Although

Table 2 Hepatocyte proliferative indices in 4-week-old and 8-month-old normal and TGF-α transgenic mice

	4 weeks old		8 months old	
	Control	*Transgenic*	*Control*	*Transgenic*
Labelling index (3 day infusion)[a]	19±0.9	43±7	0.8±0.0	6±3
Labelling index (7 day infusion)[a]	42±5	81±5	3±0.4	25±3
PCNA staining[b]	8±0.8	14±3	0.8±0.3	3±0.7
Mitotic index[c]	0.8±0.2	2.1±0.6	—	0.5±0.4

[a]Expressed as percentage of hepatocytes labelled with [³H]thymidine.
[b]Expressed as percentage of hepatcytes stained with PCNA.
[c]Expressed as percentage of mitotic figures detected in hepatocytes.

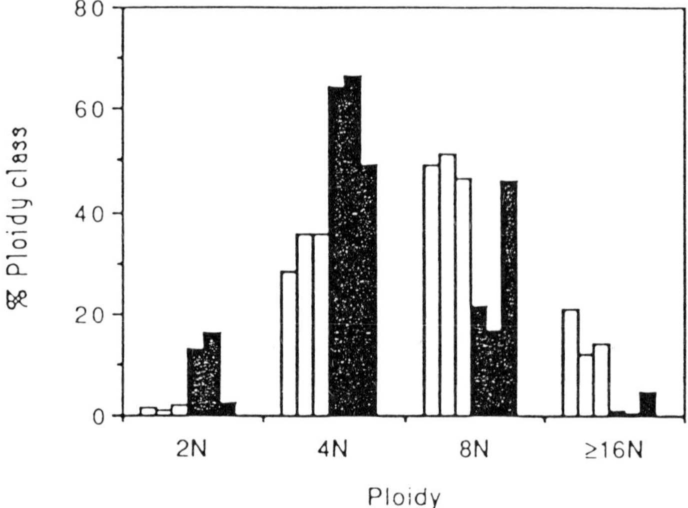

Fig. 2 Ploidy distribution of hepatocytes in young (4 to 5-week-old) normal and TGF-α transgenic mice. Hepatocytes were isolated from the livers of normal (□) and transgenic mice (■) treated with RNAase, stained with propidium iodide and analysed by flow cytometry using a Coulter EPICS 700 instrument. For each set of three animals, the percentage of the cell population comprising diploid (2N), tetraploid (4N), octaploid (8N) and higher ploidy (≥16N) classes is shown

overexpression of IGF-II may be a general property of hepatocellular carcinomas, the mechanisms responsible for increased IGF-II expression in these tumours, as well as the role of IGF-II in the transformation process, remain to be elucidated. One possibility is that continuous cell proliferation causes genomic aberrations leading to the unregulated expression of growth genes, including IGF-II. An alternative explanation is that IGF-II, which is a fetal liver product, is expressed by diploid hepatocytes which have retained a programme of gene expression similar to that of fetal hepatocytes.

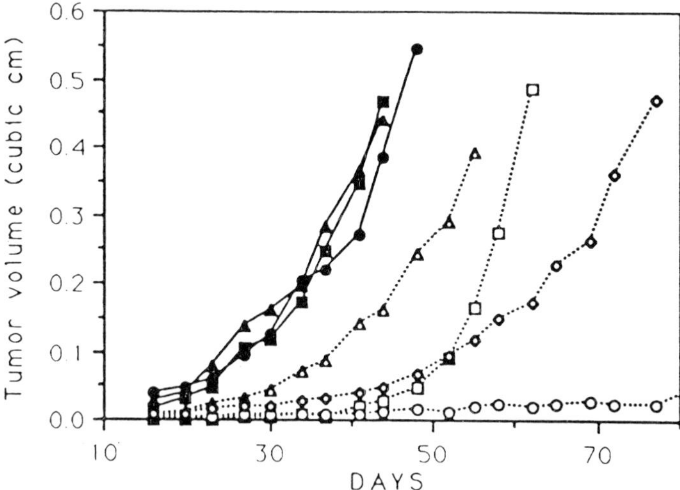

Fig. 3 Effect of antisense TGFα on tumour growth in nude mice. (**A**) 2×10^5 cells were injected into nude mice (six sites per line) and tumour volumes were measured at the indicated times. Symbols: C1, ■; C2, ▲; AS3, ●; AS1, □; AS2, △; AS3, ○; AS4, ◇. The data were analysed using single factor ANOVA and significance was assessed using Fisher's PLSD test: AS1, AS3 and AS4 inhibited relative to pooled control tumours at all time points ($p < 0.005$); AS2 inhibited relative to pooled control tumours, $p < 0.005$ except at day 4 ($p < 0.01$), day 44 ($p < 0.02$) and day 48 ($p < 0.04$)

INHIBITION OF TUMOUR GROWTH BY A TGF-α ANTISENSE GENE

Antisense genes and oligonucleotides have been used recently to inhibit the expression of oncogenes which may be required for tumour development[29]. We have made use of antisense gene sequences to block the expression of growth factors in liver cells. Plasmids that carry TGF-α sequences in the antisense orientation were constructed and transfected into cultured liver epithelial cells which overexpress TGF-α and which are highly tumorigenic when injected into nude mice[30]. The purpose of these experiments was to test whether inhibition of TGF-α expression by the antisense gene would inhibit the tumorigenicity of these cells. Cells of the LE2 line (an oval cell line) were used in these experiments because they overexpress TGF-α upon transformation in culture and produce hepatocellular carcinomas when injected into nude mice. Transfection of an antisense TGF-α cDNA fragment into these cells caused a 4- to 6-fold decrease in TGF-α secretion compared with cells which were transfected with a plasmid that did not contain the TGF-α antisense gene. Inoculation into nude mice of 2×10^5 cells transfected with the control plasmids led to formation of large hepatocellular tumours at the site of injection after 5–6 weeks[30]. In contrast, there was a delay of 30 days or more in the growth in nude mice of various cell clones that had been transfected with the TGF-α antisense gene (Fig. 3). Inhibition of tumour growth also occurred when 2×10^6 cells were injected, but the growth delay was approximately 20 days. Further experiments revealed that the TGF-α antisense gene was being actively transcribed during the delay phase but when tumour growth started after the lag phase the antisense gene was no longer active. Cessation of transcription of the gene occurred even though the plasmid carrying the construct was present in the cells. We conclude from these experiments that, in this system, continuous expression of TGF-α is required for growth of hepatocellular carcinomas in vivo[30]. Furthermore, the experiments indicate that it is possible to block hepatocellular carcinoma growth from highly tumorigenic cells by inhibiting TGF-α expression as long as the antisense gene remains active. Future work should aim at developing TGF-α antisense constructs which maintain transcriptional activity for long periods of time in vivo.

In this chapter we have briefly examined two aspects of the process of liver regeneration after partial hepatectomy: the very early events associated with the entry of hepatocytes into the cell cycle and the effects of TGF-α on hepatocyte proliferation. We conclude that in the first 30 min after partial hepatectomy post-translational modification of NFkB leading to DNA binding takes place. We hypothesize that the signal(s) mediating these changes could be: (a) oxidative changes in hepatocytes caused by metabolic overload; (b) intracellular oxidative changes caused by tumour necrosis factor release at the time of the operation; (c) growth factor signalling. The two first alternatives are the most plausible because both tumour necrosis factor and direct oxidative agents are known inducers of NFkB binding[31]. In addition, injection of antibodies to tumour necrosis factor into partially hepatectomized rats decreases DNA replication by approximately 50%[32]. The second part of this chapter demonstrates that the constitutive overexpression of TGF-α which is transiently expressed during liver regeneration, leads to liver hyperplasia, and eventually to tumorigenesis. From these experiments we conclude that: (a) TGF-α is a physiological stimulator of hepatocyte replication; (b) it leads to tumorigenesis only after repeated rounds of replication have taken place and (c) other genes, and in particular IGF-II, may be required for hepatocyte transformation. Work in all of these areas is being actively carried out in many laboratories.

References

1. Fausto N, Webber EM. Liver regeneration. In: Arias IM, Boyer JL, Fausto N, Jacoby WB, Schachter D, Shafritz DA, editors. The liver: biology and pathobiology, 3rd edn. New York: Raven Press. 1994;1059–84.
2. Higgins GM, Anderson RM. Experimental pathology of the liver. I. Restoration of the liver of the white rat following partial surgical removal. Arch Pathol. 1931;12:186–202.
3. Fausto N, Webber EM. Mechanisms of growth regulation in liver regeneration and hepatic carcinogenesis. In: Boyer JL, Ockner RK, editors. Progress in liver diseases. Philadelphia: Saunders. 1993;11:115–37.
4. Yamanaka N, Okamoto E, Kawamura E et al. Dynamics of normal and injured liver regeneration after partial hepatectomy as assessed on the basis of computed tomography and liver function. Hepatology. 1993;18:79–85.
5. Martinez-Hernandez A, Delgado FM, Amenta PS. The extracellular matrix in hepatic regeneration: localization of collagen types I, III, IV, laminin, and fibronectin. Lab Invest. 1991;64:157–66.
6. Van Thiel DH, Gavaler JS, Kam I et al. Rapid growth of an intact human liver transplanted into a recipient larger than the donor. Gastroenterology. 1987;93:1414–9.

7. Francavilla A, Zeng Q, Polimeno L et al. Small-for-size liver transplanted into larger recipient: a model of hepatic regeneration. Hepatology. 1994;19:210–16.
8. Czaja MJ, Flanders KC, Biempica L, Klein C, Zern MA, Weiner FR. Expression of tumor necrosis factor-α and transforming growth factor-β1 in acute rat liver injury. Growth Factors. 1989;1:219–26.
9. Rojkind M. From regeneration to scar formation: the collagen way. Lab Invest. 1991;64:131–3.
10. Rojkind M, Greenwel P. The liver as a bioecological system. In: Arias IM, Jakoby WB, Popper H, Schachter D, Shafritz A, editors. The liver: biology and pathology. New York: Raven Press. 1988:1269–85.
11. Morello D, FitzGerald M, Babinet MJ, Fausto N. c-*myc*, c-*fos*, and c-*jun* regulation in the regenerating livers of normal and H-2K/c-myc transgenic mice. Mol Cell Biol. 1990;10: 3185–93.
12. Haber AH, Mohn KL, Diamond RH, Taub R. Induction patterns of 70 genes during nine days after hepatectomy define the temporal course of liver regeneration. J Clin Invest. 1993;91: 1319–26.
13. Herschman HR. Primary response genes induced by growth factors and tumor promoters. Annu Rev Biochem. 1991;60:281–319.
14. Tewari M, Dobrzanski P, Mohn KL et al. Rapid induction in regenerating liver of RL/IF-1 (an IkB that inhibits NF-kB, RelB-p50, and c-Rel-p50) and PHF, a novel kB site-binding complex. Mol Cell Biol. 1992;2898–908.
15. Lenardo MJ, Baltimore D. NF-kB: a pleiotropic mediator of inducible and tissue-specific gene control. Cell. 1989;58:227–9.
16. FitzGerald MJ, Webber EM, Donovan JR, Fausto N. Rapid DNA binding by NF-kB in hepatocytes of regenerating liver. Cell Growth Different. (in press).
17. Bucher NLR. Regeneration of mammalian liver. In: Bourne GH, Danielli JF, editors. International Review of Cytology. New York: Academic Press. 1963:245–30.
18. Mead JE, Braun L, Martin DA, Fausto N. Induction of replicative competence ('priming') in normal liver. Cancer Res. 1990;50:7023–30.
19. Webber EM, Godowski PJ, Fausto N. In vivo response of hepatocytes to growth factors requires an initial priming stimulus. Hepatology. 1994;19:489–97.
20. Mead JE, Fausto N. Transforming growth factor a may be a physiological regulator of liver regeneration by means of an autocrine mechanism. Proc Natl Acad Sci USA. 1989;86:1558–62.
21. Webber EM, FitzGerald MJ, Brown PI, Bartlett MH, Fausto N. TGFα expression during liver regeneration after partial hepatectomy and toxic injury, and potential interactions between transforming growth factor-α and hepatocyte growth factor. Hepatology. 1993;18:1422–31.
22. Evarts RP, Nakatsukasa H, Marsden ER, Hu Z, Thorgeirsson SS. Expression of transforming growth factor-alpha in regenerating liver and during hepatic differentiation. Mol Carcinog. 1992;5:25–31.
23. Russell WE, Dempsey PJ, Sitaric S, Peck AJ, Coffey RJ Jr. Transforming growth factor-α (TGF-α) concentrations increase in regenerating rat liver: evidence for a delayed accumulation of mature TGFα. Endocrinology. 1993;133:1731–8.
24. Webber EM, Wu JC, Wang L, Merlino G, Fausto N. Overexpression of transforming growth factor alpha causes liver enlargement and increased hepatocyte proliferation in transgenic mice. Am J Pathol. 1994;145:398–408.
25. Jhappan C, Stahle C, Harkins RN, Fausto N, Smith GH, Merlino GT. TGFα overexpression in transgenic mice induces liver neoplasia and abnormal development of the mammary gland and pancreas. Cell. 1990;61:1137–46.
26. Lee G-H, Merlino G, Fausto N. Development of liver tumors in transforming growth factor α transgenic mice. Cancer Res. 1992;52:5162–70.
27. Takagi H, Sharp R, Hammermeister C et al. Molecular and genetic analysis of liver oncogenesis in transforming growth factor α transgenic mice. Cancer Res. 1992;52:5171–7.
28. Lassene C, Canani E, Zindy F, Lamas E, Bréchot C. Insulin-like growth factor II and human primary liver cancer. In: Bréchot C, editor. Primary liver cancer: etiological and progression factors. Boca Raton: CRC Press. 1994:283–97.
29. van der Krol AR, Mol JNM, Stuitje AR. Modulation of eukaryotic gene expression by complementary RNA or DNA sequences. Biotechniques. 1988;6:958–76.
30. Laird AD, Brown PI, Fausto N. Inhibition of tumor growth in liver epithelial cells transfected with a transforming growth factor α antisense gene. Cancer Res. 1994:54:4224–32.

31. Schreck R, Rieber P, Baverle PA. Reactive oxygen intermediates as apparently widely used messengers in the activation of the NF-kB transcription factor and HIV-1. EMBO J.1991;10:2247–58.
32. Akerman P, Cote P, Yang SQ et al. Antibodies to tumor necrosis factor-α inhibit liver regeneration after partial hepatectomy. Am J Phys. 1992;263:G579–G585.

9
Role of HGF in liver regeneration

G. K. MICHALOPOULOS, W. M. MARS and M.-L. LIU

INTRODUCTION

Liver regeneration has been studied for several decades, following the introduction of well-defined animal models and observations in humans. Indeed, observations from the days of antiquity (Greek myth of Prometheus, clay reliefs of liver shapes from Babylon, etc.) have amply demonstrated that the regenerative capacities of the liver have been observed since ancient times. The tremendous capacity of the liver to regenerate is a result of natural evolution which ensures that hepatic structure and mass becomes restored after injury resulting from accidental ingestion of toxins in the diet. Although the most common cause of hepatic injury in real life is probably chemical, the best studied model of liver regeneration is that which is induced by surgical resection. Chemical injury is followed not only by regenerative events but also by events associated with inflammation required to remove the dead tissue. Surgical removal of two-thirds of the liver in rodents is an easy surgical process, first described in 1931 by Higgins and Anderson[1]. Subsequent studies of liver regeneration utilizing this procedure have defined two interesting phenomena that relate to liver regeneration.

The first set of observations relates to response of grafted hepatic tissue in extrahepatic sites. Partial hepatectomy of the liver in situ stimulates regeneration not only in the normal liver but also of the ectopic hepatic tissue[2]. In parallel studies involving rats joined by parabiotic circulation, hepatectomy in one member of the pair resulted in stimulation of liver regeneration in the other member[3]. Transplantation into the adipose tissue of hepatocytes isolated from rat livers has been used as a model to demonstrate that stimulation of regeneration of the liver in situ results in the DNA synthesis of cells in the transplanted sites in the adipose tissue. This has conclusively demonstrated that liver regeneration is associated with rapid appearance in the plasma of substance(s) associated with stimulation of mitogenesis and hepatocytes[4].

Secondly, stimulation of liver regeneration by surgical resection results in the emergence of new populations of mRNAs deriving from more than 50 newly transcribed genes. Some of these genes are novel and are in the process of being characterized[5]. The rapidity of the reprogramming of gene expression in hepatocytes very shortly after partial hepatectomy is a very interesting phenomenon. Whatever the nature of the stimulus for liver regeneration, its emergence and its effects are rapid.

These two sets of phenomena have defined some of the fundamental aspects of the growth control mechanisms of hepatic regeneration that operate to initiate this complex process. The definition and further exploration of these phenomena is easier to perform in regeneration stimulated by hepatic resection since this process is not complicated by hepatic tissue injury, necrosis or inflammation, as is unavoidable in studies of regeneration following chemical injury models.

Studies from several laboratories have now identified and fully characterized the structure of a protein known as hepatocyte growth factor (HGF), the agent which is associated with the blood-borne factors stimulating liver regeneration. Following its original identification in 1982[6] and its subsequent cloning and sequence characterization[7,8], several studies demonstrated that HGF also binds to two high affinity sites[9]. The binding sites with the highest affinity are now known to be the HGF receptor encoded by the proto-oncogene c-*met*[10]. In addition to the high affinity binding sites, there are other lower affinity sites (at the nanomolar range) associated with glycosaminogycans[11]. It is now abundantly clear that HGF is expressed in mesenchymal cells in multiple tissues and organs and that it acts in a paracrine or endocrine model to stimulate different effects in epithelial cell types. The mitogenic targets of HGF include hepatocytes, bile duct cells, bronchial epithelium, mammary duct epithelial cells, skin squamous cells, melanocytes, endothelial cells, skeletal muscle and multiple neoplastic cell lines[12]. Given its high mol. wt, and low effective range of concentration (5–20 ng/ml) HGF is a very powerful mitogen: for most susceptible cell types it appears to be the most powerful mitogen identified. In addition to stimulating mitogenesis, HGF was also shown to be a powerful stimulator of mitogenesis, originally in endothelial cells and also in mammary carcinoma cell lines, where it exhibited mitogenesis under the influence of what was then known as scatter factor[13]. The motogenic effects were subsequently demonstrated for a variety of other cell targets. Our experience with hepatocytes indicates that both EGF and HGF are relatively powerful motogens, but HGF is a more powerful motogen in all of the assays that these two agents have been tested with so far[14].

HGF mRNA and protein have been found in essentially every tissue in the body, including liver, lungs, brain, kidney, spleen, eye and testis[15]. The receptor for HGF is present in all mucosal cells of the gastrointestinal tract, as well as tubular and duct-like structures, selective groups of neurones, hepatocytes and adrenal cortical cells[16]. Concurrent expression of HGF as well as its receptor in mesenchymal cells leads to cellular transformation which is often associated with the induction of tumours that have epithelioid appearance[17].

Given the multifunctional aspects of HGF in multiple sites and organs, the issue has been raised as to whether or not there is any specificity of the effects of HGF on the liver. An additional correlate to the question is whether HGF functions in the same way towards all tissues or whether it has any special functions at all associated toward liver regeneration that would not be relevant to its effects on other tissues. If HGF is a blood-borne factor, what mechanism imparts any specificity at all towards its function as a liver growth agent? The evidence for such specific effects of HGF in liver has been accumulated from a variety of in vivo and in vitro studies. The following is a summary of the studies that appeared in the literature in recent years which document some of the organ specific as well as the endocrine effects of HGF on liver.

CHANGES IN PLASMA HGF FOLLOWING HEPATIC RESECTION

Plasma levels of HGF rise dramatically within 30–60 min of hepatic resection in the rat[18]. The rise reaches the maximum peak within 1–2 h followed by a period of decline to a half maximal level. Elevated (above control) levels of HGF persist following hepatic resection for more than 24 h. Similar findings have been documented following hepatic resection in humans[19]. The studies also correlate with the well documented very high levels of HGF in the plasma in individuals with terminal stages of fatal hepatic disease (fulminant hepatitis)[20]. During the terminal stages of this disease most hepatocytes have already died and the actual functional hepatic mass represents a minimal fraction of the total original. Other studies have also shown that in conditions where hepatocyte proliferation has been stimulated, HGF levels in the peripheral blood also rise.

DISTRIBUTION AND UPTAKE OF HGF IN TISSUES

The pathways by which HGF is sequestrated after systemic injection are also very interesting. When radiolabelled HGF is injected through the systemic circulation, a high proportion of the injected HGF (30–40%) localizes to the liver within 15 min after injection[21]. Other tissues are much less active in taking up HGF. The only exception is the adrenal glands which seem to match the liver uptake per gram weight. The kidney also actively takes up HGF. A large proportion (50–60%) of the injected HGF localizes in low affinity, high capacity binding sites in musculoskeletal and connective tissue. While all of those tissues contain cells that express the HGF receptor (MET), comparison of the binding of HGF as documented by autoradiography with the distribution of the expression of MET protein as documented by immunohistochemistry reveals a pattern of expression of convergence or divergence in some tissues. In liver, the injected HGF predominantly localizes in the periportal sites. On the other hand, histochemical studies have shown that MET (the HGF receptor protein) is distributed throughout the cells of the hepatic lobule. Most of the HGF localizing in kidneys accumulates in the glomerulus (M. -L. Liu and G. K. Michalopoulos, unpublished), although MET receptors are predominantly expressed on the kidney tubular epithelium. There is complete convergence between MET expression and HGF binding in the adrenal glands as well as in the lungs and in the gastrointestinal tract. The above results suggest that sites other than the high affinity receptor exist which have high capacity for HGF. The abundance of those sites in comparison to MET more than compensates for their lower affinity and results in sequestering HGF in high capacity in connective tissue sites[22]. The physiological importance of these sites is not currently clear, but they appear to be the primary determinant for the amount of HGF sequestered in the liver and in other tissues.

UPTAKE AND PROCESSING OF HGF IN LIVER

Part of the HGF taken up in the liver is excreted intact in the bile[21]: an estimated 25–30% of HGF is excreted intact after a bolus injection through the portal vein. The same methodology has also demonstrated that regenerating liver is more active in taking up HGF. A measurable increase in HGF uptake/g tissue has been documented in the generating liver[22]. Overall the total capacity of liver to take up HGF is substantial, reaching a maximal total level of $0.157\pm0.012\,\mu g$ of HGF/g liver in the rat[21]. The localization of HGF in periportal sites in the liver lobule parallels that shown in previous studies shown for EGF[23]. It is of interest that the two primary mitogens for hepatocytes (EGF and HGF) localize in common sites and that these sites are exactly those that have been shown in previous reports to be associated with the initiation with DNA synthesis during liver regeneration. A wave of mitogenesis seems to proceed from the portal triads towards the central veins and this traverses the hepatic lobule over the course of 48 h following partial hepatectomy[24]. The above evidence strongly indicates that HGF has a key role to play in liver regeneration. Many questions remain, however, regarding the precise sequence of steps that lead to HGF release and the initiation of the regeneration process.

HGF CLEARANCE AND HEPATIC UPTAKE FOLLOWING PARTIAL HEPATECTOMY

Precise measurements of the clearance of HGF by liver have indicated that there is only a two-fold decrease in HGF clearance after partial hepatectomy although there is a 66% reduction in hepatic mass[22]. It has also been shown that the uptake of HGF/g of liver is increased by 20–50% following partial hepatectomy. Thus, although the evidence for the rise of HGF in the liver is dramatic and well-documented by several groups, the stoichiometry between liver mass and HGF levels is not proportionate.

The direct logical projection between the rise of HGF after early partial hepatectomy and the onset of DNA synthesis in the liver 12 h after hepatectomy is that HGF rise is responsible for onset of DNA synthesis. To further investigate this postulate, we infused increasing concentrations of HGF through the portal vein over 48 h. Similar experiments were also performed for TGF-α. In both cases initiation of DNA synthesis was stimulated by both of these growth factors, but only in the hepatocytes that immediately surround the portal triads[25].

From studies in cell culture, we have also observed that hepatocytes maintained sandwiched between collagen gel layers become unresponsive to growth factors. These hepatocytes acquire the capacity to respond to growth factors after the gels have been treated with collagenase[26]. Several studies have shown that during collagenase perfusion and shortly after digestion of the liver by collagenase, hepatocytes in primary culture express cell cycle enzymes, even though they are not stimulated to enter into DNA synthesis by growth factors or other stimuli[27–29]. Those studies have suggested that collagenase treatment can render hepatocytes responsive to growth factors. We therefore repeated the perfusion of liver by HGF but preceded the HGF perfusion by a short-term infusion of a low concentration of collagenase to the portal vein. This had a dramatic effect on the DNA synthesis response obtained. Stimulation of DNA synthesis by HGF and TGF-α, if preceded by collagenase pretreatment, was seen in 60–70% of hepatocytes. This degree of stimulation of DNA synthesis is comparable to that induced by liver regeneration[25]. These results indicate that we cannot assume that normal hepatocytes in the G0 phase of the cell cycle are responsive to growth factors. Although the level of HGF in the plasma rises, it may not be by itself a sufficient cause to stimulate the full regenerative response. Early events need to precede the elevation of HGF and render hepatocytes responsive to HGF. These phenomena may be similar to the infusion of collagenase and be composed of proteolytic events.

ROLE OF UROKINASE IN HGF ACTIVATION AND MATRIX DEGRADATION IN THE EARLIEST STAGES OF HEPATIC REGENERATION

Recent observations from our laboratory clearly suggest that urokinase plays a key role in both HGF activation and the regenerative response[30]. Urokinase may be the in vivo correlate of the collagenase treatment that was required to stimulate responsiveness to growth factors, both in vitro as well as in perfused liver. Urokinase[31,32] has been associated with several functions, including conversion of plasminogen to plasmin. Plasmin further activates fibrinolysis, several enzymes which degrade connective tissue biomatrix (stromelysin, matrilysin, collagenases, etc.) and the conversion of latent TGF-β1 into active TGF-β1. Urokinse also directly activates type IV collagenase into its active form[33] and activates single chain inactive HGF to two-chain active HGF[30,34]. The earliest measured event after partial hepatectomy (within 1 min after the operation) is the rapid elevation of urokinase activity associated with the appearance of the urokinase receptor in the plasma membrane of the hepatocytes (W. M. Mars and G. K. Michalopoulos, unpublished). Given the functions of the urokinase described above, activation as a result of the appearance of the urokinase receptor may lead both to HGF activation as well as to activation of a cascade of events leading to degradation of hepatic biomatrix rapidly after initiation of the regenerative events. Such degradation of the matrix would also lead to release of matrix components into the peripheral blood. We have recently measured high levels of hyaluronic acid in peripheral blood, these increases rapidly following partial hepatectomy (W. M. Mars and G. K. Michalopoulos, unpublished). Other components known to be associated with the biomatrix, such as TGF-β also increase rapidly within the peripheral blood following partial hepatectomy (R. L. Jirtle et al., unpublished). If degradation of matrix occurs early (within 1 min) after partial hepatectomy it may activate HGF through urokinase and release of active HGF into plasma. The active HGF may return to the liver and initiate hepatocyte DNA synthesis. It may also result in release of matrix-bound TGF-β into plasma. This would be bound by α_2-macroglobulin[35] and thus be rendered inactive, removing mitoinhibitory influences of TGF-β on hepatocytes. Removal of TGF-β bound to matrix as well as matrix components per se will also confer responsiveness of hepatocytes to the circulating growth factors. If degradation of matrix is essential to allow cells to respond to HGF, and if a rise in HGF levels in the plasma is due to its release from the liver following a rapid breakdown of hepatic biomatrix, then hepatocytes would be the only cells in the body to respond to the circulating HGF since the biomatrix in the other organs (kidney, skin, etc.) would be intact. These events together, along with co-mitogenic effects of agents such as norepinephrine, a substance also increasing following partial hepatectomy and known to be co-mitogenic to hepatocytes[36] may be ultimately responsible for shifting hepatocytes from the G0 to the G1 phase of the cycle. Hepatocytes in G1 are known to fully produce autocrine and paracrine growth factors such as TGF-α[37] aFGF[38], ALR[39] and also stimulate further production of HGF by non-parenchymal cells in the liver.

Despite the recent progress in elucidation of the early events of liver regeneration, much remains to be further understood. The phenomenon is complex yet clearly defined by simple manipulations both in vivo and in vitro. The stage has now perhaps been reached whereby these observations may be extrapolated into phenomena of clinical relevance in relation to regeneration such as fulminant hepatitis, chronic active hepatitis and hepatocellular carcinoma.

References

1. Higgins GM, Anderson RM. Experimental pathology of the liver: I. Restoration of the liver of the white rat following partial surgical removal. Arch Pathol. 1931;12:186–202.
2. Grisham JW, Leong GF, Hole BC. Heterotopic partial autotransplantation of rat liver. Technique and demonstration of structure and function of the graft. Cancer Res. 1964;24:1474–82.
3. Jirtle RL, Michalopoulos G. Effects of partial hepatectomy on transplanted hepatocytes. Cancer Res. 1982;42:3000–4.
4. Fischer B, Szuch P, Levine M, Fisher ER. A portal blood factor as the humoral agent in liver regeneration. Science. 1971;171:575–77.
5. Haber BA, Mohn KL, Diamond RH, Taub R. Induction patterns of 70 genes during nine days after hepatectomy define the temporal course of liver regeneration. J Clin Invest. 1993;1:1319–26.
6. Zarnegar R, Muga S, Enghild J, Michalopoulos G. NH2-terminal amino acid sequence of rabbit hepatopoietin A, a heparin-binding polypeptide growth factor for hepatocytes. Biochem Biophys Res Commun. 1989;163:1370–6.
7. Miyazawa K, Tsubouchi H, Naka D et al. Molecular cloning and sequence analysis of cDNA for human hepatocyte growth factor. Biochem Biophys Res Commun. 1989;163:967–73.
8. Nakamura T, Nishizawa T, Hagiya M et al. Molecular cloning and expression of human hepatocyte growth factor. Nature. 1989;342:440–3.
9. Zarnegar R, DeFrances MC, Oliver L, Michalopoulos G. Identification and partial characterization of receptor binding sites for HGF on rat hepatocytes. Biochem Biophys Res Commun. 1990;173:1179–85.
10. Naldini L, Vigna E, Narsimhan RP et al. Hepatocyte growth factor (HGF) stimulates the tyrosine kinase activity of the receptor encoded by the proto-oncogene c-MET. Oncogene. 1991;6:501–4.
11. Arakaki N, Hirono S, Ishii T et al. Identification and partial characterization of two classes of receptors for human hepatocyte growth factor on adult rat hepatocytes in primary culture. J Biol Chem. 1992;267:7101–7.
12. Michalopoulos G. HGF and liver regeneration. Gastroenterol Jpn. 1993;2(Suppl. 4):36–9.
13. Weidner M, Arakaki N, Hartmann G et al. Evidence for the identity of human scatter factor and human hepatocyte growth factor. Proc Natl Acad Sci USA. 1991;88:7001–5.
14. Beer-Stolz D, Michalopoulos GK. Comparative motogenic and mitogenic effects on rat and human hepatocytes. J Cell Biochem. 1994;55:445–64.
15. Tashiro K, Hagiya M, Nishizawa T et al. Deduced primary structure of rat hepatocyte growth factor and expression of the mRNA in rat tissues. Proc Natl Acad Sci USA. 1990;87:3200–4.

16. Liu ML, Li JM, Mars WM, Becich M, Michalopoulos GK. Tissue localization of hepatocyte growth factor (HGF) and its receptors in rats and humans (Submitted).
17. Tsarfaty I, Rong S, Resau JH, Rulong S, da Silva PP, Vande Woude GF. The Met proto-oncogene mesenchymal to epithelial cell conversion. Science. 1994;263:98–101.
18. Lindroos PM, Zarnegar R, Michalopoulos GK. Hepatocyte growth factor (hepatopoietin A) rapidly increases in plasma before DNA synthesis and liver regeneration stimulated by partial hepatectomy and carbon tetrachloride administration. Hepatology. 1991;3:743–50.
19. Tomiya T, Tani M, Yamada S, Hayashi S, Umeda N, Fujiwara K. Serum hepatocyte growth factor levels in hepatectomized and nonhepatectomized surgical patients. Gastroenterology. 1992;103:1621–4.
20. Tsubouchi H, Horono S, Gohda E et al. Clinical significance of human hepatocyte growth factor in blood from patients with fulminant hepatic failure. Hepatology. 1989;9:875–81.
21. Liu ML, Mars WM, Zarnegar R, Michalopoulos GK. Uptake and distribution of hepatocyte growth factor in normal and regenerating adult rat liver. Am J Pathol. 1994;144:129–40.
22. Appasamy R, Tanabe M, Murase N et al. Hepatocyte growth factor, blood clearance, organ uptake, and biliary excretion in normal and partially hepatectomized rats. Lab Invest. 1993;68:270–6.
23. St Hilaire RJ, Hradek GT, Jones AL. Hepatic sequestration and biliary secretion of epidermal growth factor: evidence for a high-capacity uptake system. Proc Natl Acad Sci USA. 1983;80:3797–801.
24. Rabes HM, Wirsching R, Tuczek HV, Iseler G. Analysis of cell cycle compartments of hepatocytes after partial hepatectomy. Cell Tissue Kinet. 1976;6:517–32.
25. Liu ML, Mars WM, Zarnegar R, Michalopoulos GK. Collagenase pretreatment and the mitogenic effects of hepatocyte growth factor and transforming factor alpha in adult rat liver. Hepatology. 1994;19:1521–7.
26. Michalopoulos GK, Bowen W, Nussler AK, Becich MJ, Howard TA. Comparative analysis of mitogeic and morphogenic effects of HGF and EGF on rat and human hepatocytes maintained in collagen gels. J Cell Physiol. 1993;156:443–52.
27. Ikeda T, Sawada N, Fujinaga K, Minase T, Mori M. H-*ras* gene is expressed at the G1 phase in primary cultures of hepatocytes. Exp Cell Res. 1989;185:292–6.
28. Kost DP, Michalopoulos GK. Effect of epidermal growth factor on the expression of protooncogenes c-*myc* and c-Ha-*ras* in short-term primary hepatocyte culture. J Cell Physiol. 1990;144:122–7.
29. Etienne PL, Baffet G, Desvergne B, Boisnard-Rissel M, Glaise D, Guguen-Guillouzo C. Transient expression of c-*fos* and constant expression of c-*myc* in freshly isolated and cultured normal adult rat hepatocytes. Oncogene Res. 1988;3:255–62.
30. Mars WM, Zarnegar R, Michalopoulos GK. Activation of hepatocyte growth factor by the plasminogen activators uPA and tPA. Am J Pathol. 1993;143:949–58.
31. Blasi F. Urokinase and urokinase receptor: a paracrine/autocrine system regulating cell migration and invasiveness. BioEssays. 1993;15:105–33.
32. Duffy MJ. Urokinase type plasminogen activator and malignancy. Fibrinolysis. 1993;7:295–302.
33. Keski-Oja J, Lohi J, Tuuttila A, Tryggvason K, Vartio T. Proteolytic processing of the 72,000-Da type IV collagenase by urokinase plasminogen activator. Exp Cell Res. 1992;171–6.
34. Naldini L, Tamagnone L, Vigna E et al. Extracellular proteolytic cleavage by urokinase is required for activation of hepatocyte growth factor/scatter factor. EMBO J. 1992;11:4825–33.
35. LaMarre J, Hayes MA, Wollenberg GK, Hussaini I, Hall SW, Gonias SL. An alpha 2-macro-globulin receptor-dependent mechanism for the plasma clearance of transforming growth factor-beta 1 in mice. J Clin Invest. 1991;87:39–44.
36. Cruise JL, Knechtle SJ, Bollinger RR, Kuhn C, Michalopoulos G. Alpha 1-adrenergic effects and liver regeneration. Hepatology. 1987;7:1189–94.
37. Webber EM, FitzGerald MJ, Brown PI, Bartlett MH, Fausto N. Transforming growth factor-alpha expression during liver regeneration after partial hepatectomy and toxic injury, and potential interactions between transforming growth factor-alpha and hepatocyte growth factor. Hepatology. 1993;18:1422–31.
38. Kan M, Huan J, Mansson P, Yasumitsu H, Carr B, McKeehan W. Heparin-binding growth factor type 1 (acidic fibroblast growth factor): A potential biphasic autocrine and paracrine regulator of hepatocyte regeneration. Proc Natl Acad Sci USA. 1989;86:7432–6.
39. Francavilla A, Polimeno L, Barone M, Azzarone A, Starzl TE. Hepatic regeneration and growth factors. J Surg Oncol. 1993;3(Suppl):1–7.

Part C
Clinical implications

Section V
Hepatitis and cirrhosis

10
Kupffer cell processing of bacterial lipopolysaccharide

E. S. FOX and P. THOMAS

INTRODUCTION

Kupffer cells are the largest population of fixed macrophages in the body and represent nearly 15% of rat liver cell number and 3% of its mass[1]. Kupffer cells are derived from bone marrow progenitors[2] and reach final differentiation within the liver[3]. They are located in the liver sinusoids, largely in the periportal region, but can extend pseudopodia through the fenestrations in the endothelial cell lining into the space of Disse and make direct contact with the hepatocytes[2]. Their number and orientation within the portal sinusoids are ideally suited for their role in clearance of gut-derived antigens and a presumed role in the surveillance[4] and killing[5] of cancer cells.

While the role of the liver in the clearance and detoxification of gut-derived endotoxin is well known[6,7], the role of the Kupffer cell has only recently been examined in any detail. In rodents, Kupffer cells are the major cell population implicated in clearance of endotoxin[8,9]. A recent study based on immuno-histochemical staining with factor C has also suggested that sinusoidal endothelial cells can clear endotoxin[10]. Studies with isolated rat Kupffer cells have demonstrated that endotoxin uptake is largely through absorptive pinocytosis, while peritoneal macrophages isolated from the same animals possessed a saturable receptor mediated system for endotoxin uptake[11,12]. Catabolism of bacterial endotoxin by rat Kupffer cells is mainly by deglycosylation[13] while other monocytic cells catabolize endotoxin through deacylation[14]. The hepatocyte has been implicated in the further processing of this Kupffer cell-modified endotoxin[8,15,16]. Incubation of isolated hepatocytes with Kupffer cell-modified LPS showed a 4 to 5-fold increase in uptake over native LPS. Furthermore the modified LPS was 5 to 6-fold less capable of eliciting a TNF-α response from peritoneal macrophages, implying detoxification[17].

Bacterial endotoxin is used as an in vitro stimulatory agent to activate monocyte and macrophage populations. Recently a photoaffinity labelling technique has been developed[18] which has allowed identification of endotoxin binding moieties on the cell surface. A 73 kDa protein has been identified on the surfaces of splenic lymphocytes, splenic and peritoneal macrophages and peripheral monocytes from endotoxin sensitive species[19–22]. Monoclonal antibodies against this protein activate peritoneal macrophages to become tumoricidal[23], suggesting that various effects of endotoxin stimulation may be manifested through its action. Two proteins of 55 and 65 kDa have also been implicated as potential LPS receptors since they have been detected on the macrophage-like cell line J774.1 but not on an LPS-resistant mutant derived from this cell line[24]. The CD18 complex of human macrophages has also been implicated in endotoxin binding[25]; however, binding to this complex is not involved in activation[26]. Multiple binding sites for the lipid A component of LPS have been reported on murine macrophage-like cell lines and human phagocytes[27,28], but no evidence has been presented that they are involved in activation. The aim of this study was to investigate the presence of putative endotoxin receptors on the Kupffer cell surface and to determine the molecular response to endotoxin activation. We present data which demonstrate that under similar labelling conditions to those used for other cell types the 80 kDa protein or other potential endotoxin binding proteins were not detectable on Kupffer cells. We were also unable to recover this LPS binding protein by affinity chromatography. However, using a ligand blot assay with labelled endotoxin we showed specific endotoxin binding to two other proteins (34 and 31 kDa). Northern blot analysis of interleukin-1 (IL-1) and tumour necrosis factor-α (TNF-α) mRNA expression by Kupffer cells demonstrates that expression of these genes differs from that in murine peritoneal macrophages.

MATERIALS AND METHODS

Animals

Male Sprague Dawley rats weighing 200–250 g or male C57BL/6 mice (10–12 weeks of age; Harlen–Sprague Dawley, Indianapolis, IN) were used in all experiments. Animals were housed in a temperature and light controlled room and allowed standard lab chow and water ad libitum. Germ-free Fisher 344 rats were obtained from the University of Wisconsin Gnotobiotic Lab (Madison WI). Kupffer cells were isolated from these animals immediately upon receipt. Animal protocols for these studies were approved by the animal care committee, New England Deaconess Hospital.

Lipopolysaccharides

Salmonella minnesota LPS, *Escherichia coli* 011B4 LPS, *S. Typhimurium* TB119 (Ra) and *S. minnesota* Re595 LPS were obtained from Sigma Chemical Co (St Louis, MO).

LPS modification and radioiodination

Synthesis of the photoactivatable LPS cross-linker complex was achieved by covalent modification of *E. coli* 0114B4 LPS with sulphosuccinimidyl 2-(p-azidosalicylamido)-1,3′-dithiopropinate (SASD), (Pierce, Rockford, IL) as previously described[16]. SASD–LPS was iodinated by the chloramine T procedure[29]. The mean specific activity for [^{125}I]SASD–LPS was 0.5 μCi/μg. *E. coli* wild type and Re LPS used for ligand blotting was labelled as previously described[11].

Kupffer cell and peritoneal macrophage isolation

Kupffer cells were isolated from fasted rats by collagenase perfusion of the liver. Kupffer cells were purified from the cell suspension by differential centrifugation and metrizamide density gradient centrifugation as previously described[10]. Peritoneal macrophages were elicited in rats or C57BL/6 mice with thioglycolate (4%) and isolated 72h later by lavage of the peritoneum with PBS. Macrophages were purified by adherence to plastic dishes. Identification of macrophages was determined by staining for endogenous peroxidase activity and phagocytosis of 1.0 μm latex beads as described previously[10]. Preparations of hepatic non-parenchymal cells contained >75% Kupffer cells and peritoneal lavage cells contained >85% macrophages by these criteria. Cell viability exceeded 90% as determined by trypan blue staining.

Cross-linking of macrophage populations

Cross-linking of isolated macrophage populations was performed as previously described[17]. Briefly, 10^7 Kupffer cells isolated directly or following overnight culture or rat peritoneal macrophages were reacted with 5 μg of [^{125}I]SASD–LPS at 37°C for 30min in the dark. After cross-linking with short wave UV light for 10min, the cells were washed twice with PBS and reduced in 0.5% SDS, 5% 2-mercaptoethanol, 1mM phenylmethylsulphonyl fluoride (PMSF) and 1 μg/ml leupeptin in Tris-buffered saline; (TBS; pH 7.4). Samples were dialysed extensively against 0.5% SDS in TBS and concentrated by Centricon 3 micro-concentration (Amicon, Danvers, MA). Detergent extracts were analysed on 10% SDS–polyacrylamide gels, stained with Coomassie blue, dried and exposed to X-ray film at −70°C.

Surface labelling of isolated Kupffer cells

Kupffer cells were isolated as described and labelled directly or cultured overnight in RPMI 1640 with 10% fetal calf serum, glutamate and penicillin/streptomycin. Cultured cells were isolated by scraping and washed three times in PBS prior to labelling. Cell surfaces were labelled with 1mCi of Na^{125}I by the lactoperoxidase method. Labelled cells were washed and surface proteins solubilized in 0.5% Triton X-100, 2mM PMSF and 1 μg/ml leupeptin in TBS. The detergent extracts were dialysed extensively against 0.5% Triton X-100 in TBS. Labelled preparations were aliquoted and stored at −70°C.

Preparation of LPS affinity columns

Affinity columns were generated by coupling purified LPS isolated from *S. minnesota* wild type or strain Re595 LPS to cyanogen bromide-activated agarose (Sigma Chemical Corp., St Louis, MO). Briefly the gel was swelled and washed in 1 mM HCl. Following washing in 0.5 M NaCl in 0.1 M bicarbonate buffer (pH 8.3) coupling to the two LPS chemotypes was achieved at 4°C. After incubation, the matrices were washed in the same buffer and then incubated for 2 h in 1 M glycine (pH 8.0). Following incubation, the matrices were washed alternately with 0.1 M acetate buffer (pH 4.0) and 0.1 M borate buffer (pH 8.5). Column matrices were stored in PBS with azide at 4°C.

Isolation of LPS binding proteins by affinity chromatography

Matrices were poured into disposable chromatography columns (Bio-Rad, Richmond, CA) and washed with several vol of PBS followed by 0.5% Triton X-100 in PBS. Approximately 1.5×10^6 cpm of extracted proteins was applied to each column. Void volume was collected as 10 1 ml fraction of 0.5% Triton X-100 in PBS and bound activity was eluted with 10 1 ml fraction of 0.5 M NaCl, 0.5% Triton X-100 in 0.1 M phosphate buffer (pH 7.4. More than 95% of the applied radioactivity could be accounted for in these fractions. Peak activity in the high salt fraction was pooled and dialysed against 0.1% SDS or Triton X-100 in TBS (pH 7.4) and concentrated in Centricon 10 microconcentrators (Amicon, Danvers, MA). Samples were analysed by either 10% SDS–PAGE or two dimensional electrophoresis[30]. The first dimension was an isoelectric focusing tube which resolves proteins in the range of pH 5–8. After equilibration, the IEF gel was applied to a standard 10% SDS–PAGE. Gels were dried and autoradiographed at −70°C.

Ligand blotting with ^{125}I-labelled Re LPS

Isolated Kupffer cells were extracted with 1% SDS, 2 mM PMSF, 1 µg/ml leupeptin and aprotinin in TBS. After centrifugation the extracts were run on 10% SDS–polyacrylamide gels and the separated proteins were electro-phoretically transferred to nitrocellulose membranes. The membranes were blocked with 5% BSA in TBS washed and exposed to ^{125}I-labelled Re LPS (*S. minnesota* Re595) in both the absence and presence of excess (100 µg/ml) unlabelled wild-type or Re LPS. After incubation the membranes were extensively washed in TBS and exposed to X-ray film.

RNA extraction and Northern blot analysis

Isolated Kupffer cells were incubated overnight in RPMI 1640 with 5% fetal calf serum and antibiotics. Murine peritoneal cells were allowed to adhere to culture dishes and non-adherent cells were removed. Both macrophage populations were stimulated with 20 ng/ml *E. coli* 011B4 LPS, *S. typhimurium* TB119 (Ra) and

S. minnesota Re595 LPS for a total of 3.0 h. RNA was isolated by a modified rapid procedure[31]. The cell pellet was solubilized in 8 M guanidine hydrochloride, 1% sarkosyl, 0.3 M sodium acetate (pH 5.2), and 20 mM ribonucleoside vanadyl complexes and centrifuged. RNA was isolated from the supernatant by precipitation with ethanol. Nucleic acids in the pellet were resuspended in 8 M guanidine hydrochloride with 0.3 M sodium acetate (pH 5.2) and reprecipitated with ethanol. RNA in the pellet was quantitated by its absorbance at 260 nm. Isolated RNA (20 μg) was separated in 1.0% agarose gels with 0.66 M formaldehyde and transferred to a nylon membrane (NEN, Boston, MA) by capillary blotting techniques[32]. cDNA probes for the rat glyceraldehyde-3-phosphate dehydrogenase (GAP-DH)[33] and the murine cytokines IL-1α and β[34] were kindly provided by Dr Matthew Fenton, Boston University School of Medicine. cDNA probe fragments were isolated by standard techniques[30] and labelled with [^{32}P]dCTP ($> 10^8$ cpm/μg) by a commercially available random priming procedure (US Biochemical, Cleveland, OH). Blotted macrophage RNA was prehybridized in 50% formamide, 1 M NaCl, 1% SDS and 10% dextran sulphate at 37°C for 6 h when 0.1 mg/ml denatured salmon sperm DNA as well as the denatured labelled cDNA probe (10^6 cpm/ml) were added. Blots were hybridized overnight at 37°C. Hybridized blots were rinsed twice in 0.5% SDS in 2×SSC (0.3 M sodium chloride, 0.3 M sodium citrate) then washed twice at room temperature in 0.5% SDS in 2×SSC and then 0.5% SDS in 0.5×SSC. The final wash was at 37°C in 0.5% SDS in 0.2×SSC. Washed blots were wrapped in Saranwrap and exposed to X-ray film. After autoradiography, the blot was regenerated by repeated washing in boiling 0.1% SDS in 0.1×SSC and reprobed as described. Equal loading of RNA at the beginning of the experiment and the integrity of the blotted RNA after three separate probings was determined by hybridization to the housekeeping gene GAP-DH.

RESULTS

To determine whether endotoxin-specific binding proteins are present on the surface of isolated Kupffer cells we utilized the photoactivatable, iodinatable cross-linker, SASD, covalently bound to LPS. This complex has been used previously to identify an endotoxin-specific 73 kDa protein on the surface of isolated murine spleen cells[17,18] and peritoneal macrophages[19]. Under similar conditions to those described previously[17–19] both rat Kupffer cells and peritoneal macrophages were reacted with the [^{125}I]SASD–LPS complex. Figure 1 shows an autoradiogram of a 10% SDS–PAGE gel comparing cross-linking with SASD–LPS between isolated rat Kupffer cells and peritoneal macrophages. No detectable cross-linking occurred with Kupffer cells while a single protein of approximately 80 kDa was detected on the peritoneal macrophages. Similarly, incubation of Kupffer cells overnight did not result in identification of the 80 kDa protein as determined by photoaffinity labelling. The 80 kDa protein could not be detected on Kupffer cells isolated from germ-free animals. These results suggest that chronic exposure to normal flora endotoxins does not down-regulate expression of the 80 kDa endotoxin-binding protein in the Kupffer cell population. Attempts were also made to isolate this protein from Kupffer cells

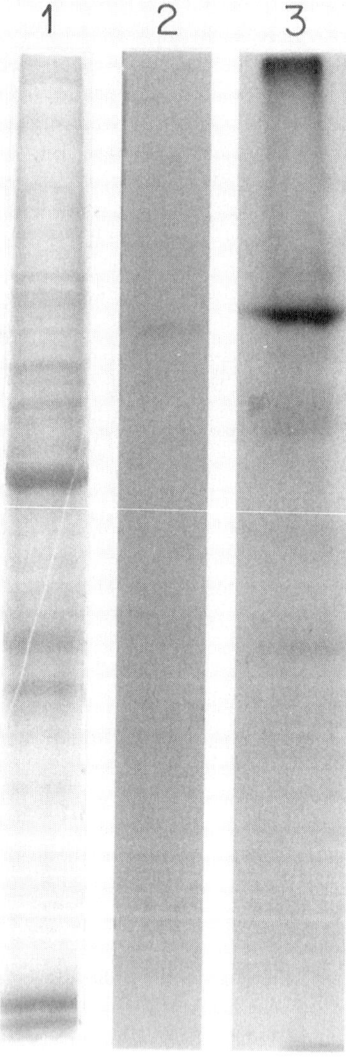

Fig. 1 Cross-linking of isolated rat Kupffer cells and peritoneal macrophages. Kupffer cells and peritoneal macrophages were isolated and cross-linked to [^{125}I]SASD–LPS. After photoactivation and reduction, total cell protein was extracted and separated on 10% SDS–PAGE gels. Lane 1, Coomassie blue stained total Kupffer cell protein. Lane 2, cross-linked Kupffer cells. Lane 3, cross-linked peritoneal macrophages

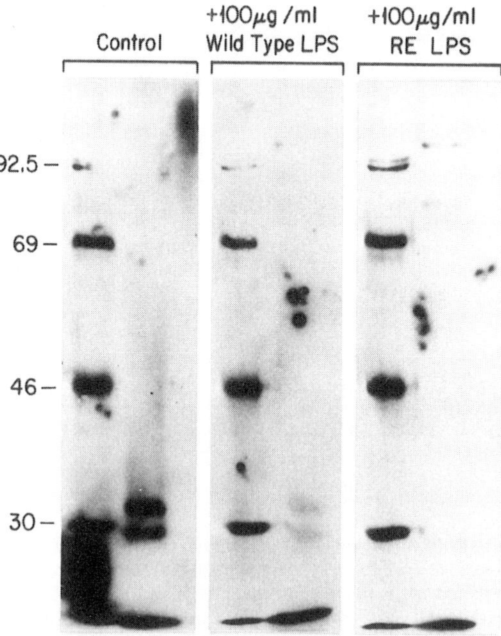

Fig. 2 Ligand blots of SDS extracts of rat Kupffer cells. Membranes were blotted with ^{125}I-Re LPS. Blot 1: Control, no additions. Blot 2: As blot 1, but blotting carried out in the presence of excess unlabelled wild-type LPS (100 μg/ml). Blot 3: As blot 1, but blotting carried out in the presence of excess unlabelled Re LPS (100 μg/ml). In each blot lane 1 contains MW standards, lane 2 Kupffer cell extracts

by affinity chromatography. A single protein band was seen on 10% SDS–PAGE; however, when repeated samples were applied to a two-dimensional gel this signal had an isoelectric point and molecular weight characteristic of albumin and probably resulted from non-specific binding of LPS to albumin absorbed to the Kupffer cell surface after culture. No difference was detected in cells which were labelled directly or incubated overnight except for this albumin species. Thus we were unable to detect the putative endotoxin receptor on Kupffer cells under conditions which detected its presence on peritoneal macrophages. However, preliminary data using a ligand blotting technique on Western blots of Kupffer cell detergent extracts showed two putative endotoxin binding proteins of 34 and 31 kDa (Fig. 2). The blotting with ^{125}I-labelled LPS could be totally inhibited by the presence of excess wild-type or Re endotoxin (see Fig. 2). These proteins were only detected in SDS extracts and were absent, for example, when the cells were extracted with octylglucoside (data not shown). This suggests that these proteins are either internal or transmembrane proteins that have a cytoplasmic domain. It is possible, therefore that one of these proteins may be involved in the cytokine response to LPS in Kupffer cells[35].

Lipopolysaccharides isolated from mutant bacterial strains have also been used to activate peritoneal macrophages isolated from normally endotoxin-

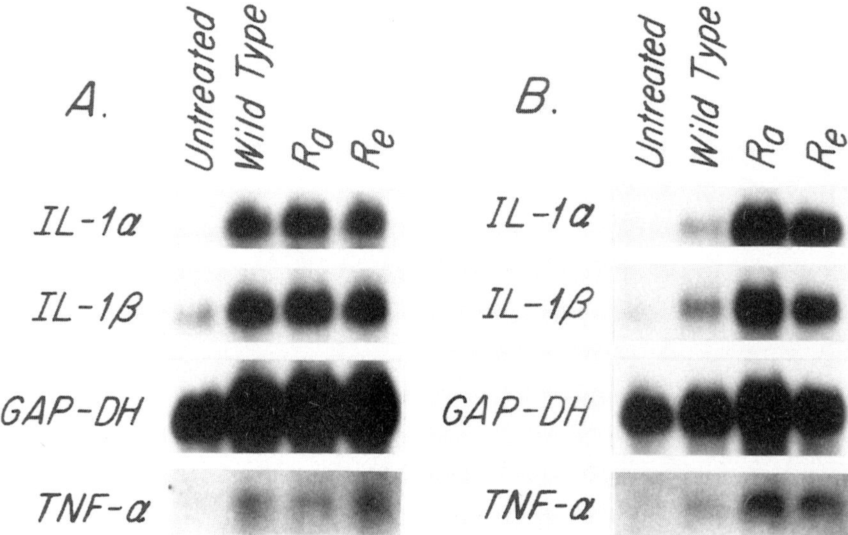

Fig. 3 IL-1 expression following activation of rat Kupffer cells and murine peritoneal macrophages by wild-type and rough strain LPS. RNA was isolated from Kupffer cells (**A**) or peritoneal macrophages (**B**) treated with 20 ng/ml of wild-type or rough strain LPS. 20 μg total RNA was probed for expression of IL-1α, IL-1β, TNF-α and GAP-DH by northern blot analysis

resistant mice[36]. The presence of the putative endotoxin receptor on splenocytes isolated from both responder and non-responder mice has also been shown[18]. We therefore investigated the response of the Kupffer cell, a macrophage population which lacks this protein, to these mutant forms of LPS. Endotoxin stimulation of macrophage populations, amongst many other changes, results in the production of the cytokine IL-1. Isolated rat Kupffer cells or murine peritoneal macrophages were stimulated with 20 ng/ml of *E. coli* 011B4 wild-type LPS or equivalent amounts of the Ra and Re chemotypes. After 3 h of stimulation the cells were harvested and total RNA was isolated. Relative induction of the IL-1α and β genes was determined by Northern blot analysis. As shown in Figure 3A Kupffer cells express IL-1β mRNA constitutively. Both IL-1 genes were up-regulated by stimulation with all three forms of LPS. Densitometric scanning did not reveal any difference in signal strength among treated cells. However, unlike Kupffer cells, murine peritoneal macrophages did not express these genes without prior stimulation and responded differentially to the lipid-rich rough strains (Fig. 3B). Similar responses to LPS stimulation were seen with TNF-α mRNA (Figs 3A,B). Densitometric scanning of stimulated peritoneal macrophages when adjusted for even loading based on GAP-DH results, revealed a 6-fold difference in stimulation with the rough strain LPS versus the wild-type.

DISCUSSION

Lipopolysaccharide activation of peritoneal macrophages to kill tumour cells and an associated TNF release is mediated through a 73 kDa surface protein[21]. A similar protein has been detected on splenocytes isolated from endotoxin responding and non-responding mice[17] and monocytes from endotoxin-sensitive species[20]. Using a similar labelling protocol we were unable to detect this protein on Kupffer cell plasma membranes, while it could be clearly identified on peritoneal macrophages isolated from the same animals. Furthermore, this protein could not be isolated from Kupffer cells by affinity chromatography on LPS–Sepharose columns. Due to its orientation in the portal sinusoids, the Kupffer cell is chronically exposed to gut-derived endotoxins. It is possible that this chronic exposure to endotoxin may down-regulate expression of this putative receptor. For example, multiple exposure of macrophages to LPS leads to internalization and sequestration of the receptor for TNF[37]. However, experiments with Kupffer cells isolated from germ-free rats also failed to detect the presence of this 80 kDa receptor or any other potential binding protein. This absence of specific binding proteins cannot be due to down regulation by the chronic endotoxaemia of the portal vein in the normal animal and is not an adaptation to environmental exposure. These data suggest that signals derived from endotoxin activation are mediated differently in the Kupffer cell. In support of this idea, endotoxin activation of isolated Kupffer cells leads to different levels of endotoxin responsive gene induction to those in similarly treated inflammatory peritoneal macrophages.

In vitro, LPS stimulation of Kupffer cells can lead to the production of IL-1[38], IL-6[39,40] and tumor necrosis factor[41] as well as a multitude of other peptide and non-protein mediators. The byproducts of Kupffer cell activation have been the subject of a recent review[1]. The molecular basis and the time course of expression of these particular cytokines by Kupffer cells is unknown. Northern blot analysis of stimulated and unstimulated rat Kupffer cells (Fig. 3A) demonstrate that these cells constitutively express mRNA for IL-1α and β. The positioning of the Kupffer cell in the liver leads to a chronic exposure to gut-derived endotoxins and other gut-derived antigens. This exposure may account for this low state of activation. Repeated exposure of other monocytic cells to endotoxin stimulation leads to a state of hyporesponsiveness. A recent study in RAW 264.7 cells has suggested that the initial exposure to LPS is the source of the hyporesponsiveness to subsequent stimulation regardless of LPS concentration[42]. Thus the presence of these mRNAs is not consistent with studies of other monocytes[43–45]. Stimulation of Kupffer cells with different chemical forms of LPS leads to similar levels of gene induction. This is different to that seen with inflammatory peritoneal macrophages (Fig. 3B). The level of IL-1 mRNA is considerably greater when peritoneal macrophages are stimulated with rough strain LPS than when stimulated with a similar amount of wild-type LPS. This is consistent with a previous report which studied tumour necrosis factor release[33].

Previous studies have suggested that Kupffer cells have a much greater capacity for uptake and processing of endotoxins than other macrophages. It is likely that most endotoxin is taken up by non-specific pinocytosis, where the lipid A component inserts into the plasma membrane and is internalized when the membrane pinches off[11]. A receptor capable of transducing a signal that results in a cytokine response in these cells has so far not been identified. We have provided evidence that the putative endotoxin receptor on Kupffer cells is not the 73 kDa protein previously identified on other macrophages and monocytes[19,20] as this protein seems to be absent from Kupffer cells. We have, however, identified two major endotoxin binding proteins (34 kDa, 31 kDa) by ligand blotting that may serve as the receptor for the cytokine response. Studies are continuing to determine whether these proteins are indeed involved in this process.

These results suggest the presence of a regulatory mechanism which controls the degree of the Kupffer cell response to the chronic stimulus of gut-derived endotoxin. This relative hyporesponsiveness to LPS may be a component of a tolerance mechanism to gut-derived endotoxin and other immunoreactive antigens. Previous studies of the steady-state TNF mRNA level and TNF secretion in the RAW 264.7 cell line have shown that a secondary challenge with LPS leads to no change in either the steady-state mRNA level or TNF activity in the supernatant[39]. Similar hyporesponsiveness has been observed in peritoneal macrophages in terms of release of TNF and procoagulant activity[42]. These studies suggest that macrophages may be responsible for induction and prolongation of the tolerant state. Kupffer cells, the largest pool of macrophages in the body, are chronically endotoxin stimulated and have a constitutive level of IL-1 mRNA yet respond differently to LPS stimulation than do inflammatory peritoneal macrophages. These results may illustrate mechanisms designed to regulate Kupffer cell immune responsiveness in the face of chronic gut-derived stimulatory signals.

ACKNOWLEDGEMENTS

Supported by grants CA44583 from the National Cancer Institute and DK44305 from the National Institute of Diabetes and Digestive and Kidney Diseases. Its contents are solely the responsibility of the authors and do not necessarily represent the official views of the above institutes.

References

1. Decker K. Biologically active products of stimulated liver macrophages (Kupffer cells). Eur J Biochem. 1990;192:245–61.
2. Gale RP, Sparkes RS, Golde DW. Bone marrow origin of hepatic macrophages (Kupffer cells). Science. 1978;201:937–8.
3. Diesselhoff-den Dulk MMC, Crofton RW, van Furth R. Origin and kinetics of Kupffer cells during an acute inflammatory response. Immunology. 1979;37:7–14.
4. Whitworth PW, Pak CC, Esgro J, Kleinerman ES, Fidler IJ. Macrophages and cancer. Cancer Metastasis Rev. 1990;8:319–51.
5. Cohen SA, Salazar D, Nolan JP. Natural cytotoxicity of isolated rat liver cells. J Immunol. 1982;129:495–51.
6. Ravin HA, Rowley D, Jenkins C, Fine J. On the absorption of bacterial endotoxin from the gastrointestinal tract of the normal and shocked animal. J Exp Med. 1960;112:783–92.
7. Farrar WE, Corwin LM. The essential role of liver in detoxification of endotoxin. Ann NY Acad Sci. 1966;133:668–84.
8. Freudenberg MA, Freudenberg N, Galanos C. Time course of cellular distribution of endotoxin in liver, lung and kidney of rats. Br J Exp Pathol. 1982;63:56–64.
9. Praaning van-Dalen DP, Brouwer A, Knook DL. Clearance capacity of rat liver Kupffer, endothelial and parenchymal cells. Gastroenterology. 1981;81:1036–44.

10. Knack A, Take S, Ace M et al. The fate of intravenously injected endotoxin in normal rats and in rats with liver failure. Hepatology. 1994;19:1251–6.
11. Fox ES, Thomas P, Broitman SA. Comparative studies of endotoxin uptake by isolated rat Kupffer and peritoneal cells. Infect Immun. 1987;55:2962–6.
12. Heffner-Cavaillon N, Chaby R, Cavaillon JM, Szabo L. Lipopolysaccharide receptor on rabbit peritoneal macrophages: binding characteristics. J Immunol. 1982;128:1950–4.
13. Fox ES, Thomas P, Broitman SA. Clearance of gut derived endotoxins by the liver. Release and modification of ^{3}H,^{14}C-lipopolysaccharide by isolated rat Kupffer cells. Gastroenterology. 1989;96:456–61.
14. Munford RS, Hall RL. Uptake and deacylation of bacterial lipopolysaccharide from normal and endotoxin hyporesponsive mice. Infect Immun. 1985;48:464–73.
15. Fukuda I, Tanamoto K, Kanegasaki S, Yajima Y, Goto Y. Deacylation of bacterial lipopolysaccharide by rat hepatocytes in vitro. Br J Exp Pathol. 1989;70:267–74.
16. Fox ES, Thomas P, Broitman SA. Lipopolysaccharide processing by Kupffer cells releases a modified LPS with increased hepatocyte binding and decreased tumor necrosis factor-α stimulatory capacity. Proc Soc Exp Biol Med. 1993;102:153–8.
17. Treon SP, Thomas P, Broitman SA. Lipopolysaccharide processing by Kupffer cells releases a modified LPS with increased hepatocyte binding and decreased tumor necrosis factor-α stimulatory capacity. Proc Soc Exp Biol Med. 1993;202:153–8.
18. Wollenwber HW, Morrison DC. Synthesis and biochemical characterization of a photoactivatable, iodinatable, cleavage bacterial lipopolysaccharide derivative. J Biol Chem. 1985;260:15068–74.
19. Lei MG, Morrison DC. Specific endotoxic lipopolysaccharide binding protein on murine splenocytes. I. Detection of lipopolysaccharide binding sites on splenocytes and splenocyte subpopulation. J Immunol. 1988;141:996–1005.
20. Lei MG, Morrison DC. Specific endotoxic lipopolysaccharide binding protein on murine splenocytes. II. Membrane localization and binding characteristics. J Immunol. 1988;141:1006–11.
21. Hunt JS, Soares MJ, Lei MG. Products of lipopolysaccharide activated macrophages (tumor necrosis factor-α, transforming growth factor-β) but not lipopolysaccharide modify DNA synthesis by rat trophoblast cells exhibiting the 80 kDa lipopolysaccharide binding protein. J Immunol. 1989;143:1606–13.
22. Roeder DJ, Lei MG, Morrison DC. Endotoxic-lipopolysaccharide-specific binding proteins on lymphoid cells of various animal species: association with endotoxin susceptibility. Infect Immun. 1989;57:1054–58.
23. Chen TY, Bright SW, Pace JL, Russell SW, Morrison DC. Induction of macrophage mediated tumor cytotoxicity by a hamster monoclonal antibody with specificity for lipopolysaccharide receptor. J Immunol. 1990;145:8–12.
24. Hara-Kuge S, Amano F, Nishijima M, Akamatsu Y. Isolation of a lipopolysaccharide (LPS) resistant mutant, with defective LPS binding, of cultured macrophage like cells. J Biol Chem. 1990;265:6606–10.
25. Wright SD, Jong MTC. Adhesion-promoting receptor on human macrophages recognize *E. coli* binding to lipopolysaccharide. J Exp Med. 1986;164:1876–88.
26. Wright SD, Detmers PA, Aida Y et al. CD18-deficient cells respond to lipopolysaccharide in vitro. J Immunol. 1990;144:2566–71.
27. Hampton RY, Golenbock DT, Raetz CRH. Lipid A binding sites in membranes of macrophage tumor cells. J Biol Chem. 1988;263:14802–7.
28. Golenback DT, Hampton RY, Raetz CRH, Wright SD. Human phagocytes have multiple lipid A-binding sites. Infect Immun. 1990;58:4069–75.
29. Greenwood F, Hunter W, Glover J. The preparation of ^{125}I-labeled human growth hormone of high specific activity. Biochem J. 1963;58:114–29.
30. Dunbar BS. Two dimensional electrophoresis and immunological techniques. Plenum Press, New York. 1987.
31. Fox ES, Thomas P. Modification of the rapid method of Evans and Kamdar for application to isolation of mRNA from Kupffer cells. Biotechniques. 1991;10:182–4.
32. Sambrook J, Fritsch EF, Maniatis T. Molecular cloning. A laboratory manual. 2nd Edn. Cold Spring Harbor: Cold Spring Harbor Laboratory. 1989.
33. Fort PH, Marty L, Piechacyk M et al. Various rat adult tissues express only one major mRNA species from the glyceraldehyde-3-phosphate dehydrogenase multigenic family. Nucleic Acids Res. 1985;13:1431–42.

34. Gray PW, Glaister D, Chen E, Goeddel DV, Pennica D. Two interleukin 1 genes in the mouse: Cloning and expression of the cDNA for murine interleukin 1β. J Immunol. 1986;137:3644–8.
35. Fox ES, Broitman SA, Thomas P. Identification of lipopolysaccharide binding proteins on isolated rat Kupffer cells. Hepatology. 1991;14:126A.
36. Flebbe LM, Chapes SK, Morrison DC. Activation of C3H/HeJ macrophage tumoricidal activity and cytokine release by R-chemotype lipopolysaccharide preparations. J Immunol. 1990;145:1505–11.
37. Ding AH, Sanchez S, Srimal S, Nathan CF. Macrophages rapidly internalize their tumor necrosis factor receptors in response to bacterial lipopolysaccharide. J Biol Chem. 1989;264:3924–9.
38. Shirahama M, Ishibashi H, Tsuchiya Y et al. Kupffer cells may autoregulate interleukin 1 production by producing interleukin 1 inhibitor and prostaglandin E_2. Scand J Immunol. 1988;28:719–25.
39. Bauer J, Birmelin M, Northoff G-H et al. Induction of rat α_2-macroglobulin in vivo and in hepatocyte primary cultures: synergistic action of glucocorticoids and a Kupffer cell-derived factor. FEBS Lett. 1984;177:89–94.
40. Busam KJ, Homfeld A, Zawatzky R et al. Virus- vs endotoxin-induced activation of liver macrophages. Eur J Biochem. 1990;191:577–82.
41. Karck U, Peters T, Decker K. The release of tumor necrosis factor from endotoxin stimulated rat Kupffer cells is regulated by prostaglandin E2 and dexamethasone. J Hepatol. 1988;7:352–61.
42. Virca GD, Kim SY, Glaser KB, Ulevitch RJ. Lipopolysaccharide induces hyporesponsiveness to its own action in RAW 264.7 cells. J Biol Chem. 1989;264:21951–6.
43. Fenton MA, Clark BD, Collins KL, Webb AC, Rich A, Auron PE. Transcriptional regulation of the human prointerleukin 1β gene. J Immunol. 1987;138:3972–9.
44. Fenton MJ, Vermeulen MW, Clark BD, Webb AC, Auron PE. Human pro-IL-1β gene expression in monocytic cells is regulated by two distinct pathways. J Immunol. 1988;140:2267–73.
45. Haslberger A, Sayers T, Reiter H, Chung J, Schutze E. Reduced release of TNF and PCA from macrophages of tolerant mice. Circ Shock. 1988;26:185–92.

11
Cytokines in alcoholic liver cirrhosis

J. DÉVIÈRE, O. LE MOINE, M. GOLDMAN and E. DUPONT

INTRODUCTION

Cytokines are polypeptides involved in cell to cell communication via specific membrane receptors. Some act as proinflammatory or growth factors while others have immunosuppressive and antiinflammatory properties[1]. These substances are produced by a variety of cells. Among them, of particular relevance to alcoholic liver disease, are endothelial cells, hepatocytes, Ito cells, Kupffer cells and peripheral blood mononuclear cells (PBMC). Cytokines are produced in response to a variety of stimuli, of which endotoxin (LPS) is the most frequently used in experimental studies. Endotoxin is also involved in many models of liver injury[2–4], acting synergistically with various hepatotoxins.

Interleukin (IL)-1, tumour necrosis factor-α (TNF-α), IL-6 and IL-8 have many overlapping biologic activities[5]. They often act synergistically to produce their physiological or pathological effects and can stimulate one another. Their biological effects help explain well known manifestations of alcoholic liver cirrhosis (ALC) or hepatitis, including anorexia, muscle wasting, fever, hypotension, stimulation of the acute phase reaction, neutrophilia, decreased albumin synthesis, increased triglyceride levels and collagen synthesis[1,6]. IL-10 has recently emerged as a potent anti-inflammatory cytokine mainly produced by monomacrophagic, T and B cells. A main effect of IL-10 on monomacrophagic cells is strong inhibition of proinflammatory cytokine (IL-1, IL-6, IL-8 and TNF-α) synthesis after LPS stimulation at both mRNA and protein levels. IL-10 may therefore counterbalance the inflammatory processes[7].

The present review will focus on disturbances of cytokine synthesis, at the peripheral level. These can potentially explain the clinical complications of ALC and the mechanisms of alcohol-induced hepatic injury. Cytokine measurement for diagnostic purposes in humans and the potential development of 'anticytokine' therapy will also be discussed.

ALTERATIONS OF CYTOKINE PRODUCTION IN ALCOHOLIC LIVER DISEASE

Interleukin 1, tumour necrosis factor and interleukin 6

Besides their implication in T and B cell activation, these monokines might play some role in the development of hepatotoxicity, liver fibrosis and immune abnormalities associated with ALC such as hypergammaglobulinaemia. IL-1, known as 'endogenous pyrogen', induces collagen secretion by fibroblasts and has major effects on vascular endothelium, including expression of adhesion molecules and increased endothelial cell permeability[8]. Moreover, it acts as a potent inducer of other cytokines such as TNF-α, IL-6 and IL-8. TNF-α has cytopathic and cytotoxic properties[9] and is one of the major mediators implicated in septic shock manifestations, and in the development of experimental liver injury induced by galactosamine injection, reperfusion injury, CCl_4, alcohol, concanavalin A, liver transplantation and *Corynebacterium parvum* infection[2–4,10–12]. A recent review by McClain[12] emphasized the concepts of sensitization and priming as important factors in understanding TNF-α mediated liver injury. Sensitization is the mechanism by which the hepatocyte is made hypersensitive to normally inocuous amounts of TNF-α: a classic model is liver injury induced by galactosamine[3]. The latter inhibits hepatic uridine synthesis (and ultimately blocks RNA production), a mechanism by which the liver is made sensitive to very low doses of LPS. After priming, monocytes of Kupffer cells, when stimulated, are capable of secreting massive amounts of TNF-α, potentiating hepatocyte injury. The classic animal model of priming is that of *Corynebacterium parvum* infection[10]. This microorganism induces massive liver infiltration by primed mononuclear cells. In this condition, injection of a normally inocuous amount of endotoxin leads to massive TNF-α release with consequent fulminant liver injury. In both models, anti-TNF-α antibodies block or attenuate liver injury[10,13]. IL-6 plays a pivotal role in the terminal differentiation of B lymphocytes and their maturation to immunoglobulin (Ig)-secreting plasma cells. Its essential role in the development of hypergammaglobulinaemia has been demonstrated in numerous human diseases[14,15]. IL-6, or hepatocyte stimulating factor, is the major inducer of acute phase proteins secretion by hepatocytes[16]. It also stimulates collagen secretion by activated Ito cells and is involved in the development of liver fibrosis in experimental animals[17].

The first cytokine whose biological activity was shown to be increased in the serum of patients with ALC was IL-1[18]. However, the thymocyte proliferation assay used at that time was subsequently demonstrated to detect IL-6 as well[19]. In vitro, secretion of IL-1 by PBMC from cirrhotics and challenged with LPS was shown to be elevated using more specific assays[20]. Circulating IL-1 was not consistently found in ALC patients' sera, except in some cases of severe alcoholic hepatitis[21,22]. However, IL-1 measurement is hampered by the presence of multiple IL-1 inhibitors in this condition. Increased production of IL-1 in ALC could participate in T lymphocyte activation reported in this disease, as evidenced by the presence of in vivo activation markers on T lymphocytes[23]. The interest of investigators was next focused on TNF-α and IL-6, whose synthesis and secretion by monocytes was shown to be increased in ALC both in the basal state and after LPS stimulation[24,25]. Further investigations demonstrated that basal overproduction, when present, was very limited if extensive precautions were taken to avoid contamination with endotoxin during manipulations[20]. The major finding is LPS-induced TNF-α and IL-6 overproduction which is reversible when cells are allowed to rest in vitro for one day before stimulation[20]. This suggests that monocytes from ALC patients are primed for TNF-α and IL-6 secretion in vivo. The priming factor remains to be determined. Monomacrophage responsiveness to LPS can be modulated by interferon-γ (IFNγ), the principal macrophage activating factor[26,27]. Lined hepatic sinusoidal IgAs might also be potent priming factors for TNF-α release after endotoxin challenge[28]. On the other hand, a defective anti-inflammatory response (i.e. IL-10 synthesis) could be implicated in TNF-α overproduction[29,30]. Increased circulating TNF-α and IL-6 levels are also found in ALC[20–22,31–34]. The increase is moderate in compensated cirrhosis and greater in alcoholic hepatitis. In the latter, persistently elevated TNF-α serum levels correlate with a poor prognosis[22,31,33]. Increased IL-6 activity has also been found in alcoholic hepatitis and correlates with clinical outcome, bilirubin levels and markers of hepatic acute phase response[34]. Even if it is clear that patients with ALC have increased plasma and monocyte IL-1, IL-6 and TNF activity, the exact relationship to ethanol remains unclear. Chronic endotoxin exposure related to an ethanol-induced increase in gut permeability might act as a continuous stimulus. However, endotoxaemia, even when measured in the portal vein, is very limited and cannot account for monocyte priming[35–38]. In vitro, ethanol inhibits TNF-α secretion in a dose-dependent fashion[39]. In animal studies, acute alcohol intoxication inhibits LPS-induced TNF-α production while chronic alcohol administration enhances this process[40]. This suggests a chronic and indirect phenomenon, possibly related to alcohol induced glutathione (GSH) depletion, thus decreasing a potential TNF-α inhibitor[41,42].

Interleukin 8

IL-8 (neutrophil activating peptide) is secreted by a variety of immune and non-immune cells, including hepatocytes[43]. It stimulates neutrophil chemotaxis, adherence, degranulation and tissue invasion. The major stimuli for IL-8 secretion are endotoxin, IL-1 and TNF-α. Studies on IL-8 in alcoholic hepatitis were prompted by the clinical observation of characteristic neutrophilia and liver infiltration by polymorphonuclear cells (PMN) in this disease. Dramatically increased IL-8 serum levels were found in patients with alcoholic hepatitis when compared with normal controls or patients with 'inactive' alcoholic cirrhosis and liver injury of other aetiologies[44,45]. Quantification in liver biopsies confirmed that IL-8 is produced locally and serial measurements showed that decreased serum levels correlated with clinical improvement. Moreover, in both studies, moderate increases of serum levels were found in active alcoholics without liver disease, suggesting that ethanol can trigger a mechanism stimulating IL-8 production.

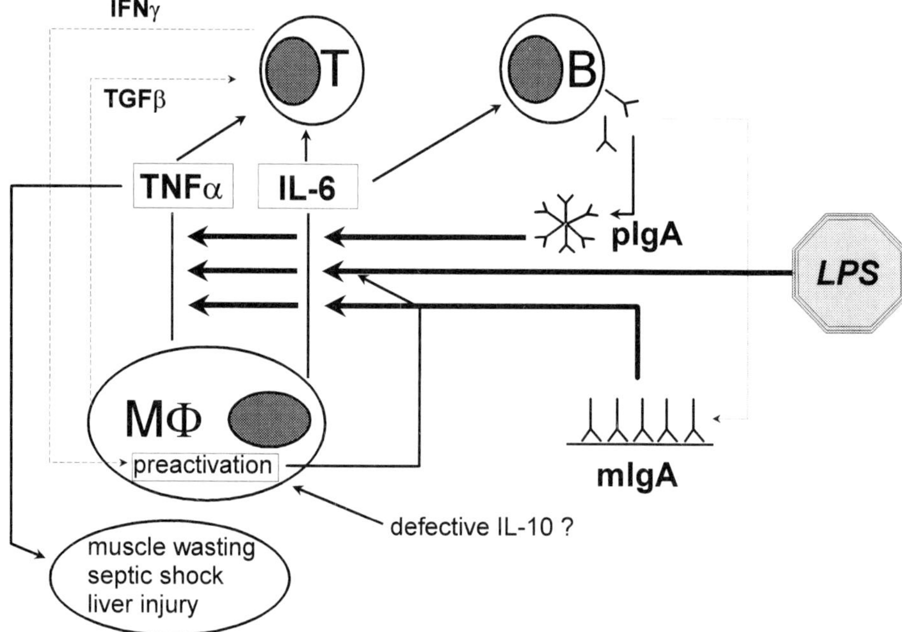

Fig. 1 Summary of immune disturbances affecting the monocytes (M) in ALC. T = T lymphocyte; B = B lymphocyte

Interleukin 10

IL-10 is a cytokine which plays a major role in the regulation of inflammatory processes and in tolerogenesis. It is a potent inhibitor of monocyte pro-inflammatory cytokine secretion[7,29] and has a major regulatory role in TNF-α synthesis, as illustrated by the enhancement of in vivo and in vitro TNF-α production by anti-IL-10 monoclonal antibodies[46,47]. TNF-α induces IL-10 mRNA and protein synthesis in vitro, a phenomenon further enhanced by LPS[7]. In animals, IL-10 pretreatment was shown to reduce TNF-α release and prevent lethality of experimental septic shock[47]. This effect remains obvious when IL-10 treatment is delayed for 1 h after LPS injection[48]. IL-10 production can be modulated by cyclosporin[49] or chlorpromazin[50] and this could explain many effects of these drugs. In humans, elevated circulating levels of IL-10 have been demonstrated in sepsis[51], after OKT3 treatment or, most dramatically, after unclamping the portal vein in the course of liver transplantation[52]. In the latter case, local production by the grafted liver has been demonstrated. Recent data from our laboratory suggest defective monocyte IL-10 secretion in ALC; this could be involved in the increased production of proinflammatory cytokines after LPS stimulation (Le Moine et al., submitted).

Briefly, it is well established that monomacrophages from ALC patients produce higher amounts of proinflammatory cytokines after stimulation (Fig. 1). These cytokines (particularly TNF-α) are involved in many models of experimental liver injury. Both increased synthesis and decreased catabolism (at the hepatocyte level) contribute to elevated circulating levels. These proinflammatory cytokines certainly explain many complications of alcoholic cirrhosis, including cachexia, muscle wasting and ascites. It also seems highly probable that they play a major role in the development of liver injury. Increased, though less pronounced, serum or monocyte cytokine activity has also been observed in other types of liver disease. Of all cytokine disturbances, probably only those concerning IL-8 are specific to ALC. This brings us to focus on a more specific, ALC related immune disturbance, namely alterations of the IgA system and their relationship to monocyte activation.

IMMUNOGLOBULIN A AND CYTOKINES IN ALCOHOLIC LIVER DISEASE

Disturbances of IgA metabolism are so characteristic of ALC that the disease has been suggested to be IgA related[53–57]. Elevation of serum IgA levels have been reported in both alcoholic and non-alcoholic liver disease but are much more pronounced in the former[56]. Serum IgA levels are increased in early alcoholic liver damage, long before cirrhosis is apparent[55–57]. Factors involved in this elevation of serum Iga levels include reduction of polymeric IgA catabolism[54], and increased IgA producing capacity by B lymphocytes (see ref. 57 for review). Of particular interest is the finding that monomeric (m)IgA$_1$ is frequently observed along the sinusoids of patients with ALC and those with steatosis, before the development of overt fibrosis[55,56]. Lined IgAs on the surface of hepatocytes, Kupffer cells and endothelial cells have been reported as possible markers of progression of fatty liver to cirrhosis and they are possible co-factors mediating liver injury[53,57]. We have studied the effect of different IgA forms on monocytes by culturing cells either in the presence of monomeric, soluble IgA1 (msIgA), polymeric soluble IgA1 (psIgA) or monomeric IgA1 coated on the culture plates (mcIgA). The two latter situations are those in which IgA attachment to Fcα receptors might induce FCαR cross-linking. In these conditions, both pIgA and coated mIgA are capable of inducing IL-6 and TNF-α secretion by monocytes[28,58]. Coated mIgA and LPS also act synergistically to induce TNF-α secretion in normal cells and cells from individuals with alcoholic cirrhosis (Fig. 2). Coated mIgA could be considered the in vitro correlate of sinusoidal IgA deposits present in ALC. Release of TNF-α by monocytes might be the mechanism by which IgA contributes to the pathogenesis of ALC. In addition, since IL-6 stimulates IgA production, IgA-induced IL-6 secretion by monocytes may initiate a positive feedback loop, further enhancing IgA synthesis and promoting development of polyclonal hypergammaglobulinaemia. Further investigations are necessary to determine which alcohol-related mechanisms provoke IgA1 attachment to the hepatocyte surface in liver sinusoids.

USE OF CYTOKINE MEASUREMENT AS A DIAGNOSTIC MARKER IN SEPTIC COMPLICATIONS OF LIVER CIRRHOSIS

Bacterial infections occur as a life-threatening complication in 25–50% of cirrhotic patients and have a high morbidity and mortality[59]. Cirrhotic patients

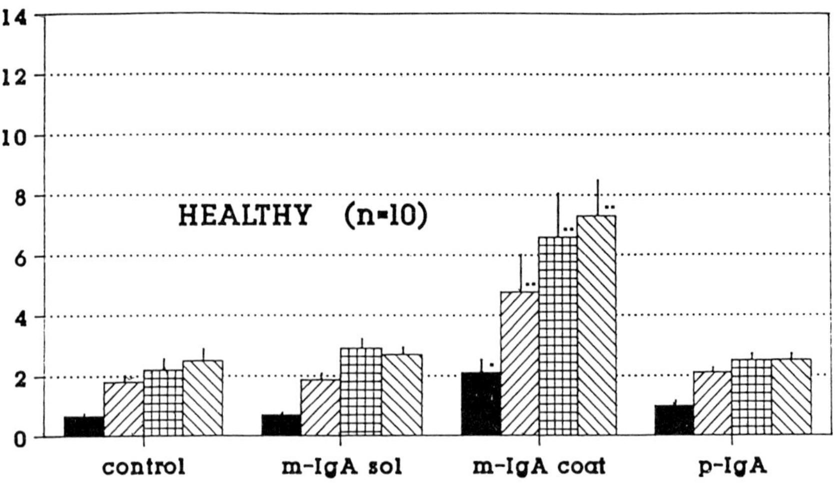

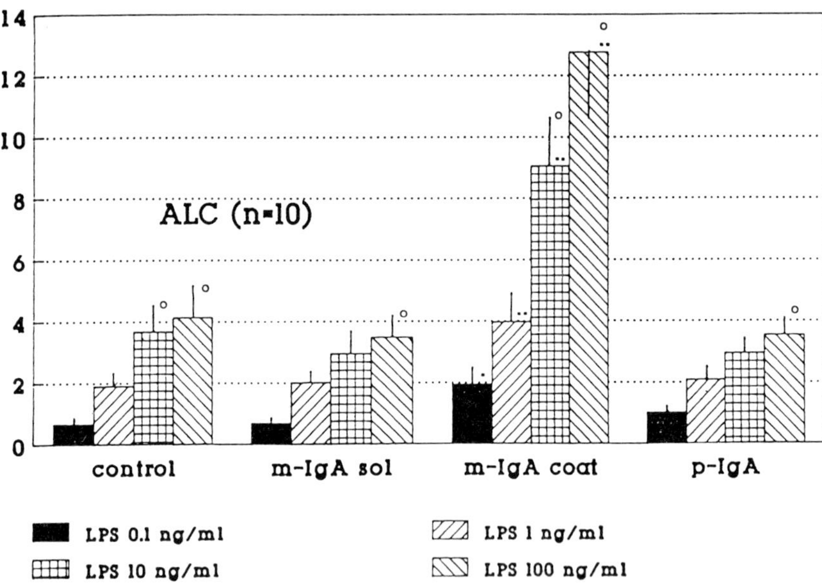

Fig. 2 TNF-α secretion (mean±SEM) by PBMC of healthy subjects or alcoholic liver cirrhosis (ALC) patients cultured for 24h with LPS concentrations varying from 0.1 to 100ng/ml in the presence of various forms of IgA. °$p < 0.05$ between healthy subjects and alcoholic cirrhotics; ·$p < 0.01$ and ··$p < 0.001$ between TNF-α secretion in the presence of m-IgA and under control conditions with the corresponding LPS concentration (from Ref. 28)

with septicaemia have circulating levels of TNF-α and IL-6 5 – 10 times higher than septic patients without underlying liver disease[60]. This probably reflects increased production and decreased catabolism of these cytokines. While peak TNF-α levels are transient and return to normal within 6 – 12 h in patients with normal liver function, levels are sustained for several days in patients with cirrhosis[60]. These observations, in addition to the increased mortality associated with sepsis in cirrhosis, make these patients a unique population in which to assess the efficacy of anti-TNF-α antibodies and TNF-α-inhibiting cytokines such as IL-10 in reducing mortality and/or morbidity. Trials using anti-TNF-α antibodies in the management of septic shock have been disappointing as TNF-α peak levels are transient, and antibodies were usually given when levels of TNF-α in the serum had returned to normal[61]. Ascites, jaundice and encephalopathy are common clinical features of decompensation in cirrhosis, whatever its cause: variceal haemorrhage, bacterial infection, alcoholic hepatitis or the development of a hepatocarcinoma. The diagnosis of infection at presentation is difficult as clinical or biological features such as fever are often absent in cirrhosis[59]. Treatment may therefore be delayed pending the results of bacterial cultures. An early, sensitive and specific marker of infection could improve the diagnosis and management of these patients. IL-6 and TNF-α produced during infection are major hepatocyte stimulating factors, contributing to the acute phase response. Their plasma levels are exquisitely sensitive to infection in cirrhotics while acute phase protein secretion is defective in this setting, related to hepatocellular insufficiency. A recent prospective study analysed the sensitivity and specificity of early clinical or biological signs of bacterial infections (including IL-6 and TNF-α levels) in 57 patients presenting with decompensated cirrhosis[62]. Bacterial screening demonstrated infection in one third of the study population. Fever, polymorphonuclear cell count, fibrinogen or C-reactive protein levels were found to be of no or little benefit in the diagnosis of bacterial infection on admission. IL-6 was the most sensitive parameter to differentiate infected from non-infected patients. At cut-off value of 200 pg/ml, sensitivity and specificity were 100% and 74%, respectively. Given that rapid immunoenzymatic tests will soon become available, IL-6 measurement could become an important part of the diagnostic armamentarium in this condition (Fig. 3).

PROSPECTS FOR 'CYTOKINE-RELATED' THERAPY IN ALCOHOLIC LIVER DISEASE

One may question whether a better knowledge of cytokine-related mechanisms would help predict the development of liver disease or improve its treatment. At present, preventive treatment is limited by our inability to recognize which alcoholic patients will progress to cirrhosis. Once the disease is established, our incomplete knowledge of its pathogenesis impairs assessment of treatment efficacy. Most current therapies influence cytokine metabolism. Glucocorticoids are potent inhibitors of proinflammatory cytokine production[63], while colchicin also inhibits cytokine production, and protects against TNF-α toxicity in vivo[64]. Drugs and foods that maintain gut integrity, can improve glutathione stores and

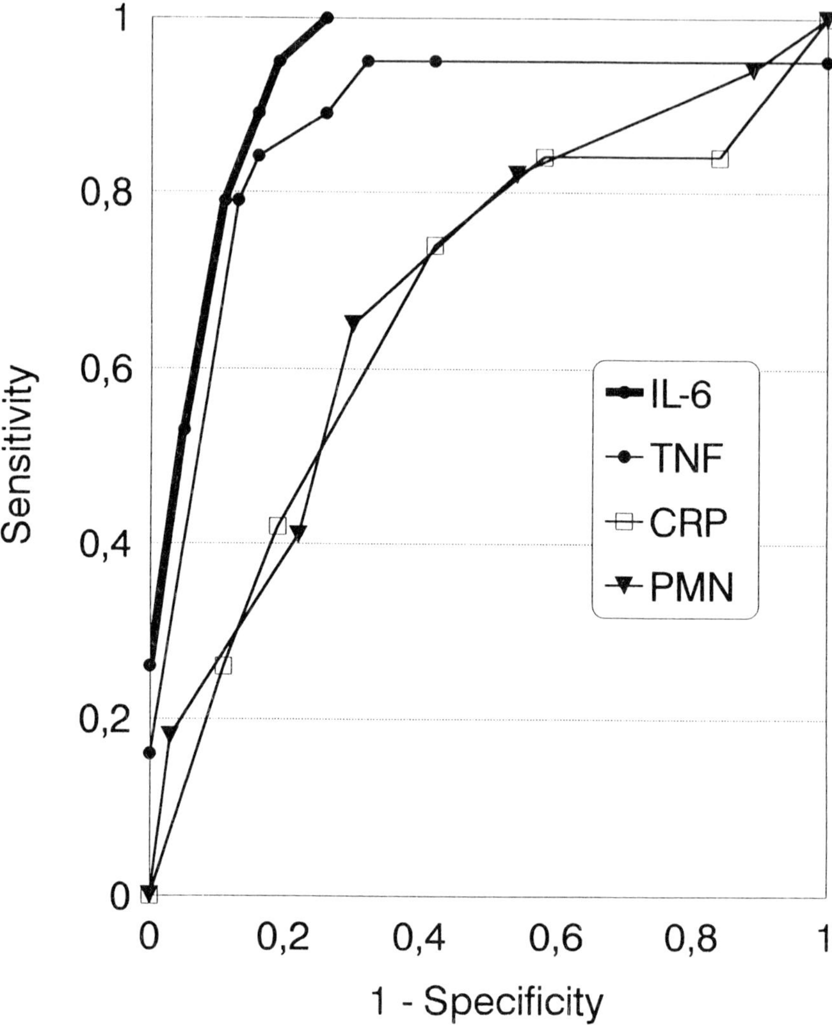

Fig. 3 Receiver operating curves of PMN count, C reactive protein, TNF-α and IL-6 levels for the diagnosis of bacterial infection on admission in 57 decompensated cirrhotics (19 infected, 38 non-infected). Each point represents the sensitivity and the specificity of the assay for a given threshold. The area under the curve represents the power of the test (from Ref. 62)

inhibit TNF-α secretion. Phosphatidylcholine, which has been shown to protect against cirrhosis in alcohol-fed non-human primates decreases the activation of Ito cells to transitional cells (which is cytokine dependent). It could be suggested that increased levels of collagenase observed in this condition are also cytokine mediated[65].

Numerous agents have been developed for anticytokine therapy and the mechanisms of action (at the cytokine level) of known immunosuppressive drugs have become better understood. Cytokine inhibitors such as antibodies against cytokines, soluble receptors and receptor antagonists were initially developed to prevent lethality of septic shock and have since been used to treat more chronic inflammatory processes such as rheumatoid arthritis or inflammatory bowel disease. These cytokine blockers act following cytokine production and their clinical use will probably be restricted to acute conditions such as sepsis, and very limited in the treatment of chronic diseases such as ALC. In our opinion, anti-inflammatory cytokines, of which IL-10 is the best described, have important therapeutic potential, either when administered directly or used to monitor drug therapies. A better knowledge of the effect of IL-10 on Ito cells and on the fibrotic process of cirrhotics might initiate studies on immunomodulation in experimental models of hepatotoxicity. It is now apparent that IL-10 mediates some effects of immunosuppressive drugs such as glucocorticoids and cyclosporin. It is therefore likely that monitoring of IL-10 might improve the monitoring of drug effects on cytokine metabolism. It is clear that the knowledge of cytokine network in ALC could help to discover new drugs or agents able to modulate the disease course or complications.

References

1. Le J, Vilcek J. Biology of disease: tumor necrosis factor and interleukin 1: cytokines with multiple overlapping biological activities. Lab Invest. 1987;56:234–48.
2. Chojkier M, Fierer J. D-Galactosamine hepatotoxicity is associated with endotoxin sensitivity and mediated by lymphoreticular cells in mice. Gastroenterology. 1985;88:114–21.
3. Lehmann V, Freudenberg MA, Galanos C. Lethal toxicity of lipopolysaccharide and tumor necrosis factor in normal and D-galactosamine treated mice. J Exp Med. 1987;165:657–63.
4. Hansen J, Cherwitz DL, Allen JL. The role of tumor necrosis factor α in acute endotoxin-induced hepatotoxicity in ethanol-fed rats. Hepatology. 1994;20;461–74.
5. Decker K. The macrophages and their signal products. In Bianchi L, Gerok W, Maier KP, Deinhardt F, editors. Infectious diseases of the liver. Dordrecht: Kluwer Academic Publishers; 1990:49–71.
6. Kishimoto T. The biology of interleukin 6. Blood. 1989;74:1–10.
7. Moore KW, O'Garra A, De Waal Malefyt R et al. Interleukin-10. Annu Rev Immunol. 1993;11:165–90.
8. Dinarello CA. Biology of interleukin 1. FASEB J. 1988;2:108–15.
9. Tracey KJ, Vlassara H, Cerami A. Cachectin/tumor necrosis factor. Lancet. 1989;ii:1122–6.
10. Nagakawa J, Hishinuma I, Hirota K et al. Involvement of tumor necrosis factor α in the pathogenesis of activated macrophage mediated hepatitis. Gastroenterology. 1990;99:758–65.
11. Mizuhara H, O'Neill E, Seki N et al. T cell activation associated hepatic injury: metabolism by tumor necrosis factors and protection by interleukin 6. J Exp Med. 1994;179:1529–37.
12. McClain CJ, Hill D, Schmidt J, Diehl AM. Cytokines and alcoholic liver disease. Semin Liver Dis. 1993;13:170–82.
13. Hishinuma I, Nagakawa J, Hirota K et al. Tumor necrosis factor α in galactosamine induced hepatitis. Hepatology. 1990;12:1187–91.
14. Kawano M, Hirano T, Matsuda T et al. Autocrine generation and essential requirement of BSF-2/IL-6 for human multiple myelomas. Nature. 1988;332:83–5.
15. Kishimoto T, Hirano T. Molecular regulation of B lymphocytes response. Annu Rev Immuol. 1988;6:485–512.
16. Gauldie J, Richards C, Harnish D et al. Interferon α2/B cell stimulatory factor type 2 share identity with monocyte derived hepatocyte stimulating factor and regulates the major acute phase protein response in liver cells. Proc Natl Acad Sci USA. 1987;84:7251–5.
17. Choi I, Kang HS, Pyun KH. IL-6 induces hepatic inflammation and collagen synthesis in vivo. Clin Exp Immunol. 1994;95:530–5.
18. McClain CJ, Cohen DA, Dinarello CA et al. Serum interleukin-1 (IL-1) activity in alcoholic hepatitis. Life Sci. 1986;39:1479–85.

19. Houssiau FA, Coulie PG, Olive D et al. Synergistic activation of human T cells by interleukin 1 and interleukin 6. Eur J Immunol. 1988;18:653–6.
20. Deviere J, Content J, Denys C et al. Excessive bacterial lipopolysaccharide-induced production of monokines in cirrhosis. Hepatology. 1990;11:628–34.
21. Khoruts A, Stahnke L, McClain CJ et al. Circulating tumor necrosis factor, interleukin-1 and interleukin-6 concentrations in chronic alcoholic patients. Hepatology. 1991;13:267–76.
22. Felver ME, Mezey E, McGuire M et al. Plasma tumor necrosis factor α predicts decreased long term survival in severe alcoholic hepatitis. Alcohol Clin Exp Res. 1990;14:255–9.
23. Deviere J, Denys C, Schandene L et al. Decreased proliferative activity associated with activation markers in patients with alcoholic liver cirrhosis. Clin Exp Immunol. 1988;72:377–82.
24. McClain CJ, Cohen DA. Increased tumor necrosis factor production by monocytes in alcoholic hepatitis. Hepatology. 1989;9:349–51.
25. Deviere J, Content J, Denys C et al. High interleukin-6 serum levels and increased production by leucocytes in alcoholic liver cirrhosis. Correlation with IgA serum levels and lymphokines production. Clin Exp Immunol. 1989;77:221–5.
26. Hamilton TA, Adams DO. Molecular mechanism of signal transduction in macrophages. Immunol Today. 1987;8:151–8.
27. Schultz RM, Kleinschmidt WJ. Functional identity between murine interferon and macrophage activating factor. Nature. 1983;305:239–40.
28. Deviere J, Vaerman JP, Content J et al. IgA triggers tumor necrosis factor α secretion by monocytes: a study in normal subjects and patients with alcoholic cirrhosis. Hepatology. 1991;13:670–5.
29. de Waal Malefyt R, Abrams J, Bennett B et al. Interleukin-10 (IL-10) inhibits cytokine synthesis by human monocytes: an autoregulatory role of IL-10 produced by monocytes. J Exp Med. 1992;174:1209–20.
30. Ishida H, Hastings R, Thompson-Snipes L et al. Modified immunological status of anti-IL-10 treated mice. Cell Immunol. 1993;148:371–84.
31. Bird GLA, Sheron N, Goka AKJ et al. Increased plasma tumor necrosis factor in severe alcoholic hepatitis. Ann Intern Med. 1990;112:917–20.
32. Tilg H, Wilmer A, Vogel W et al. Serum levels of cytokines in chronic liver diseases. Gastroenterology. 1992;103:264–74.
33. Sheron N, Bird G, Goka J et al. Elevated plasma interleukin-6 and increased severity and mortality in alcoholic hepatitis. Clin Exp Immunol. 1991;84:449–53.
34. Hill D, Marsano L, Cohen D et al. Increased plasma interleukin 6 activity in alcoholic hepatitis. J Lab Clin Med. 1992;119:547–52.
35. Bode C, Kugler V, Bode JC. Endotoxemia in patients with alcoholic and non-alcoholic cirrhosis and subjects with no evidence of chronic liver disease following acute alcohol excess. J Hepatol. 1988;4:8–14.
36. Fukui H, Brauner B, Bode JC et al. Plasma endotoxin concentrations in patients with alcoholic and non-alcoholic liver disease: reevaluation with an improved chromogenic assay. J Hepatol. 1992;12:162–9.
37. Bigatello LM, Broitman SA, Fattori L et al. Endotoxemia, encephalopathy, and mortality in cirrhotic patients. Am J Gastroenterol. 1987;82:11–15.
38. Fulenwider JT, Sibley C, Stein SF et al. Endotoxemia of cirrhosis: an observation not substantiated. Gastroenterology. 1980;78:1001–4.
39. D'Souza NB, Bagby CJ, Nelson S. Acute alcohol infusion suppresses endotoxin-induced serum tumor necrosis factor. Alcohol Clin Exp Res. 1989;13:295–8.
40. Honchel R, Ray M, Marsano L et al. Tumor necrosis factor in alcohol enhanced endotoxin liver injury. Alcohol Clin Exp Res. 1992;16:665–9.
41. Peristeris P, Clark B, Gatti S et al. N-acetylcystein and glutathione as inhibitors of tumor necrosis factor production. Cell Immunol. 1992;140:390–99.
42. Mitchell MC, Raiford DS, Mallat A. Effect of ethanol on glutathione metabolism. In: Watson RR, editor. Drug and alcohol abuse. Reviews, 2: Liver pathology and alcohol. Clifton, NJ: Humana Press; 1991.
43. Baggiolini M Walz A, Kunkel SL. Neutrophil-activating peptide/interleukin 8 a novel cytokine that activates neutrophils. J Clin Invest. 1989;84:1045–9.
44. Hill DB, Marsano LS, McClain CJ. Increased plasma interleukin 8 concentrations in alcoholic hepatitis. Hepatology. 1993;18:576–80.

45. Sheron N, Bird G, Koskinas J et al. Circulating and tissue levels of the neutrophil chemotoxin interleukin 8 are elevated in severe acute alcoholic hepatitis and tissue levels correlated with neutrophil infiltration. Hepatology. 1993;18:41–6.
46. Marchant A, Bruyns C, Vandenabeele P et al. IL-10 controls IFN-γ and TNF production during experimental endotoxemia. Eur J Immunol. 1994;24:1167–71.
47. Gerard C, Bruyns C, Marchant A et al. Interleukin-10 reduces the release of tumor necrosis factor and prevents lethality in experimental endotoxemia. J Exp Med. 1993;177:547–50.
48. Howard M, Muchamuel T, Andrade S et al. Interleukin-10 protects mice from lethal endotoxemia. J Exp Med. 1993;177:1205–8.
49. Durez P, Abramowicz D, Gerard C et al. In vivo induction of interleukin 10 by anti-CD3 monoclonal antibody or bacterial lipopolysaccharide: differential modulation by cyclosporin. J Exp Med. 1993;177:551–5.
50. Mengozzi M, Fantuzzi G, Faggioni R et al. Chlorpromazine specifically inhibits peripheral and brain TNF production, and upregulates IL-10 production, in mice. Immunology. 1994;82:207–10.
51. Marchant A, Deviere J, Byl B et al. Interleukin-10 production during septicaemia. Lancet. 1994;343:707–8.
52. Le Moine O, Marchant A, Durand F et al. Systemic release of interleukin-10 during orthotopic liver transplantation. Hepatology. 1994;20:889–92.
53. Van De Wiel A, Schuurman HJ, Kater L. Alcoholic liver disease: an IgA associated disorder. Scand J Gastroenterol. 1987;22:1025–30.
54. Delacroix DL, Elkon KB, Geubel AP et al. Changes in size, subclass and metabolic properties of serum immunoglobin A in liver diseases and in other diseases with high serum immunoglobin A. J Clin Invest. 1983;71:358–67.
55. Van De Wiel A, Schuurman HJ, Van Riessen D et al. Characteristics of IgA deposits in liver and skin of patients with liver diseases. Am J Clin Pathol. 1986;86:724–30.
56. Swerdlow MA, Chowdhury LN, Horn T. Patterns of IgA deposition in liver tissues in alcoholic liver disease. Am J Clin Pathol. 1982;77:259–66.
57. Brown WR, Kloppel TM. Liver and IgA: immunological, cell biological and clinical implications. Hepatology. 1989;9:763–84.
58. Deviere J, Content J, Denys C et al. Immunoglobin A and interleukin 6 form a positive secretory feedback loop: a study of normal subjects and alcoholic cirrhotics. Gastroenterology. 1992;103:1296–301.
59. Wycke RJ. Problems of bacterial infection in patients with liver disease. Gut. 1987;28:623–41.
60. Byl B, Roucloux I, Crusiaux A et al. Tumor necrosis factor α and interleukin-6 plasma levels in infected cirrhotic patients. Gastroenterology. 1993;104:1492–7.
61. Michie HR, Manogue KR, Spriggs DR et al. Detection of circulating tumor necrosis factor after endotoxin administration. N Engl J Med. 1988;318:1481–6.
62. Le Moine O, Deviere J, Devaster JM et al. Interleukin-6: an early marker of bacterial infection in decompensated cirrhosis. J Hepatol. 1994;20:819–24.
63. De Forge LE, Nguyen DT, Kunkel SL, Remick DG. Regulation of the pathophysiology of tumor necrosis factor. J Clin Lab Med. 1990;116:429–38.
64. Ding AH, Porteu F, Sanchez E, Nathan CF. Down regulation of tumor necrosis factor receptors on macrophages and endothelial cells by microtubule depolymerizing agents. J Exp Med. 1990;171:715–27.
65. Lieber CS, Robins SJ, Li J et al. Phosphatydylcholine protects against fibrosis and cirrhosis in the baboon. Gastroenterology. 1994;106:152–9.

12
Autoimmune hepatitis and cytokines

C. TRAUTWEIN and M. P. MANNS

INTRODUCTION

Autoimmune hepatitis (AIH) comprises a group of chronic hepatitis syndromes in which patients appear to lose immunological tolerance to the liver itself. AIH is a chronic necro-inflammatory disorder of the liver of unknown aetiology, devoid of evidence of antecedent viral infection, that is characterized by immune and autoimmune features, including the presence of circulating autoantibodies, hypergammaglobulinaemia, a female predominance, typical major HLA types and the association with other autoimmune diseases[1]. At the present time three types of AIH can be distinguished based upon serological findings. AIH type I is associated with high titres of antinuclear antibodies (ANA) or smooth muscle antibodies (SMA), type II is characterized by liver kidney microsomal (LKM-1) antibodies directed against cytochrome P450 IID6. In type III AIH soluble liver antigen (SLA) or other antibodies without ANA or anti-LKM are found (Table 1)[2]. Standardization of the diagnosis of AIH has been achieved through the use of a combination of clinical, serum biological and serological findings established by the nomenclature groups of the international association for the study of the liver (IASL)[2].

ROLE FOR CYTOKINES IN AUTOIMMUNE HEPATITIS

There are different hypotheses relating to how the autoimmune process is triggered and then becomes a self-perpetuating disease. Factors which may play a role include molecular mimicry between viruses, endogenous retroviruses, genetic factors and host factors or various environmental factors[3–6]. Each factor may independently enhance the immunogenicity of autoantigens, by increasing either their processing and presentation by B lymphocytes and macrophages or by increasing the chance for recognition by autoreactive T and B lymphocytes[3–6]. One of the main routes of communication between these different cells of the defence system is the cytokines[7,8]. Dysregulation of certain cytokines could mediate the course of autoimmunity and by blocking the pathway could have an impact on the therapy of the disease. At the present time little is known about the

Table 1 Classification of chronic hepatitis on the basis of aetiology

Hepatitis type	HBsAg	HBV DNA	HDV antibody (HDV RNA)	HCV antibody (HCV RNA)	Autoantibodies
B	+	±	–	–	—
D	+	–	+	–	~10% anti-LKM-3
C	–	–	–	+	~2% anti-LKM-1
Autoimmune					
type 1	–	–	–	–	ANA
type 2	–	–	–	–	LKM-1
type 3	–	–	–	–	SLA/LP
Drug-induced	–	–	–	–	Some: ANA, LKM, LM
Cryptogenic	–	–	–	–	—

SLA, soluble liver antigen antibody; LP, liver-pancreas antigen antibody; LM, liver microsomal antibody
According to ref. 3

regulation of cytokines during the course of AIH. Therefore the main therapy of AIH is a more general suppression of the immune system by glucocorticosteroids or a combination of glucocorticosteroids and azathioprine[1,2].

INTERFERON AND AUTOIMMUNE HEPATITIS

Interferon-α (IFN-α) is at the present time the only effective therapy in viral hepatitis, which may lead to the elimination of the virus. IFN-α modulates the immune system and renders cells resistant to certain viral infections and therefore increases the defence mechanisms of the host. Known mechanisms are, for example, the induction of proteins such as class I and II MHC molecules or intercellular adhesion molecule 1 (ICAM-1)[9]. On the other hand, viral replication is decreased by increasing proteins which are involved in the viral response, such as 2′,5′-oligoisoadenylate synthetase[7]. LKM-1 autoantibodies are known to occur in AIH type II[10,11]. Before the standardization of AIH a distinction between type IIa and IIb was made by the presence of markers for HCV-infection in type IIb infection[12]. Type IIb is considered to be a viral infection which triggers the immune system towards the production of LKM-1 autoantibodies. The administration of IFN in both type II forms of AIH may therefore have different effects on the course of the disease. In type IIb IFN may lead to elimination of the HCV virus and a consequent decrease in LKM-1 antibodies titres. In contrast IFN has been shown to lead to a dramatic deterioration of AIH type IIa, with increase in ALT level and LKM-1 antibodies (Fig. 1)[13]. At the present time it is unclear which mechanisms are responsible for the progression of the disease and how interferon leads to the deterioration of autoimmune hepatitis. Since autoimmune hepatitis type IIb clinically resembles viral hepatitis it is regarded as chronic hepatitis C with associated autoimmunity rather than an autoimmune liver disease. However controlled trials are necessary to evaluate whether IFN is of benefit or may prove hazardous in patients with hepatitis C and LKM antibodies. In this context it is worth mentioning that the epitopes recognized by LKM antibodies in HCV-negative AIH type II differ from those in chronic hepatitis C-associated autoimmunity.

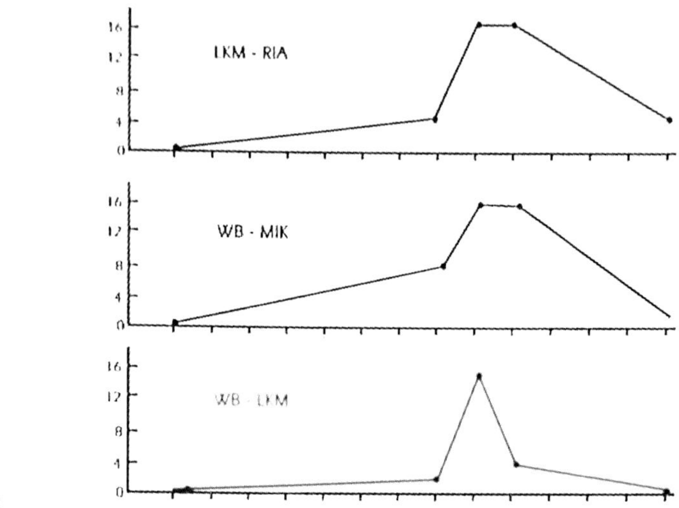

(a)

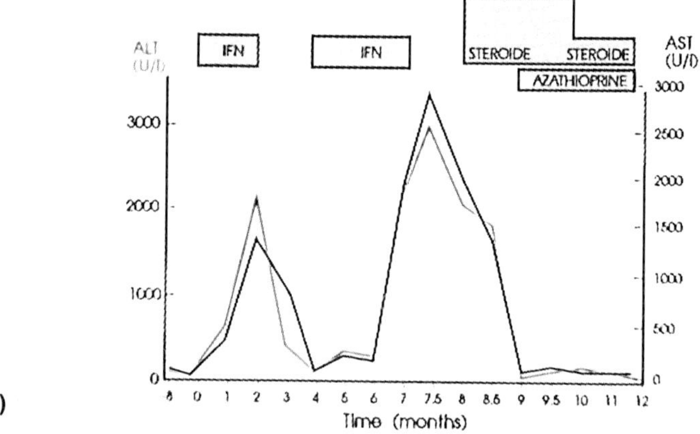

(b)

Fig. 1 Manifestation of autoimmune hepatitis type 2 during interferon medication. (**B**) Drug therapy and ALT-levels. (**A**) LKM-1 antibody titres as determined by RIA or Western blot (WB) with human liver microsomes or human recombinant LKM-1 (rLKM) antigen

REGULATION OF AUTOANTIGENS BY CYTOKINES

Regulation of the expression of the autoantigen itself could explain the progression of the disease. For example, tissue expression of Sp 100, an autoantigen of primary biliary cirrhosis (PBC), increases after IFN administration[14]. Higher levels of expression and presentation of the autoantigen to the immune system could then contribute to progression of the disease. The major LKM-1 autoantigen cytochrome P450 2D6 is also responsive to regulation by cytokines. The acute phase cytokines IL1, IL6 and tumour necrosis factor-α (TNF-α) lead to a decrease in LKM-1 autoantigen expression in a mouse in vivo model. Six hours after cytokine injection only 10% of the original level is detected at the RNA level (Fig. 2), and a rebound phenomenon is seen 24h after cytokine administration, with levels higher than the original P450 2D6 level[15] This is especially intriguing as patients with autoimmune liver disease have been shown to have decreased mRNA levels for IL1, IL6 and TNF-α in the liver compared with normal individuals[16]. Additionally, differences in the serum concentration of IL6 and TNF-α have been observed in children with AIH type 1 and 2[17]. Children suffering from lupoid type 1 AIH have higher levels of IL6 and TNF-α than children with AIH type 2, who have serum levels comparable to those of healthy controls[17]. Further studies are needed to investigate whether IFN and other cytokines also influence the expression of the LKM-1 autoantigen. Regulation of autoantigen expression by cytokines could potentially play a role in the course of AIH, especially if the surface expression on the hepatocyte membrane can be triggered by cytokines[18,19].

LIVER-INFILTRATING T-CELLS AND CYTOKINES

Striking evidence shows that liver-infiltrating T-cells are pivotal in the course of autoimmune liver disease and PBC. CD4$^+$ positive T-helper cells specifically recognize autoantigens and proliferate in a MHC II-restricted pattern[20,21]. T-helper cells can be differentiated into T-helper 1 (TH1) and T-helper 2 (TH2) cells by their ability to produce a different cytokine panel. In the mouse model, differentiation of naive TH cells into TH1 cells is mainly triggered by IL-12 and IFN-γ. Mature TH1 produce IL-2 and IFN-γ, and are involved in cell-mediated immune responses. Naive TH cells differentiate into TH2 cells in an IL4-dependent fashion and TH2 produce IL-4, IL-5 and IL-10 and are important for antibody production in the humoral immune response[22]. This model of two different T-helper cell subsets also has some implications in humans. An additional subset of TH0 cells, which can secrete both panels of cytokines and therefore could have implications for both pathways, makes the picture less clear. However, the fine tuning between these cytokines could be important in determining the antigen-specific response of TH cells in the liver. Purified peripheral blood mononuclear cells produce high levels of IL-4 in AIH, in contrast to patients suffering from chronic hepatitis B, where high levels of IL-2 and IFN-γ are found[22]. Similar results were found with liver-infiltrating T-cells from patients with chronic viral hepatitis B and AIH type 1: the former show high levels of IFN-γ while the latter have high levels of IL-4. Therefore CD4$^+$ cells in AIH type 1 are preferentially TH2 cells, which are mainly implicated in mediating antibody production in the humoral immune response[23]. Results obtained from liver-infiltrating T-cells of patients with AIH type 2 are less clear. Preliminary results for AIH type 2 indicate a role of mainly TH1 with a higher

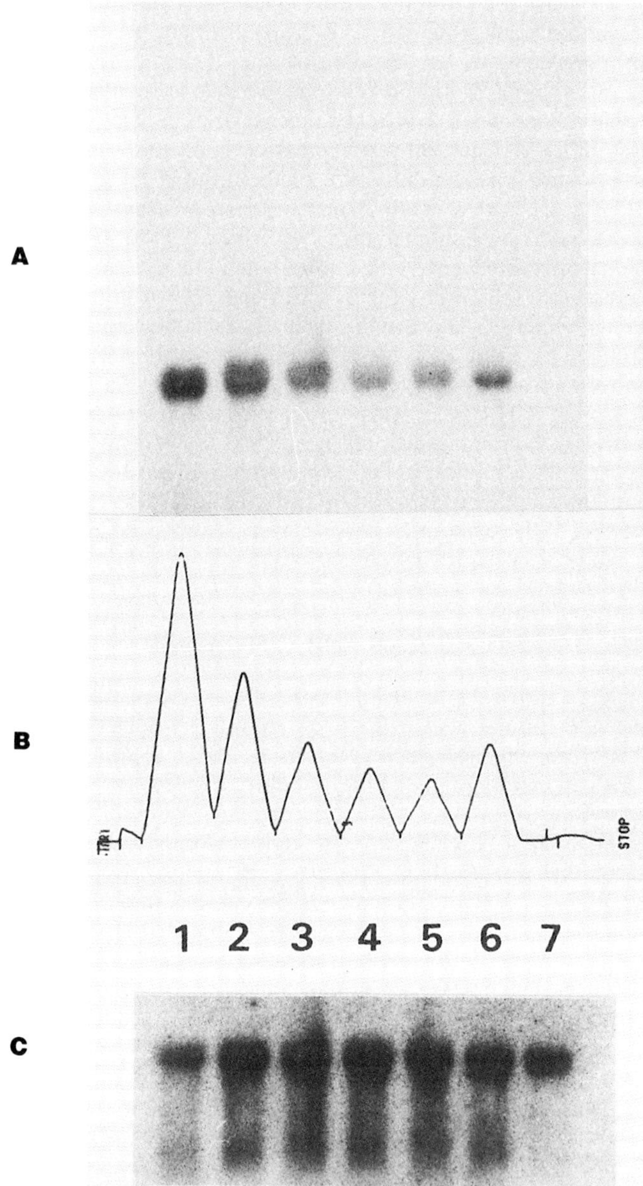

Fig. 2 Regulation of cytochrome P450 2D6 by TNF-α. TNF-α was injected i.p. into C3H/HeJ mice and the change in level of 2D6 RNA was determined by Northern blot analysis. Lane 1 represents the solvent alone, lanes 2–5 different amounts of TNF-α (0.01, 0.1, 1 and 2 μg). In lane 6 and 7 control experiments are shown; lane 6 liver of C3H mice 16h after the injection of 15 μg endotoxin, lane 7 macrophage line U 937 which lacks the expression of 2D6. (**A**) hybridization with the labelled probe of cytochrome P450 2D6; (**B**) respective densitometric evaluation; (**C**) hybridization with a labelled 28s probe

level of IFN-γ secretion and a minor role for TH2 cells[21,23]. The numbers of patients in these studies is low, and the results should be confirmed using a larger group of patients. However these differences in T-cell level and in the expression of acute phase cytokines raises the question of differences in the aetiology of AIH types 1 and 2. As TH1 cells are mainly induced in patients suffering from viral infections a role of virus-induced autoimmunity could be important not only for AIH type 2b but also for AIH type 2a. It may be that cross reactivities – as shown between the B-cell epitope of cytochrome P450 2D6 and herpes simplex virus (HSV) – are involved in triggering autoimmunity and thus in the development of AIH type 2[6].

OUTLOOK

Increasing evidence points to the role of different panels of cytokines in the aetiology and course of AIH. There are differences in cytokine level between the different types of AIH and in patients with viral hepatitis. Further research is needed to locate the exact mechanisms which may be important in triggering autoimmunity in the liver. This may lead to new and more sophisticated therapeutic approaches in which certain pathways are blocked specifically as opposed to the currently used non-specific immunosuppression. In this context the heterogeneous syndrome of chronic hepatitis could serve as a good model to study the role of cytokines in autoimmune disease compared with chronic viral infection.

References

1. Johnson PJ, McFarlane IG. Meeting report: international autoimmune hepatitis group. Hepatology. 1993;18:998–1008.
2. Desmet VJ, Gerber M, Hoffnagle JH, Manns M, Scheuer PJ. Classification of chronic hepatitis. Hepatology. 1994;19:1513–20.
3. Barnett LA, Fujinami RS. Molecular mimicry: a mechanism for autoimmune hepatitis. FASEB J. 1992;6:840–4.
4. Carson DS. Genetic factors in the etiology and pathogenesis of autoimmunity. FASEB J. 1992;6:2800–5.
5. Krieg AM, Gourly MK, Perl A. Endogenous retroviruses. potential etiologic agents in autoimmunity. FASEB J. 1992;6:2537–44.
6. Manns M, Griffin KJ, Sullivan KF, Johnson EF. LKM-1 autoantibodies recognize a short linear sequence in P450IID6, a cytochrome P-450 monooxygenase. J Clin Invest. 1991;88:1370–8.
7. Staehli P. Interferon-induced proteins and the antiviral state. Adv Virus Res. 1990;38:147–56.
8. Scott P. IL-12: Initiation cytokine for cell-mediated immunity. Science. 1993;260:496–7.
9. Wallach DM, Fellous M, Revel M. Preferential effect of gamma interferon on the synthesis of HLA antigens and their mRNAs in human cells. Nature. 1982;299:833–6.
10. Homberg JC, Abauf N, Bernard O et al. Chronic active hepatitis associated with antiliver/kidney microsomal antibody type I: a second type of 'autoimmune hepatitis'. Hepatology. 1987;7:1333–9.
11. Manns M, Johnson EF, Griffin KJ, Tan E, Sullivan KF. Major antigen of liver kidney microsomal autoantibodies in idiopathic autoimmune hepatitis is cytochrome P450db1. J Clin Invest. 1989;83:1066–72.
12. Michel G, Ritter A, Gerken G, Meyer zum Büschenfelde KH, Decker R, Manns MP. Anti-GOR and hepatitis C virus in autoimmune liver disease. Lancet. 1991;339:267–9.
13. Ruiz-Moreno M, Rua MJ, Carreno V, Quiroga JA, Manns M, Meyer zum Büschenfelde K-H.

Autoimmune hepatitis type 2 manifested during interferon therapy in children. J Hepatol. 1991;12:265–6.

14. Guldner HH, Szostecki C, Grötzinger T, Will H. IFN enhance expression of Sp 100, an autoantigen in primary biliary cirrhosis. J Immunol. 1992;149:4067–73.

15. Trautwein C, Ramadori G, Gerken G, Meyer zum Büschenfelde K-H, Manns M. Regulation of cytochrome P450 IID by acute phase mediators in C3H/HeJ mice. Biochem Biophys Res Commun. 1992;182:617–23.

16. Tovey MG, Gugenheim J, Guymarho J et al. Genes for interleukin-1, interleukin-6, and tumor necrosis factor are expressed at markedly reduced levels in the livers of patients with severe liver disease. Autoimmunity. 1991;10:297–310.

17. Maggiore G, de Benedetti F, Massa M, Pignatti P, Martini A. Circulating levels of interleukin 6, interleukin 8 and tumor necrosis factor-a in children with autoimmune hepatitis. In press.

18. Loeper J, Descatoire V, Maurice M et al. Presence of functional cytochrome P450 on isolated rat hepatocyte plasma membrane. Hepatology. 1990;11:850–8.

19. Trautwein C, Gerken G, Löhr H, Meyer zum Büschenfelde K-H, Manns M. Lack of surface expression for the B-cell autoepitope of cytochrome P450 IID6 evidenced by flow cytometry. Z Gastroenterol. 1993;31:225–30.

20. Löhr H, Manns M, Kyriatsoulis A et al. Clonal analysis of liver infiltrating T cells in patients with LKM-1 antibody positive autoimmune chronic hepatitis. Clin Exp Immunol. 1991;84: 297–302.

21. Löhr HF, Schlaak JF, Fleischer B, Dienes H-P, Meyer zum Büschenfelde K-H. Phenotypical analysis and cytokine release of liver-infiltrating and peripheral blood T lymphocytes from patients with chronic hepatitis of different etiology. Liver. 1994;14:161–6.

22. Al-Wabel A, Mansour A-J, Raziuddin S. Cytokine profile of viral and autoimmune chronic hepatitis. J Allergy Clin Immunol. 1993;92:902–8.

23. Schlaak JF, Löhr H, Gallati H, Meyer zum Büschenfelde K-H, Fleischer B. Analysis of the in vitro cytokine production by liver infiltrating T cells of patients with autoimmune hepatitis. Clin Exp Immunol. 1993;94:168–73.

13
Cytokine profiles in primary biliary cirrhosis: an approach to define the underlying immunoreactivity

P. A. BERG, R. KLEIN, M. LEUSCHNER and U. LEUSCHNER

INTRODUCTION

Two arms of the immune response are regulated by distinct subsets of CD4[+] T-helper cells termed TH1 and TH2 which are characterized by the release of defined cytokines[1-3]. All of the regulatory and direct effector functions of TH cells are mediated by the cytokines they secrete. The distinct array of cytokines produced by each subset of TH cells dictates their effector function and their role in inhibiting the induction and effector function of the reciprocal subset[4-6]. The release of cytokines by TH1 cells is generally elevated in response to a variety of intracellular and viral pathogens and can be related to the cellular immune response[7-14]. TH2-related cytokines are released predominantly during allergic conditions and helminthic infections and are responsible for B-cell activation, especially IgE production[15,16]. A dynamic, finely regulated balance between different types of immune response may also be involved in regulatory responses to self antigens. Thus, studies in experimentally induced autoimmune diseases have revealed that distinct cytokine profiles are apparent during cell-mediated reactions to autoantigens[17,18]. Preferential activation of the TH1 response is central to the pathogenesis of some of these diseases. Thus, spontaneous recovery of rats and mice with experimental allergic encephalomyelitis (EAE), a CD4[+] T-cell mediated disease correlated with an expansion of TH2-like cells and cytokines, while progression was associated with increased production of TH1-related cytokines[18]. There is also evidence of TH1 involvement in insulin-dependent diabetes mellitus in man and in animal models[19].

PBC is also believed to be an autoimmune disorder and is characterized by pronounced B-cell activation as shown by the pronounced elevation of IgM. We were, therefore, interested in studying cytokine profiles in these patients, and it is postulated that TH2-specific cytokines are preferentially produced.

PATIENTS

Sera and peripheral blood monocytes (PBMC) were obtained from 47 PBC patients seen at the Department of Gastroenterology, University of Frankfurt. Diagnosis was confirmed by clinical, histological, and serological data; 37 patients were in stage I/II, 10 patients in stage III/IV. All were anti-M2 positive. Supernatants of PBMC from 26 healthy controls were used as controls. Sera from 49 patients with autoimmune hepatitis, 31 patients with primary sclerosing cholangitis (PSC), 52 patients with rheumatoid arthritis, and 50 blood donors were also analysed.

METHODS

Lymphocyte cultures

PBMC from PBC patients and controls were separated from heparinized blood by standard Ficoll–Hypaque gradient centrifugation[20]. The cells were aspirated from the interface, washed three times, and resuspended in RPMI supplemented with gentamicin ($50\,\mu g/ml$) and glutamine ($2\,mmol/l$)[21]. The mononuclear cells ($3\times10^6\,ml$) were supplemented with 25% autologous serum and cultured for 7 days under three different conditions: non-stimulated, stimulated with pokeweed mitogen (PWM; $10\,\mu g/3\times10^5$ cells), or stimulated with M2 (ATPase fraction) prepared from beef heart mitochondria[22], consisting of the five major subunits of the α-ketoacid dehydrogenase complex recently defined as the target antigen of anti-M2 antibodies in PBC[23,24], and pyruvate dehydrogenase (PDC) from pig heart (Sigma, St Louis) corresponding to M2a ($70\,kDa$) (concentrations for both antigens ranging from 0.1 to $1000\,\mu g/ml$).

Lymphocyte supernatants were drawn at day 7 and kept frozen at -20°C.

Cytokine assays

The following cytokines were determined by enzyme-linked immunosorbent assay (ELISA): interleukin (IL)-1, -2, -4, -5, -6, -10, tumour necrosis factor-α (TNFα), interferon-γ (INF-γ) and granulocyte–macrophage colony stimulating factor (GM-CSF). All assays have been established by our own. Briefly, microtitre plates (Nunc, Wiesbaden) were coated with monoclonal anti-human cytokine antibodies diluted in bicarbonate buffer ($0.1\,M$, pH 9.6) for 16 h at 4°C. Patients' sera and supernatants of PBMC were added undiluted. As standards recombinant or natural cytokines have been applied at different concentrations. After incubation for 2 h at 37°C polyclonal anti-cytokine antibodies from rabbit (for IL-1, -2, -4, -5, -10, TNFα, IFN-γ) or goat (IL-6) were added (2 h, 37°C). Afterwards, the reaction was visualized by peroxidase conjugated anti-rabbit or -goat antibodies and addition of substrate (*o*-pheylenediamine).

All assays were controlled for sensitivity and specificity using commercially available test kits.

Table 1 Subsets of TH-cells as defined by their cytokine spectrum

| | *Principal subsets of murine CD4+ T-cells* | | | *Monocytes/NK-cells/* |
	TH0	*TH1*	*TH2*	*mast cells*
Innate immune system/monocytes				
IL-1	+	−	−	++
IL-6	?	−	++	++
Differentiation				
IFN-γ	++	++	−	++
IL-4	++	−	++	+
IL-12	−	−	−	++
TH1				
IL-2	+	+	−	−
TNFα	?	++	+	++
GM-CSF	+	++	+	−
TH2				
IL-5	++	−	++	−
IL-10	+	−	++	−
IL-13	?	−	++	−

Cytokine profiles

Immune response was classified according to the different cytokines characterizing certain compartments of the immune system[1–3,5] as shown in Table 1.

AMA profiles

In all PBC patients AMA profiles were determined, sera being tested for anti-M2, -M4, -M8, -M9 by ELISA and complement fixation test (CFT) as previously described (AMA profiles A/B: anti-M9 and/or anti-M2 positive by ELISA; profile C: anti-M2/-M4 and/or -M8 positive by ELISA; profile D: anti-M2/-M4 and/or -M8 positive by ELISA and CFT)[25,26]. The presence of complement fixing antibodies to M4 and M8 in association with anti-M2 indicates an active immunological stage, and this antibody constellation (profile D) showed a significant correlation with a progressive course[25].

Statistical analysis

Statistical analysis comparing the different cytokines was performed using the Student's *t*-test; $p < 0.05$ was considered as significant.

RESULTS

Cytokine profiles in sera from patients with PBC and in healthy controls

Cytokines were analysed in sera from 47 PBC patients and 50 blood donors (in vivo situation). As shown in Figure 1, the frequency of sera containing TH1-related cytokines (IL-2, TNFα, GM-CSF) was lower (up to 20%) than in controls

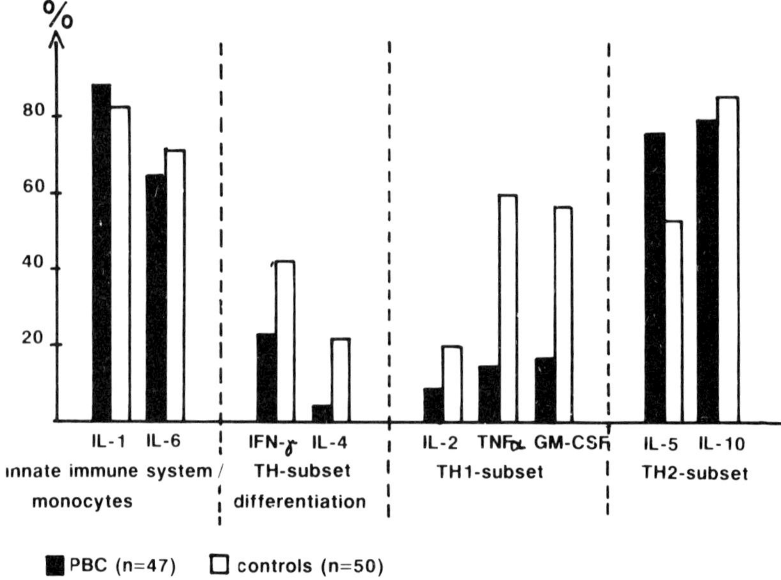

Fig. 1 Frequency of TH1 and TH2-specific regulatory cytokines in sera from patients with PBC as compared to controls (in vivo situation). TH1-related cytokines were less frequently observed in sera from patients with PBC than from controls, while IL-5 was more frequently found in PBC-sera (77%) than in healthy blood donors (54%). Monocyte/NK-cell related cytokines showed no difference in both groups

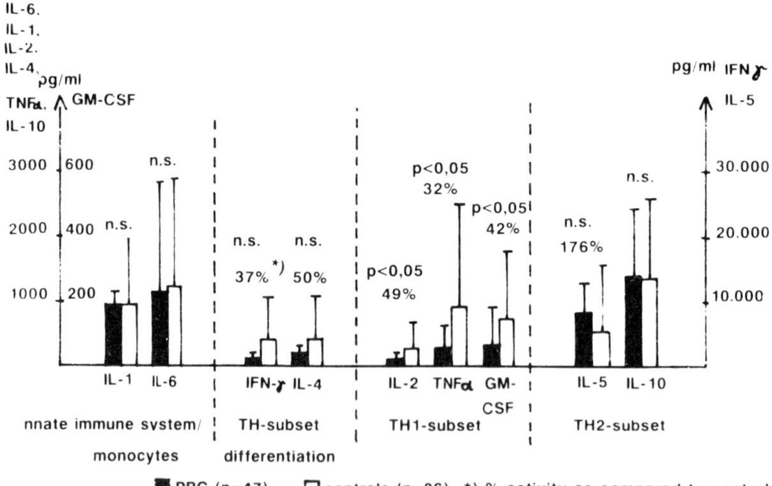

Fig. 2 Activity of TH1 and TH2-related cytokines in sera from PBC patients and healthy controls, reflecting the in vivo situation. Levels of TH1-related cytokines were significantly lower in PBC patients than in controls ($p < 0.05$). IL-5 levels were increased, but the difference was statistically not significant

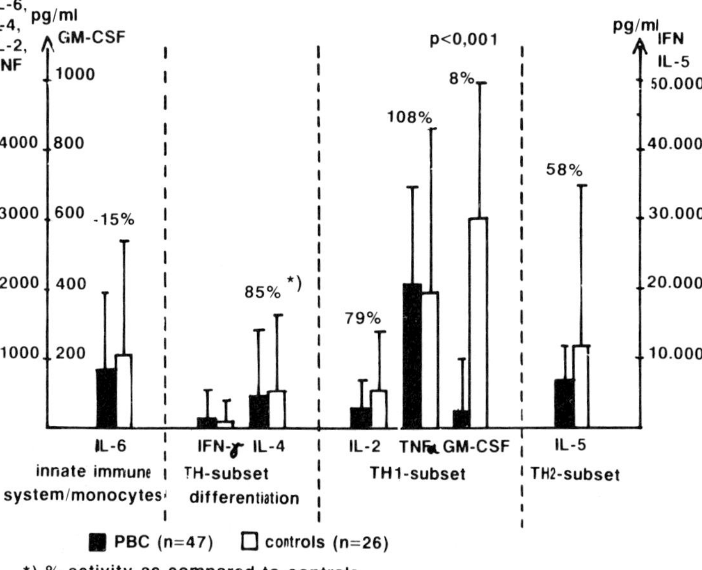

Fig. 3 Activity of cytokines in supernatants of cultured non-stimulated PBMC from PBC patients and controls. The only significant difference in the activity of the different cytokines analysed was the low GM-CSF levels in supernatants of PBMC from PBC patients ($p < 0.001$)

(up to 60%), and the activities of these cytokines were significantly lower in those with PBC ($p < 0.05$) (Fig. 2). IFN-γ and IL-4 were rarely observed. In contrast, IL-5, a TH2-cytokine, was detected in 77% of the PBC sera but only 54% of blood donors; mean activity was increased compared with controls (8.453 ± 5.199 pg/ml vs 4.874 ± 11.766 pg/ml), but this difference was statistically not significant.

Cytokine profiles in supernatants of cultured PBMC of PBC patients

Non-stimulated supernatants of PBMC derived from all 47 PBC patients and from 26 healthy controls were analysed for TH1/TH2-related cytokines. In this in vitro situation, the mean levels did not vary significantly between the two groups with the exception of GM-CSF activity which was significantly lower in PBC patients than in controls ($p < 0.001$; Fig. 3).

This phenomenon was also observed when PBMC of both groups were stimulated with pokeweed mitogen (PWM). GM-CSF concentration in supernatants of lymphocytes from PBC patients was 641.33 ± 289.21 pg/ml and from controls 934.23 ± 235.18 pg/ml (data not shown).

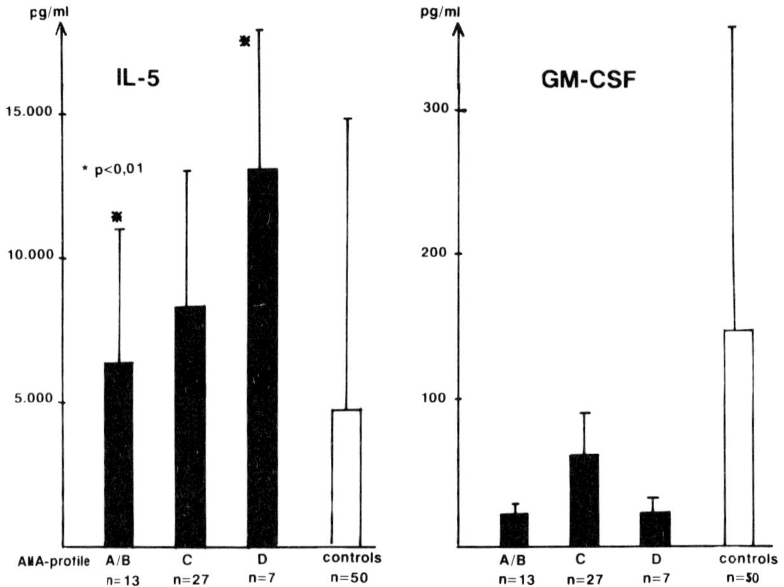

Fig. 4 Correlation between AMA-profiles and IL-5 as well as GM-CSF activity in sera from PBC patients. In patients with profile D IL-5 levels were significantly higher than in patients with profile A/B ($p<0.01$). GM-CSF levels were similar in both groups

Cytokine profiles in sera from PBC patients in relation to immunological and histological activity

Analysing the cytokine levels in sera from PBC patients in relation to the AMA profiles, which can be taken as parameter of immunological activity, a significant difference in the activity of IL-5 was observed when patients with profile A/B and D were compared ($p<0.01$; Fig. 4). In contrast, GM-CSF-levels did not vary significantly and were of low activity in all three different profiles. TH1-related cytokines and IL-6, a cytokine related to the innate immune system, showed no relationship to any AMA profile.

Similar results were obtained analysing the cytokine levels in relation to the histological stages of PBC. Thus, patients with stage III/IV had significantly higher IL-5 levels (2972.22 ± 3022.26 pg/ml) than patients with stage I/II disease (5988.89 ± 4355.87 pg/ml; $p<0.05$; data not shown).

Comparison of cytokine profiles in sera from patients with PBC and other disorders

The cytokine profiles in PBC were compared with those in patients with autoimmune hepatitis, rheumatoid arthritis, and PSC. Interestingly, patients with PSC had decreased IL-5 and normal GM-CSF levels; this observation is in accordance with the concept that PBC and PSC differ in their aetiopathogenesis. In patients with autoimmune hepatitis and rheumatoid arthritis the TH1-pattern predominated (Fig. 5).

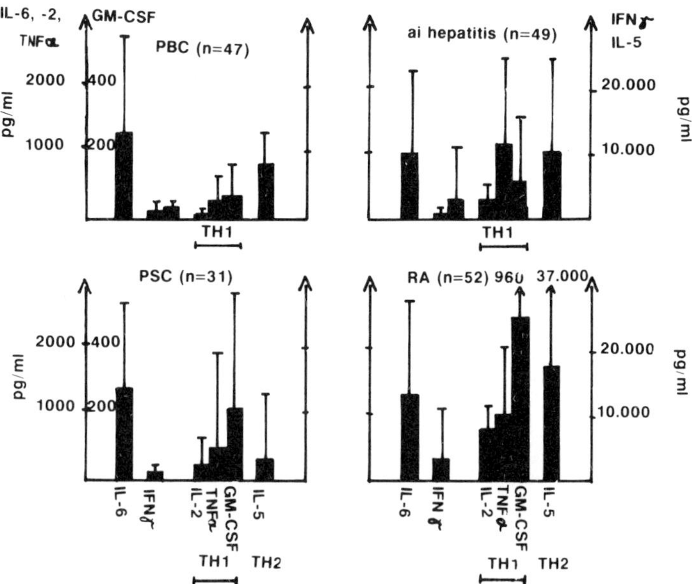

Fig. 5 Comparison of the cytokine profile in PBC with three other autoimmune disorders. In patients with PSC, GM-CSF levels were in the normal range but IL-5 activity was decreased showing a clear difference to the PBC-pattern. In patients with autoimmune hepatitis activation of TH1 cytokines predominated, and this finding also contrasts to the reduced TH1-pattern in PBC. In rheumatoid arthritis (RA) especially GM-CSF and TNFα levels were significantly increased as compared with PBC patients

Release of cytokines after stimulation of PBMC with autoantigens

In a preliminary approach, PBMC of a PBC patient and a healthy control were stimulated with M2 and PDC in different concentrations. In both instances, this antigen-stimulation led to a release of TNFα, IL-6 and GM-CSF, but not of IL-2 or IFN-γ. Increased IL-5 production was observed only in control PBMC. A typical example of these preliminary results is shown in Figure 6.

DISCUSSION

Clinical, serological and histological observations provide indirect evidence that TH2-regulated autoimmune reactions may play an important role in PBC. Thus, for instance the increased IgM levels, the eosinophilic reactions observed in some of the PBC patients, particularly in early stages, and the presence of CD8[+] T-cells (TH2-related) in bile duct lesions point toward TH2-regulated autoimmune conditions in this disease[27]. The cytokine profiles in sera and PBMC supernatants of PBC patients presented in this study support this concept. Thus, in most PBC sera the TH1/TH2-cytokine pattern was shifted towards TH2, i.e. TH2-relevant cytokines predominated (ratio of TH1 : TH2 in healthy controls, 1 : 3; in PBC patients, 1 : 9). TH1-related cytokine levels were significantly lower

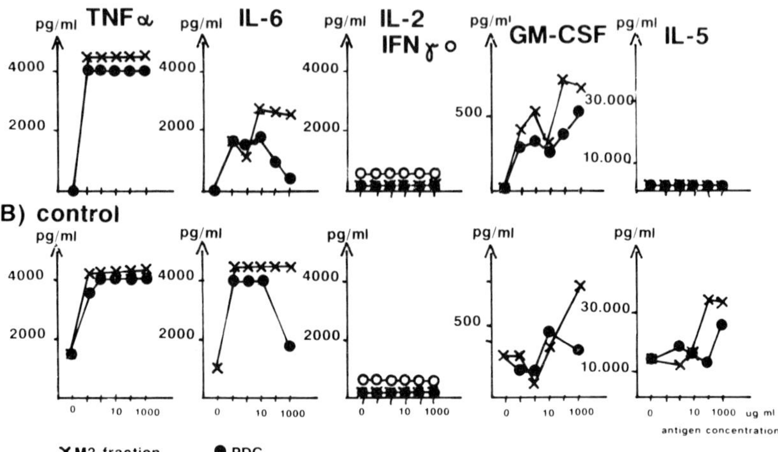

Fig. 6 Cytokine production of PBMC from a PBC patient (**A**) and a healthy control (**B**) after stimulation with the PBC-related antigens M2 (ATPase fraction) and PDC (M2a). Both antigens led to a release of TNFα, IL-6 and GM-CSF by lymphocytes of the PBC patient and the control but not of IL-2 or IFN-γ. IL-5 was only produced by lymphocytes of the control

in PBC patients than in controls. As also reported by other authors[28–30], TNFα levels were decreased in sera from PBC patients.

Analysis of cytokines in supernatants of cultured PBMC from PBC patients, however, revealed no major differences from controls with respect to their activity and frequency. This suggests that under in vitro conditions this functional parameter was not altered. This was true with the exception of GM-CSF production which was significantly decreased in PBC patients ($p < 0.001$). A selective TH1(?) defect may be responsible for this phenomenon.

Although IL-5-activity (TH2-related) was higher in PBC sera than in controls, this difference was not statistically significant. However, comparing immunological or inflammatory activity as defined by AMA-profiles or histological stages with IL-5 levels, IL-5 activity was found to be significantly higher in late stages or patients with AMA-profile D (high disease activity) than in early PBC or patients with profile A/B.

IL-6 levels were not increased in patients with late stages of the disease, and this finding is in contrast to a previous report indicating an increase of IL-6 in advanced stages[31]. The increased production of the TH2-related cytokine in active PBC may fit well with observations in experimental animal models that progression of the disease is accompanied by an activation of TH2-cells[7–15].

The clinical significance of the PBC-specific cytokine profile could be also documented by the analysis of cytokines in patients with autoimmune disorders, especially PSC, autoimmune hepatitis and rheumatoid arthritis. Thus, in patients with PSC, the TH2-related IL-5 activity was low. The inflammatory activity in patients with rheumatoid arthritis was well reflected by the cytokine pattern showing an increase of IL-2 and TNFα. Patients with autoimmune hepatitis showed an activation of TH1 pattern, but there was also evidence for an increase in IL-5 activity.

In order to determine whether the PBC-related autoantigens M2 and PDC are involved in the production of certain cytokines, PBMC of a PBC patient and a healthy control were exposed to these antigens in a 7-day culture. The cytokines released into the supernatants of both individuals revealed no difference indicating that these antigens may act predominantly as archaic antigens, stimulating preferentially cells of the innate immune system (IL-6). The fact that lymphocytes of the PBC patient produced GM-CSF after antigen stimulation also indicates that these antigens are not involved in the aetiopathogenesis of PBC.

One can, therefore, postulate that a genetically determined (MHC-related) inappropriate immune response towards a yet undefined autoantigen or exogenous antigen may be responsible for the TH2-related phenomena in PBC (IgM production, eosinophilia).

ACKNOWLEDGEMENTS

R.K. is supported by the Deutsche Forschungsgemeinschaft, Bonn-Bad Godesberg (Be 431/19).

References

1. Street NE, Schumacher JH, Fong AT et al. Heterogeneity of mouse helper T cells. Evidence from bulk cultures and limiting dilution cloning for precursors of Th1 and Th2 cells. J Immunol. 1990;144:1629–39.
2. Scott P. Selective differentiation of CD4$^+$ T helper cell subsets. Curr Opin Immunol. 1993;5: 391–7.
3. Salgame P, Abrams JS, Clayberger C et al. Differing lymphokine profiles of functional subsets of human CD4 and CD8 T cell clones. Science. 1991;254:279–82.
4. Maggi E, Parronchi P, Manetti R et al. Reciprocal regulatory effects of IFN-γ on the in vitro development of human Th1 and Th2 clones. J Immunol. 1992;148:2142–7.
5. Powrie F, Coffman RL. Cytokine regulation of T-cell function: potential for therapeutic intervention. Immunol Today. 1993;14:270–4.
6. Cavallo MG, Pozzilli P, Thorpe R. Cytokines and autoimmunity. Clin Exp Immunol. 1994,96. 1–7.
7. Kemp M, Hey AS, Kurtzhals JAI et al. Dichotomy of the human T-cell response to leishmania antigens. I. Th1-like response to *Leishmania major* promastigote antigens in individuals recovered from cutaneous leishmaniasis. Clin Exp Immunol. 1994;96:410–15.
8. Modlin RL, Nutman TB. Type 2 cytokines and negative immune regulation in human infections. Curr Opin Immunol. 1993;5:511–7.
9. Kurtzhals JAL, Hey AS, Jardim A et al. Dichotomy of the human T cell response to Leishmania antigens. II. Absence of Th2-like response to gp63 and Th1-like response to lipophosphoglycan-associated protein in cells from cured visceral leishmaniasis patients. Clin Exp Immunol. 1994;96:416–21.
10. Kullberg MC, Pearce EJ, Hieny SE, Sher A, Berzofsky JA. Infection with *Schistosoma mansoni* alters Th1/Th2 cytokine responses to a non-parasite antigen. J Immunol. 1992;148:3264–70.
11. Haanen JBAG, de Waal malefijit R, Res PCM et al. Selection of a human T helper type 1-like T cell subset by mycobacteria. J Exp Med. 1991;174:583–92.
12. Yamamura M, Yemura K, Deans RJ et al. Defining protective responses to pathogens: cytokine profiles in leprosy lesions. Science. 1991;254:277–9.

13. Bretscher PA, Wei G, Menon JN, Bielefeldt-Ohmann H. Establishment of stable, cell-mediated immunity that makes 'susceptible' mice resistant to *Leishmania major*. Science. 1992;257: 539–42.

14. Barnes PF, Abrams JS, Lu S, Sieling PA, Rea TH, Modlin RL. Patterns of cytokine production by mycobacterium-reactive human T-cell clones. Infect Immun. 1993;61:197–203.

15. Kay AB, Ying S, Varney V et al. Messenger RNA expression of the cytokine gene cluster, interleukin 3 (IL-3), IL-4, IL-5, and granulocyte/macrophage colony stimulating factor, in allergen-induced late phase cutaneous reactions in atopic subjects. J Exp Med. 1991;173:775–8.

16. Wierenga EA, Snoek M, DeGroot C et al. Evidence for compartmentalization of functional subsets of CD4[+] T lymphocytes in atopic patients. J Immunol. 1990;144:4651–6.

17. Yamamura M, Wang X-H, Ohmen JD et al. Cytokine patterns of immunologically mediated tissue damage. J Immunol. 1992;149:1470–5.

18. O'Garra A, Murphy K. T-cell subsets in autoimmunity. Curr Opin Immunol. 1993;5:880–6.

19. Fowell D, Mason D. Evidence that the T cell repertoire of normal ras contains cells with the potential to cause diabetes. Characterization of the CD4[+] T cell subset that inhibits this autoimmune potential. J Exp Med. 1993;177:627–36.

20. Boyum A. Isolation of leukocytes from blood and bone marrow. Scand J Clin Lab Med. 1968;21:97.

21. Brattig NW, Diao G-J, Berg PA. The specificity of the lymphocyte transformation test in a patient with hypersensitivity reactions to pyrazolone compounds. A 10-week follow-up study before and after rechallenge. Eur J Clin Pharmacol. 1988;35:39–45.

22. Lindenborn-fotinos J, Baum H, Berg PA. Mitochondrial antibodies in primary biliary cirrhosis. Further characterization of the M2-antigen by immunoblotting, revealing species and non-species specific determinants. Hepatology. 1985;5:763–9.

23. Bassendine MF, Fussey SPM, Mutimer DJ, James OFW, Yeaman SJ. Identification and characterization of four M2 mitochondrial autoantigens in primary biliary cirrhosis. Semin Liver Dis. 1989;9:124–31.

24. van de Water J, Surh CD, Leung PSC et al. Molecular definitions, autoepitopes and enzymatic activities of the mitochondrial autoantigens of primary biliary cirrhosis. Semin Liver Dis. 1989;9:132–7.

25. Klein R, Klöppel G, Garbe W, Fintelmann V, Berg PA. Antimitochondrial antibody profiles determined at early stages of primary biliary cirrhosis differentiate between a benign and a progressive course of the disease: a retrospective analysis of 76 patients over 6–18 years. J Hepatol. 1991;12;21–7.

26. Klein R, Huizenga JR, Gips CH, Berg PA. Antimitochondrial antibody profiles in patients with primary biliary cirrhosis before orthotopic liver transplantation and titres of antimitochondrial antibody-subtypes after transplantation. J Hepatol. 1994;20:181–9.

27. Berg PA, Klein R. Immunology of PBC. Balliéres Clin Gastroenterol. 1987;1:675–706.

28. Spengler U, Möller A, Jung MC et al. T lymphocytes from patients with primary biliary cirrhosis produce reduced amounts of lymphotoxin, tumor necrosis factor and interferon-γ upon mitogen stimulation. J Hepatol. 1992;15:129–35.

29. Tilg H, Wilmer A, Vogel W et al. Serum levels of cytokines in chronic liver diseases. Gastroenterology. 1992;103:264–74.

30. Broomé U, Eriksson LS, Sundin U, Sundqvist KG. Decreased in vitro production of tumor necrosis factor in primary biliary cirrhosis patients. Scand J Gastroenterol. 1992;27:124–8.

31. Müller C, Zielinski CC. Interleukin-6 production by peripheral blood monocytes in patients with chronic liver disease and acute viral hepatitis. J Hepatol. 1992;15:372–7.

Section VI
Responses of the challenged liver

14
Growth factors in liver disease

W. E. FLEIG

INTRODUCTION

Most liver growth factors have been identified and characterized in the simple experimental model of partial hepatectomy. However, it is very likely that such growth factors and growth inhibitors are not only operative in situations of organogenesis during development and gross regeneration after resection but also in acute and chronic liver disease in which regeneration or lack of regeneration is part of the pathogenetic processes. Table 1 compiles a list of growth factors and growth inhibitors. They act at least on hepatocytes, but many of them also on some of the non-parenchymal cells. None of them is specific for the liver, although hepatocyte growth factor/scatter factor (HGF-SF) was primarily identified by its proliferative action on hepatocytes (for review, see ref. 1). Hepatic stimulatory substance (HSS)[2,3] is not included in this list, since it is not a primary mitogen for hepatocytes and since no information whatsoever is available to date on its potential contribution to the pathophysiology of liver disease. Data regarding the clinical significance of acid fibroblast growth factor (aFGF) and hepatopoietin B[4] are also sparse. The largest body of information has been collected on EGF and TGFα as well as on HGF-SF.

EGF and TGFα are polypeptides which are synthesized in a variety of somatic cells; EGF is synthesized extrahepatically, while TGFα is also produced in hepatocytes[5]. Both peptides share the same receptor. TGFα gene expression in hepatocytes is strikingly increased after partial hepatectomy[6]. HGF-SF, a hetero-

Table 1 Some important growth factors/growth inhibitors for hepatocytes

Growth factors	Growth inhibitors
EGF; TGFα	TGFβ
Acid FGF	Activin A
HGF-SF/HPTA	IL-1
HPTB	IL-6
Norepinephrine	

dimer polypeptide with strong sequence homology to plasminogen, is produced by a wide variety of cell types in various tissues. It represents the most potent mitogen for hepatocytes, while it is inhibitory to the growth of most hepatoma cell lines. HGF is activated by plasminogen activators such as urokinase or tissue plasminogen activator[1]. Its receptor has been identified as the c-met proto-oncogene product[7]. HGF increases TGFα secretion from hepatocytes[8]. Details may be obtained from the articles by Michalopoulos and by Fausto in this book.

In the following, the potential relevance of EGF and TGFα as well as of HGF-SF in liver disease will be reviewed by asking these questions:

1. Is there a relationship between measurable growth factor levels in blood or tissue or mRNA expression and the extent of tissue loss or damage or regeneration?
2. Do growth factor levels in liver disease possess prognostic information?
3. What are the possible mechanisms of action of growth factors in the pathogenesis and pathophysiology of liver disease?
4. May growth factors/growth factor receptors have any therapeutic potential in liver disease?
5. What is the role of growth factors in hepatocarcinogenesis?

1. IS THERE A RELATIONSHIP BETWEEN MEASURABLE GROWTH FACTOR LEVELS IN BLOOD OR TISSUE OR mRNA EXPRESSION AND THE EXTENT OF TISSUE LOSS OR DAMAGE OR REGENERATION?

In experimental models of liver regeneration such as 2/3 hepatectomy or CCl_4 intoxication, blood levels of EGF do not change significantly, while HGF concentrations increase dramatically[1]. In humans, highest plasma HGF levels are found in patients with fulminant hepatic failure[9-12]. However, careful investigation of the hepatic clearance of HGF after partial hepatectomy or experimental CCl_4 intoxication in the rat[13,14] indicates that the increase of HGF in serum or plasma is probably more consequent on decreased hepatic clearance than on increased synthesis and secretion into the bloodstream. In addition, the injured liver releases a peptide called injurin, which induces HGF synthesis at distant, non-hepatic sites[15]. Obviously, systemic inflammation may also be a cause of increased serum HGF concentrations: HGF plasma levels are not only increased in patients after hepatic resection but also after surgery other than liver resection, and the increase correlates with parameters of hepatic injury and systemic inflammation[16]. Thus, the rapid increase of plasma HGF after hepatectomy or liver damage is predominantly related to reduced hepatic clearance caused by the loss of functional liver mass. This does not, however, preclude that increased plasma levels of HGF ultimately derived from extrahepatic sources stimulate liver cell proliferation. In fact, infusion of recombinant human HGF into normal animals succeeded in stimulating replicative DNA synthesis in the liver three- to thirty-fold[17].

In contrast, HGF gene expression in the liver is clearly related to the regenerative processes after various forms of experimental liver injury[18,19]. However, the response appears to be variable depending on the type of injury, with some toxins leading to regeneration in the presence of decreasing HGF gene expression[20]. Obviously, the balance between HGF and other growth stimulators and inhibitors is crucial for the regenerative response, with a decrease of inhibitors but unchanged or even reduced growth stimulators being sufficient to induce proliferation in certain experimental situations. TGFα gene expression in the rat also exhibits a striking temporal relationship to regeneration after partial hepatectomy[5]. A similar relationship between TGFα gene expression and markers of proliferation has been observed in liver tissue of patients with cirrhosis and regenerative nodules[21].

2. DO GROWTH FACTOR LEVELS IN LIVER DISEASE POSSESS PROGNOSTIC INFORMATION?

It has recently been shown that the fraction of necrotic parenchyma on liver biopsies from patients with fulminant hepatic failure is an independent predictor of survival and death and increases the predictive accuracy of the King's College prognostic index in 'borderline' patients[22]. If levels of HGF in plasma are determined by hepatic clearance as shown in the rat[13,14], they might eventually carry similar prognostic information in patients with fulminant liver failure. In fact, plasma HGF levels are significantly higher in severe acute than in chronic liver disease[12]. In this study, a significant correlation with various parameters of hepatocellular necrosis has been described[12], while others have failed to establish such a relationship[11]. In patients with acute liver failure, elevated HGF plasma levels rapidly decrease as liver function improves. Persistently elevated high HGF levels appear to indicate poor prognosis[10–12,23]. Overall, HGF levels in acute hepatitis and fulminant liver failure may reflect loss of hepatocellular function. The prognostic efficacy of HGF concentrations in serum, however, has not yet been defined and compared to more established prognostic indicators.

3. WHAT ARE THE POSSIBLE MECHANISMS OF ACTION OF GROWTH FACTORS IN THE PATHOGENESIS AND PATHOPHYSIOLOGY OF LIVER DISEASE?

In acute liver injury or after hepatectomy, activation of urokinase and subsequent activation of HGF into its active heterodimeric form within minutes may be one of the earliest events. Increasing levels of HGF due to reduced hepatic clearance and increased extrahepatic production may then induce DNA synthesis and proliferation. Furthermore, HGF may lead to a sustained proliferative response through the induction of TGFα synthesis by hepatocytes. Details of this model are described elsewhere in this book.

In chronic liver disease, HGF may be synthesized by Ito cells[24] and sinusoidal endothelial cells[19] and induce proliferation of hepatocytes via a paracrine loop. In alcoholic hepatitis, local infiltrates of granulocytes may be the source of HGF. Similarly, TGFα mRNA expression by hepatocytes and markers of proliferation have been found in biopsy specimen from patients with cirrhosis and regener-

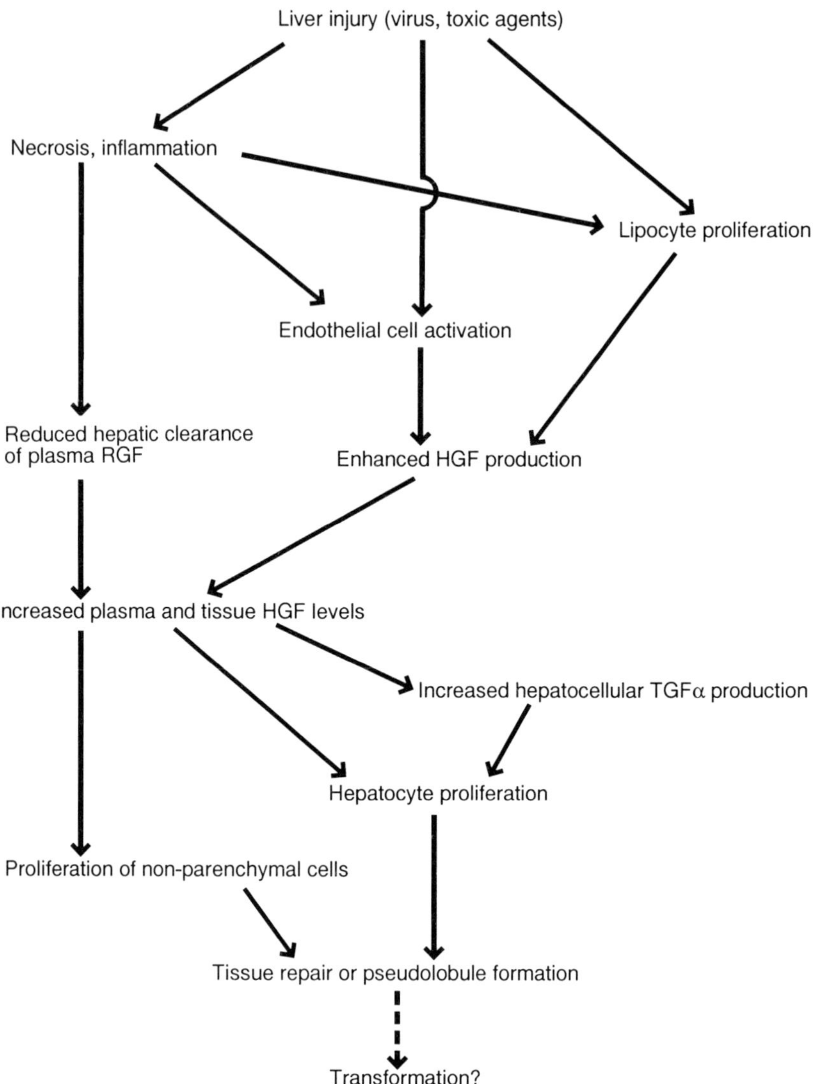

Fig. 1 Hypothetical model of the implication of HGF and TGFα in the mechanisms governing acute and chronic liver injury

ative nodules[21]. Although this latter study suffers from several weaknesses, there is considerable support to the hypothesis that both HGF and TGFα are involved in the complex cytokine network governing fibrogenesis and regeneration in chronic liver disease. A model mechanism is depicted in Fig. 1.

4. MAY GROWTH FACTORS/GROWTH FACTOR RECEPTORS HAVE ANY THERAPEUTIC POTENTIAL IN LIVER DISEASE?

To date, information on the eventual therapeutic value of growth factors in acute and chronic liver disease is sparse. Since HGF levels in fulminant hepatic failure are the highest reported, a lack of HGF does not appear to represent a significant problem, at least at the time point when massive hepatocellular necrosis has already led to fulminant functional organ failure. Similarly, remnant hepatocytes appear to be reactive to growth factors, since similar fractions of proliferating hepatocytes have been found in fulminant and uncomplicated acute hepatitis[25]. Thus, the simple infusion of HGF or TGFα does not appear to be an appealing therapeutic concept. Whether a lack of proliferative response in the early phases of hepatocellular necrosis (i.e. before the proportion of necrotic parenchyma has reached a critical threshold) due to problems of HGF or TGFα receptor expression or in HGF activation may be involved, is unknown.

Infused r-hHGF increases hepatocellular DNA synthesis in normal experimental animals 3–30-fold[17]. Infused or i.v.-injected r-hHGF and TGFα dramatically increase hepatocellular DNA synthesis in 30%-hepatectomized or CCl_4-treated animals[17,26]. Several groups have performed studies into the prevention rather than the treatment of hepatocellular necrosis and liver failure. The protocols used are closely related to the approach used in experimental acute pancreatitis with the eventual protective agent applied simultaneously with or even well before the experimental injury. HGF appears to be protective in rats and mice treated with the cholestatic agent α-naphthylisothiocyanate[27,28]; in rats, some protection could also be shown when treatment was started 12h after application of the toxin[28]. Since cholestasis caused by this compound is different from the various forms of cholestasis in human pathology, these results cannot be simply extrapolated to man. Data obtained in different experimental models are needed. Furthermore, more information about the pathogenesis of fulminant liver failure of different aetiology is required before more sophisticated approaches to treatment rather than a simple infusion of possible growth promoters can be proposed.

5. WHAT IS THE ROLE OF GROWTH FACTORS IN HEPATOCARCINOGENESIS?

The implication of HGF and TGFα and TGFβ in human hepatocarcinogenesis is unclear to date. *In vitro*, HGF is inhibitory to the growth of most[29] but not all[30] hepatoma cells. It can transform immortalized c-met-expressing mouse hepatocytes transfected with HGF[31]. In general, however, it is believed that the action of HGF is anti-tumorigenic rather than tumorigenic. One could speculate that a lack of HGF could result from abundant transformation of HGF-producing Ito cells into non-HGF-producing myofibroblasts, thus allowing the unorganized proliferation of oval cells as an important step in neoplastic transformation. On the other hand, fibroblasts, which are capable of HGF production, should be abundant in active cirrhosis, which is the major risk factor for the development of hepatocellular carcinoma in those parts of the world where hepatitis B is not endemic. Thus, the exact role of HGF in human hepatocarcinogenesis or protection from hepatocellular carcinoma remains to be clarified. Transgenic mice overexpressing TGFα develop hepatocellular adenoma and carcinoma[32]. Again, this cannot simply be transferred to human pathology.

In summary, growth factors such as HGF-SF and TGFα are implicated in the repair mechanisms of acute and chronic liver diseases. A complex interaction between these factors and other cytokines as well as between hepatocytes and non-parenchymal liver cells and between the liver and other potential sources of growth factors exists.

The role of HGF-SF and TGFα in hepatocellular carcinogenesis is not sufficiently understood. *In vitro*, most hepatocellular carcinoma cell lines are suppressed by HGF. TGFα transgenic mice develop hepatocellular tumors.

HGF plasma levels reflect tissue damage and systemic inflammatory response rather than hepatic regeneration. Persistently high HGF levels in fulminant hepatic failure correlate with poor prognosis. Fulminant hepatic failure is not caused by hepatocellular unresponsiveness to growth factors.

HGF administration in experimental situations *in vivo* induces hepatocyte proliferation and prevents or inhibits hepatotoxicity of drugs. Further investigation regarding its potential clinical use is necessary.

REFERENCES

1. Michalopoulos GK, Zarnegar R. Hepatocyte growth factor. Hepatology. 1992;15:149–55.
2. La Brecque DR. In vitro stimulation of cell growth by hepatic stimulator substance. Am J Physiol. 1982;242:G289–95.
3. Fleig WE, Lehmann H, Wagner H, et al. Hepatic regenerative stimulator substance in the rabbit. Relation to liver regeneration after partial hepatectomy. J Hepatol. 1986;3:19–26.
4. Michalopoulos G, Houck KA, Dolan ML, et al. Control of hepatocyte replication by two serum factors. Cancer Res. 1982;42:4673–82.
5. Mead JE, Fausto N. Transforming growth factor α may be a physiological regulator of liver regeneration by means of an autocrine mechanism. Proc Natl Acad Sci USA. 1989;86:1558–62.
6. Fausto N, Mead JE. Regulation of liver growth: protooncogenes and transforming growth factors. Lab Invest. 1989;60:4–13.
7. Bottaro DP, Rubin JS, Faletto DL, et al. Identification of the hepatocyte growth factor receptor as the c-*met* proto-oncogene product. Science. 1991;251:802–4.
8. Webber E, FitzGerald MJ, Brown PI, Bartlett MH, Fausto N. Transforming growth factor-α expression during liver regeneration after partial hepatectomy and toxic injury, and potential interactions between transforming growth factor-α and hepatocyte growth factor. Hepatology. 193;18:1422–31.
9. Gohda E, Tsubouchi H, Nakayama H, et al. Human hepatocyte growth factor in blood of patients with fulminant hepatic failure. Basic aspects. Dig Dis Sci. 1991;36:785–90.
10. Tsubouchi H, Hirono S, Gohda E, et al. Human hepatocyte growth factor in blood of patients with fulminant hepatic failure. Clinical aspects. Dig Dis Sci. 1991;36:780–4.
11. Tsubouchi H, Niitani Y, Hirono S, et al. Levels of human hepatocyte growth factor in serum of patients with various liver diseases determined by an enzyme-linked immunosorbent assay. Hepatology. 1991;13:1–5.
12. Tomiya T, Nagoshi S, Fujiwara K. Significance of serum human hepatocyte growth factor levels in patients with hepatic failure. Hepatology. 1992;15:1–4.
13. Appasamy R, Tanabe M, Murase N, Zarnegar R, Venkataramanan R, van Thiel D, Michalopoulos GK. Hepatocyte growth factor blood clearance, organ uptake, and biliary excretion in normal and partially hepatectomized rats. Lab Invest. 1993;68:270–6.

14. Liu K-X, Kato Y, Yamazaki M, Higuchi O, Nakamura T, Sugiyama Y. Decrease in the hepatic clearance of hepatocyte growth factor in carbon tetrachloride-intoxicated rats. Hepatology. 1993; 17:651–60.
15. Matsumoto K, Tajima H, Hamanoue M, Kohno S, Kinoshita T, Nakamura T. Identification and characterisation of 'injurin', an inducer of expression of the gene for hepatocyte growth factor. Proc Natl Acad Sci USA. 1992;89:3800–4.
16. Tomiya T, Tani M, Yamada S, Hayashi S, Umeda N, Fujiwara K. Serum hepatocyte growth factor levels in hepatectomized and nonhepatectomized surgical patients. Gastroenterology. 1992;103:1621–4.
17. Fujiwara K, Nagoshi S, Ohno A, et al. Stimulation of liver growth by exogenous human hepatocyte growth factor in normal and partially hepatectomized rats. Hepatology. 1993;18:1443–9.
18. Hamanoue M, Kawaida K, Takao S, Shimazu H, Noji S, Matsumoto K, Nakamura T. Rapid and marked induction of hepatocyte growth factor during liver regeneration after ischemic or crush injury. Hepatology. 1992;16:1485–92.
19. Maher JJ. Cell-specific expression of hepatocyte growth factor in liver. Upregulation in sinusoidal endothelial cells after carbon tetrachloride. J Clin Invest. 1993;91:2244–52.
20. Masuhara M, Katyal L, Nakamura T, Shinozuka H. Differential expression of hepatocyte growth factor, transforming growth factor-α and transforming growth factor-β_1 in two experimental models of liver cell proliferation. Hepatology. 1992;16:1241–9.
21. Castilla A, Prieto J, Fausto N. Transforming growth factors β_1 and α in chronic liver disease. Effects of interferon alfa therapy. N Engl J Med. 1991;324:933–40.
22. Donaldson BW, Gopinath R, Wanless IR, et al. The role of transjugular liver biopsy in fulminant liver failure: Relation to other prognostic indicators. Hepatology. 1993;18:1370–4.
23. Takemura M, Furuta N, Nakamura S, et al. Determination and clinical significance of human hepatocyte growth factor in serum. Rinsho-Byori. 1992;40:1168–72.
24. Schirrmacher P, Geerts A, Pietrangelo A, Dienes HP, Rogler CE. Hepatocyte growth factor/ Hepatopoietin A is expressed in fat-storing cells from rat liver but not myofibroblast-like cells derived from fat-storing cells. Hepatology. 1992;15:5–11.
25. Wolf HK, Michalopoulos GK. Hepatocyte regeneration in acute fulminant and nonfulminant hepatitis: a study of proliferating cell nuclear antigen expression. Hepatology. 1992;15:707–13.
26. Webber EM, Godowski PJ, Fausto N. In vivo response of hepatocytes to growth factors requires an initial priming stimulus. Hepatology. 1994;14:489–97.
27. Ishiki Y, Ohnishi H, Muto Y, Matsumoto K, Nakamura T. Direct evidence that hepatocyte growth factor is a hepatotrophic factor for liver regeneration and has a potent antihepatitis effect in vivo. Hepatology. 1992;16:1227–35.
28. Roos F, Terrell TG, Godowski PJ, Charnow SM, Schwall RH. Reduction of α-naphthyl-isothiocyanate-induced hepatotoxicity by recombinant human hepatocyte growth factor. Endocrinology. 1992;131:2540–4.
29. Shiota G, Rhoads DB, Wang TC, Nakamura T, Schmidt EV. Hepatocyte growth factor inhibits growth of hepatocellular carcinoma cells. Proc Natl Acad Sci USA. 1992;89:373–7.
30. Miyazaki M, Gohda E, Tsuboi S, Tsunoi H, Daikuhara Y, Namba M, Yamamoto I. Human hepatocyte growth factor stimulates the growth of HUH-6 clone 5 human hepatoblastoma cells. Cell Biol Int Rep. 1992;16:145–54.
31. Kanda H, Tajima H, Lee GH, et al. Hepatocyte growth factor transforms immortalized mouse liver epithelial cells. Oncogene. 1993;8:3047–53.
32. Jhappan C, Stahle C, Harkins RN, Fausto N, Smith GH, Merlino GT. TGF-α overexpression in transgenic mice induces liver neoplasia and abnormal development of the mammary gland and pancreas. Cell. 1990;61:1137–46.

15
Cytokine regulation of hepatic acute phase protein expression

Z. XING, C. D. RICHARDS, T. BRACIAK, V. THIBAULT and
J. GAULDIE

INTRODUCTION

The body responds to infection or trauma through a complex series of reactions aimed at stopping the initiating set of events, minimizing the ongoing tissue damage, and returning the body to normal function. This homeostatic response, termed inflammation, has a number of local and systemic aspects that are inter-related[1-3]. One of the most prominent of the responses is that of the liver, which demonstrates significantly altered gene regulation and enhanced expression of a series of hepatic derived proteins – the acute phase proteins[4-7]. This hepatic response occurs as a result of circulating mediators, released from the site of trauma or infection, interacting with specific receptors on the hepatocyte and initiating specific gene expression. Many of the functions subtended by these acute phase proteins – opsonins, coagulation components, antiproteases and scavengers – are anti-inflammatory in nature, and the molecular control of this homeostatic acute phase response can therefore be seen as the control of the anti-inflammatory response.

The fact that the liver responds to a distal inflammation indicates a systemic circulating mediator(s) and several have now been identified and cloned and are responsible for the initiation of the hepatic acute phase response. Two groups of cytokines appear to be responsible for the initiation of the hepatic response. The first group are early or acute phase cytokines, including interleukin-1 (IL-1) and tumour necrosis factor (TNF), molecules which act directly at the liver as well as indirectly by initiating a secondary cascade of cytokines. Members of the second group, the interleukin-6 (IL-6) family, which includes a diverse group of leukaemia inhibitory factor (LIF), interleukin-11 (IL-11), oncostatin M (OM) and ciliary neurotrophic factor (CNTF), are all capable of being released in a primary fashion from a variety of cells but their synthesis is stimulated in stromal cells by molecules such as IL-1 and TNF. Interleukin-6 is known to be the primary regulator of the hepatic acute phase response in vivo while the others can

Table 1 Regulation of hepatic acute phase protein production

Effectors	*APP response*
IL-1-type cytokines (IL-1α, IL-1β, TNF-α, TNF-β)	Stimulation of type-1 APP: C-reactive protein (human) serum amyloid A α_1-acid glycoprotein complement C3 haptoglobin (rat) haemopexin (rat) Inhibition of type-2 APP
IL-6-type cytokines (IL-6, IL-11, LIF, OSM, CNTF)	Stimulation of most APP Primary activator of type-2 APP: α, β and γ fibrinogen α_2-macroglobulin (rat) thiostatin (rat) α_1-antitrypsin α_1-antichymotrypsin (or contrapsin in rodents) haptoglobin (human) haemopexin (human) ceruloplasmin Synergism with IL-1-type cytokines on type-1 APP
Glucocorticoids	Minor stimulation of most APP strong stimulation of rat α_1-acid glycoprotein Strong synergistic enhancement of cytokine effects on most APP
Insulin	Reductions of IL-1- and IL-6-type cytokine effects on most APP
HGF, FGF	Minor reduction of IL-1- and IL-6-type cytokine effects on most APP Enhancement of IL-1-type cytokine effects on rat α_1-acid glycoprotein and complement C3
Hormones acting via cyclic nucleotides or calcium mobilization	No detectable regulatory effect on APP

Abbreviations: APPs, acute phase plasma proteins; IL, interleukin; TNF-α, tumor necrosis factor-α; LIF, leukemia inhibitory factor; OSM, oncostatin M; CNTF, ciliary neutrotrophic factor; HGF, hepatocyte growth factor; FGF, fibroblast growth factor

all elicit acute phase protein expression in isolated hepatocyte or hepatoma cultures[8–17].

The main effect of these mediators on the induction of the hepatic-derived acute phase proteins is summarized in Table 1. The liver responds to IL-6 by the enhanced production of type 2 or IL-6-specific acute phase proteins, mostly opsonins and antiproteases. Since the other members of the IL-6 family cause signal transduction through the common receptor gp130[18], similar qualitative patterns of gene expression are seen[19]. IL-1 and TNF regulate a distinct subgroup of the acute phase protein genes, the type 1 genes, and act in a synergistic manner with IL-6, best seen in stimulation of α1-acid glycoprotein. IL-1 does not stimulate type 2 genes and may, in some cases, interfere with IL-6 stimulation[1,6,7,12,13]. Corticosteroid, a third and required hormone for maximum

Table 2 Acute-phase protein response[20]

Treatment	Haptoglobin		α_1-AGP		SAA	
	IL-6[+/+]	IL-6[-/-]	IL-6[+/+]	IL-6[-/-]	IL-6[+/+]	IL-6[-/-]
Control						
mRNA	1.0	1.2	1.0	0.7	<0.2	<0.2
Serum (mg/ml)	<0.1	<0.1	0.4	0.3	ND	ND
Turpentine 24h						
mRNA	23.7	4.5	48.4	3.9	100	1
Serum (mg/ml)	4.0	0.9	1.2	0.3	ND	ND
Listeria 48h						
mRNA	13.9	3.9	32.9	5.2	40	1
Serum (mg/ml)	2.6	1.2	1.0	0.4	ND	ND
LPS 26h						
mRNA	16.0	7.6	27.1	10.8	55	25
Serum (mg/ml)	1.7	0.7	1.2	0.7	ND	ND
IL-7 24h						
mRNA	4.1	8.3	1.8	7.7	12	14
Serum (mg/ml)	0.5	0.9	0.6	0.6	ND	ND

stimulation of acute phase protein expression, also acts in a synergistic fashion with IL-1 and IL-6.

Recent data obtained from experiments using recombinant embryonic stem cell technology have shown that mice in which the gene for IL-6 is knocked out[20] can still demonstrate a hepatic acute phase response when the inflammatory reaction is initiated by i.v. endotoxin challenge, implying that in this system other members of the IL-6 family can be in the circulation and can initiate the response. However, if the inflammation is initiated by s.c. injection of turpentine the hepatic acute phase response is not apparent, demonstrating a purely IL-6-dependent reaction (Table 2). Undoubtedly, other trauma and infectious systems will involve multiple cytokines in the initiation and propagation of the hepatic response but IL-6 appears to be the primary and major regulator in vivo and forms the basis for many of the investigations attempting to relate the presence of IL-6 in circulation to the plasma changes seen when the liver becomes activated during inflammation.

Cytokines in vivo

A number of studies have demonstrated raised levels of IL-6 during the inflammatory response: this increased plasma level of IL-6 correlates with an increase in the level of hepatic-derived acute phase proteins in circulation[6,7]. Direct injection of recombinant IL-6 leads to initiation of hepatic synthesis of the acute phase proteins[17]. However, one of the drawbacks of investigating how cytokines work in vivo is their short half-life in the circulation. IL-6 disappears rapidly from circulation ($T_{1/2}$ between 15 and 35 min) and this does not mimic inflammatory responses, where the level of IL-6 is raised over a long period of time[10]. In various experimental models of inflammation in the rat, IL-6 levels are significantly raised over several days and this is directly associated with hepatic responses[21]. Figure 1 shows the changes seen in plasma levels of IL-6, corti-

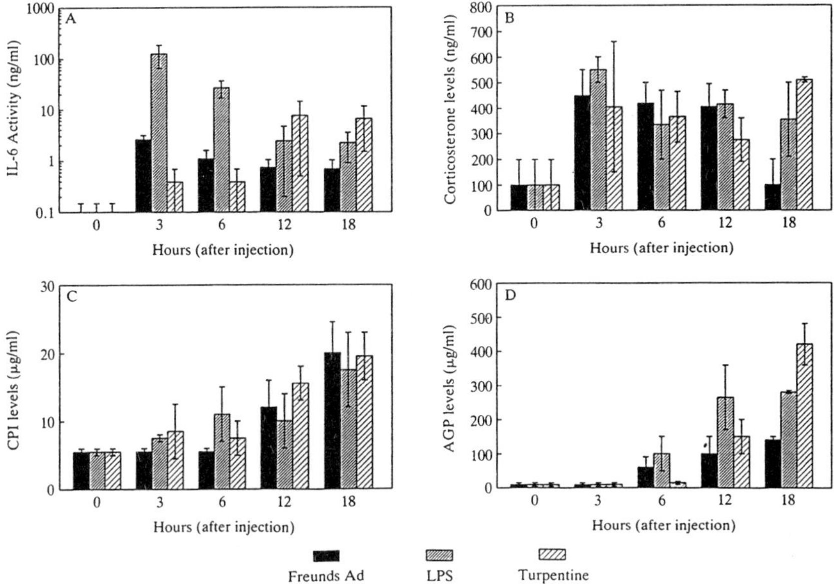

Fig. 1 Serum levels of (**A**) IL-6, (**B**) corticosterone, (**C**) cysteine proteinase inhibitor (CPI) and (**D**) α1-acid glycoprotein (AGP) of FA-, LPS- and turpentine-treated rats. Samples for each time point represent the average amount (with range) calculated from two rats injected with the eliciting agent. Adapted from Geisterfer et al.[21]

costerone and cysteine proteinase inhibitor, one of the major acute phase proteins in the rat, in three separate models of inflammation.

While it is possible to achieve raised plasma levels of cytokine over a prolonged period of time using mini-osmotic pumps[22] this is not so desirable as the pump insertion itself induces an inflammatory response. The most significant findings have occurred when new molecular biology techniques have been used to achieve constant over-expression of the IL-6 gene resulting in chronically raised levels of IL-6 in the plasma. The first studies used a transgenic mouse model in which the IL-6 gene was driven by an IgM promoter[23]. These animals showed raised IL-6 levels from birth but the response of the liver was not investigated to any great extent. It was notable that these animals died with some aspects of wasting. A second approach involves the use of recombinant retrovirus vectors to deliver the IL-6 gene and integrate the gene into the stem cell genome. Hawley succeeded in deriving bone marrow stem cells with the IL-6 gene driven by the cytomegalovirus promoter[24], and used these stem cells to reconstitute irradiated syngeneic recipients. This results in mice bearing cells that have the ability to overexpress the IL-6 gene, and significantly raised plasma levels of IL-6 are seen for as long as the mouse remains viable. Notably, there was a significant acute phase response and raised levels of acute phase proteins such as haptoglobin, but these animals appeared cachectic with various abnormalities in their haematopoietic systems. Hawley also developed a similar system with the IL-11 gene but these animals were markedly cachectic and died with severe wasting[25]. Finally, Henderson et al.[26] used a retrovirus to achieve overexpression of CNTF in tumour cells: administration of these cells to recipient mice resulted in prolonged high levels of CNTF in the circulation. Similar to previous findings, these animals died of gross cachexia within 7 days, whereas all of the appropriate controls, including one in which tumour cells were infected with a retrovirus incorporating a mutant and non-active CNTF gene, were relatively normal.

Taken together, these data imply that transgenic and permanently transfected models for overexpression of cytokines, in particular those associated with the hepatic acute phase response, yield equivocal data. It is not known whether all of these cytokines give rise to the cachectic response. However there are clearly multiple distortions in the system and the outcomes of overexpression are quite different than those expected from the physiological inflammatory response.

Adenovirus vectors for cytokine gene transfer

Given these restrictions, we have recently developed a model in which the IL-6 gene is transiently overexpressed in various tissues by the use of recombinant adenovirus vectors to deliver the IL-6 gene[27,28]. Construction of the recombinant virus involves insertion of the rodent IL-6 cDNA into either the E1 or E3 region of the human type 5 adenovirus genome. Disruption in E1 results in viral replication deficiency whereas the recombinant virus with the insertion in E3 remains replication efficient, since only the E1 region is essential for viral replication. The construction of recombinant viruses deficient in E1 or E3, nevertheless, involves similar strategies. In the instance of E1 insertion, a fragment of the murine IL-6 cDNA is ligated into the E1 multicloning site of a plasmid which accommodates a human cytomegalovirus promoter and a SV40 poly(A^+) signal in 3′ to 5′ orientation. The resulting construct containing the left 16% of the adenovirus genome is co-transfected into 293 cells, which provide the E1 function in *trans*, along with a second plasmid containing all of the adenoviral genomic sequences but the left end. The recombinant virus with murine IL-6 gene incorporated in E1 driven by the CMV promoter is rescued by homologous recombination.

Several cell types including fibroblasts and epithelial cells can be infected with the recombinant virus, producing IL-6 in vitro. For instance, upon infection of 293 cells with 10 pfu/cell of the virus carrying the IL-6 gene in the E1 or E3 region, large amounts of IL-6 are produced and released as assessed by the B9 hybridoma growth assay, while undetectable or very low levels of IL-6 are seen with non-infected or control virus-infected cells. Consistent with the nature of the E1 activities, the cells infected with E1-deficient virus appear to produce lower amounts of IL-6 and significant production seems to occur somewhat later than in those infected with the E3 virus. On average, by 72 h the E1 virus- and E3 virus-infected cells produce some 10–100 μg/ml of IL-6, respectively.

The advantage of the adenovirus system is that the gene is incorporated into cells but does not integrate into the genome, as it does with the retroviral system. When the virus is introduced into the peritoneal cavity of an animal it infects the local stromal cells as well as some of the parenchymal cells of the liver and the

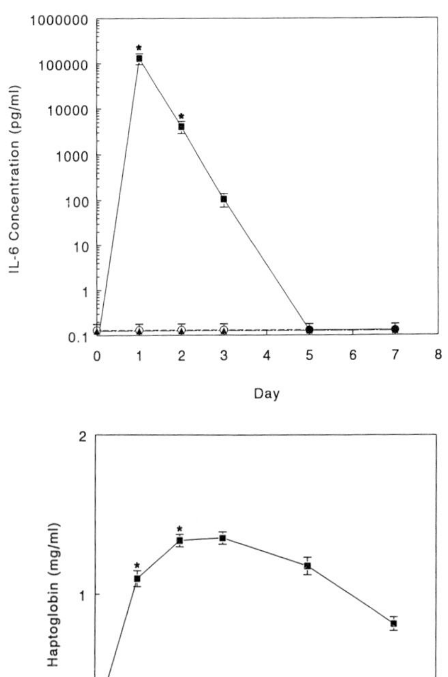

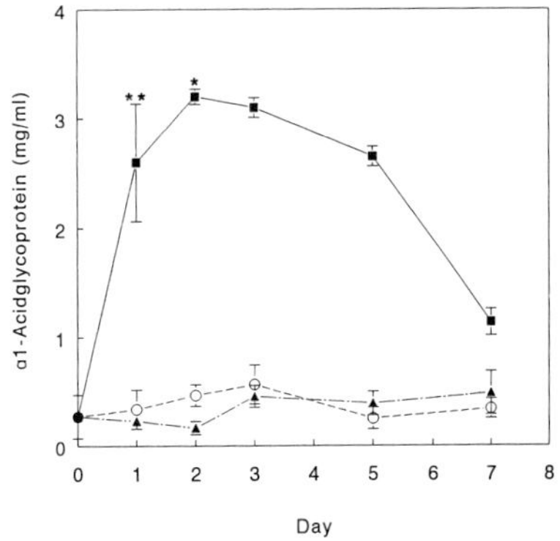

Fig. 2 Serum levels of IL-6 and acute phase proteins in mice treated with recombinant adenovirus IL-6 vector (Ad5mIL-6; ■). Control animals received a control non-cytokine adenovirus vector (AdgB8; o) or saline (▲) i.p. (**A**) IL-6 levels, (**B**) haptoglobin levels and (**C**) α1-acid glycoprotein levels. Mean±SD with $n=4$. *$p<0.01$; **$p<0.02$. Adapted from Braciak et al.[27]

spleen. Infection leads to specific cytokine gene expression since the gene is driven by the incorporated cytomegalovirus promoter. Intraperitoneal injection of the virus encoding the IL-6 gene results in a transient but prolonged raised level of IL-6 in the circulation (5–7 days) and concomitantly increased levels of the acute phase proteins, indicating that the liver has responded to the raised IL-6 levels (Fig. 2). No such changes in hepatic function are seen in animals receiving control viruses. This indicates that the system allows the investigation of single cytokine function and in the case of the IL-6-expressing virus, the data indicate that prolonged exposure to IL-6 can initiate the acute phase response and, as long as the effect is transient, no evidence of wasting or cachexia is seen and the animals fully recover after the infection has dissipated. The use of a virus which has been crippled in its ability to replicate (E_1-deficient) and one which appears to cause local expression wherever it has been introduced into the tissues is an excellent way in which the function of a single cytokine can be examined in vivo and its effect on hepatic function evaluated.

We have also made recombinant adenovirus constructs expressing the soluble form of rat IL-6 receptor. The soluble receptor appears to be present in circulation at some considerable levels, and these may be raised in pathological conditions[29,30]. This is important since the soluble receptor has been shown to be an agonist to the action of IL-6 in growth and proliferation assays and may therefore contribute to aspects of hepatic response[31]. The current viral construct was made by cloning the extracellular domain of the rat IL-6 receptor[21] coupled to a signal peptide into the adenovirus vector driven by the CMV promoter. The signal peptide allows the soluble IL-6 receptor to be exported from the cells that have been infected and the material then enters the circulation.

These reagents and recombinant virus constructs expressing other members of the IL-6 family of cytokines will be invaluable in attempting to delineate the specific role played by each cytokine in regulating the hepatic acute phase response. Thus, the data imply that a given inflammatory stimulus gives rise to a specific spectrum of cytokines which interact with specific receptors on the hepatocyte to cause acute phase and other gene regulation resulting in the acute phase response. The quantity and quality of the gene expression response depends on the amount and sequence of interaction with the various cytokines. Apparently simple systems such as a sterile abscess induced by turpentine depend on a single cytokine for regulation while others such as endotoxin activation involve several cytokines. The transient transgenic system described for the use of recombinant adenovirus to examine single cytokines roles appears to be able to restrict the interpretation to the response elicited by the specific ctyokine.

References

1. Baumann H, Gauldie J. The acute phase response. Immunol Today. 1994;15:74–80.
2. Gauldie J. Acute phase response. In: Dulbecco R, editor. The encyclopedia of human biology. San Diego: Academic Press; 1991:1–11.
3. Kushner I. The phenomenon of the acute phase response. Ann NY Acad Sci. 1982;389:39–48.
4. Fey G, Gauldie J. The acute phase response of the liver in inflammation. In: Popper H, Schaffner F, editors. Progress in Liver Diseases, vol. 89. Philadelphia: WB Saunders, 1990:89–116.
5. Koj A, Gordon AH. The acute-phase response to injury and infection (introduction). In: Dingle JT, Gordon JL, editors. Research monographs in cell and tissue pathology, Vol. 10. Amsterdam: Elsevier, 1985:xxi–xxix.
6. Richards CD, Gauldie J. The acute-phase protein response. In: Dale MM, Foreman JC, Fan T-PD, editors. Textbook of immunopharmacology. London: Blackwell Scientific Publications, 1994:269–76.
7. Richards CD, Gauldie J. Induction of inflammation: cytokines and acute-phase proteins. Xenobiotics Inflamm. 1994;4:71–96.
8. Gauldie J, Richards C, Harnish D, Lansdorp P, Baumann H. Interferon-beta2/B-cell stimulatory factor type 2 shares identity with monocyte hepatocyte-stimulating factor and regulates the major acute phase protein response in liver cells. Proc Natl Acad Sci USA. 1987;84:7251–5.
9. Baumann H, Gauldie J. Regulation of hepatic acute phase plasma protein genes by hepatocyte stimulating factors and other mediators of inflammation. Mol Biol Med. 1990;7:147–59.
10. Castell JV, Andus T, Kunz D, Heinrich PC. Interleukin-6: the major regulator of acute-phase protein synthesis in man and rat. Ann NY Acad Sci. 1989;557:86–101.
11. Andus T, Geiger T, Hirano T et al. Regulation of synthesis and secretion of major rat acute-phase proteins by recombinant human interleukin-6 (BSF-2/IL-6) in hepatocyte primary cultures. Eur J Biochem. 1988;173:287–93.
12. Baumann H, Richards C, Gauldie J. Interaction between hepatocyte-stimulating factors, interleukin-1 and glucocorticoids for regulation of acute phase proteins in human hepatoma (Hep-G2) cells. J Immunol. 1987;139:4122–8.
13. Baumann H, Onorato V, Gauldie J, Jahreis GP. Distinct sets of acute phase plasma proteins are stimulated by separate human hepatocyte-stimulating factors and monokines in rat hepatoma cells. J Biol Chem. 1987;262:9756–68.

14. Baumann H, Schendel P. Interleukin-11 regulates the hepatic expression of the same plasma protein genes as interleukin-6. J Biol Chem. 1991;266:1–4.

15. Baumann H, Wong GG. Hepatocyte-stimulating Factor III shares structural and function identity with leukemia inhibitory factor. J Immunol. 1989;13:1162–7.

16. Richards CD, Brown TJ, Shoyab M, Baumann H, Gauldie J. Recombinant oncostatin-M stimulates the production of acute phase proteins in hepatocytes in vitro. J Immunol. 1992;148:1731–6.

17. Geiger T, Andus T, Klapproth J, Hirano T, Kishimoto T, Heinrich PC. Induction of rat acute-phase proteins by interleukin 6 in vivo. Eur J Immunol. 1988;18:717–21.

18. Taga T, Kishimoto T. Cytokine receptors and signal transduction. FASEB J. 1992;6:3387–96.

19. Richards C, Gauldie J, Baumann H. Cytokine control of acute phase protein expression. Eur Cytokine Net. 1992;2:89–98.

20. Kopf M, Baumann H, Freer G et al. Impaired immune and acute-phase responses in interleukin-6-deficient mice. Nature. 1994;368:339–42.

21. Geisterfer M, Richards CD, Baumann M, Fey G, Gwynne D, Gauldie J. Regulation of IL-6 and hepatic IL-6 receptor in acute inflammation in vivo. Cytokine. 1993;5:1–7.

22. Rubbia-Brandt L, Sappino A-P, Gabbiani G. Locally applied GM-CSF induces the accumulation of α-smooth muscle actin containing myofibroblasts. Virchows Archiv B Cell Pathol. 1991;60:73–82.

23. Suematsu S, Matsuda T, Aozasa K et al. IgG1 plasmacytosis in interleukin 6 transgenic mice. Proc Natl Acad Sci USA. 1989;86:7547–51.

24. Hawley RG, Fong AZ, Burns BF, Hawley TS. Transplantable myeloproliferative disease induced in mice by an interleukin 6 retrovirus. J Exp Med. 1992;176:1149–63.

25. Hawley TS. Progenitor cell hyperplasia with rare development of myeloid leukemia in interleukin 11 bone marrow chimeras. J Exp Med. 1993;178:1175–88.

26. Henderson JT, Seniuk NA, Richardson PM, Gauldie J, Roder JC. Systemic administration of ciliary neurotrophic factor induces cachexia in rodents. J Clin Invest. 1994;93:2632–8.

27. Braciak TA, Mittal SK, Graham FL, Richards CD, Gauldie J. Construction of recombinant human type 5 adenoviruses expressing rodent IL-6 genes: an approach to investigate in vivo cytokine function. J Immunol. 1993;151:5145–53.

28. Xing Z, Braciak T, Jordana M, Croitoru K, Graham FL, Gauldie J. Adenovirus-mediated cytokine gene transfer at tissue sites: Overexpression of IL-6 induces lymphocytic hyperplasia in the lung. J Immunol. 1994;153:4059–69.

29. Honda M, Yamamoto S, Cheng M et al. Human soluble IL-6 receptor: its detection and enhanced release by HIV infection. J Immunol. 1992;148:2175–80.

30. Frieling JTM, Sauerwein RW, Wijdenes J, Hendriks T, van der Linden CJ. Soluble interleukin 6 receptor in biological fluids from human origin. Cytokine. 1994;6:376–81.

31. Mackiewicz AJ, Schooltink H, Henrich PC, Rose-John S. Complex of soluble human IL-6-receptor/IL-6 up-regulates expression of acute-phase proteins. J Immunol. 1992;149:2021–7.

16
Cytokine-induced alterations in hepatic lipid metabolism

K. R. FEINGOLD, I. HARDARDÓTTIR and C. GRUNFELD

INTRODUCTION

Infection, inflammation and trauma commonly induce changes in lipid metabolism. Many of the host's responses to injury are mediated by cytokines, such as tumour necrosis factor (TNF), the interleukins (IL), and the interferons (IFN); numerous studies have demonstrated that cytokines can alter lipid metabolism in the liver and other tissues. In this review we will describe the changes in lipid metabolism induced by cytokines, emphasizing the important role of the liver. We will also discuss the potential detrimental and/or beneficial effects of these alterations.

EFFECT OF CYTOKINES ON TRIGLYCERIDE METABOLISM

Administration of TNF, IL-1, IL-2, IFN-α and IFN-γ increases serum triglyceride levels by increasing levels of very low density lipoprotein (VLDL)[1-16]. The increase in serum triglyceride levels induced by TNF and IL-1 in rodents is rapid, with the peak occurring by 2h and triglyceride levels remaining elevated for at least 17h[2,14]. In contrast, continuous infusion of TNF or IL-1 decreases serum triglyceride levels[17,18]. However, it should be recognized that TNF and IL-1 are usually released in a pulsatile fashion in response to stimuli; thus the continuous delivery of TNF and IL-1 could have effects that differ from the usual physiological patterns. Bolus administration of TNF once or twice a day for as long as 7 days results in sustained hypertriglyceridaemia[19].

Early studies demonstrated that TNF and IL-1 decrease the activity of lipoprotein lipase in cultured adipocytes[20-22]. A decrease in activity of this enzyme in adipose tissue could produce hypertriglyceridaemia by slowing the clearance of triglyceride-rich lipoproteins. However, studies by our laboratory and others have shown that TNF and IL-1 increase serum triglyceride levels chiefly by stimulating hepatic lipoprotein secretion. First, although TNF and IL-1 decrease lipoprotein lipase activity in adipose tissue in vivo, this decrease is delayed, requiring several hours, whereas the increase in serum triglyceride levels occurs rapidly, preceding the inhibition of lipoprotein lipase activity[23,24]. Second, neither TNF nor IL-1 delay the clearance of triglyceride rich lipoproteins from the circulation[7,13,14,16,25]. Third, TNF and IL-1 rapidly stimulate triglyceride synthesis and secretion by the liver[7,14,26]. Together these results indicate that the increase in serum triglyceride levels in TNF and IL-1-treated rodents is primarily due to increased hepatic production.

There are two main sources for the fatty acids that form triglycerides in the liver; de novo hepatic fatty acid synthesis and the re-esterification of fatty acids derived from lipolysis in adipose tissue. In intact animals, TNF, IFN-α and IFN-γ acutely stimulate lipolysis, raising serum free fatty acid levels[2,7,14,27–29]. In cultured adipocytes, TNF, IL-1 and IFN-α, -β and -γ stimulate lipolysis[21,22,30–32]. These peripherally derived fatty acids may contribute to the cytokine induced increase in hepatic VLDL secretion.

TNF-α, lymphotoxin (TNF-β), IL-1, IL-6 and IFN-α stimulate de novo fatty acid synthesis in the liver, while IL-2 and IFN-γ do not affect hepatic acid synthesis under similar conditions[2,7,14,26,33,34]. In vitro studies have demonstrated that TNF, IL-1 and IFN-α (but not IFN-γ) increase lipid synthesis and secretion in HepG2 cells, although exposure for 24h is needed for this effect[35]. The increase in hepatic fatty acid synthesis induced by TNF in vivo is observed under a variety of diets ranging from high sucrose to high fat[36]. Only prolonged starvation prevents the TNF-induced increase in hepatic fatty acid synthesis[36]. This stimulation of hepatic fatty acid could provide fatty acids for the cytokine-induced increase in hepatic triglyceride secretion.

TNF, IL-1 and IL-6 stimulate hepatic fatty acid synthesis by increasing hepatic levels of citrate, an allosteric activator of acetyl CoA carboxylase, the rate limiting enzyme in fatty acid synthesis[34,37,38]. In contrast, IFN-α has no effect on hepatic citrate levels; the mechanism by which IFN-α stimulates fatty acid synthesis in the liver is unknown[38].

These observations suggest that there are two classes of cytokines that stimulate hepatic fatty acid synthesis; TNF, IL-1, and IL-6 in one class and IFN-α in another. Additional support for these two classes has been provided by experiments using a combination of cytokines. When IFN-α is administered simultaneously with either TNF or IL-1, they act synergistically in stimulating hepatic lipogenesis[38]. In contrast, maximum doses of TNF and IL-1 are not additive when given simultaneously and doses that are ineffective alone do not show synergy when given in combination[38]. Furthermore, IL-4, an inhibitory anti-inflammatory cytokine, by itself has no effect on hepatic fatty acid synthesis; it does, however, inhibit the stimulation of hepatic lipogenesis induced by TNF, IL-1, and IL-6[39]. IL-4 blocks the ability of these cytokines to stimulate fatty acid synthesis in the liver by preventing the increase in hepatic citrate levels[39]. However, IL-4 has no effect on the ability of IFN-α to stimulate hepatic fatty acid synthesis[39]. These findings provide additional support for the hypothesis that there are at least two classes of cytokines that stimulate hepatic fatty acid synthesis. Moreover, these results demonstrate that complex inter-relationships exist between cytokines in regulating hepatic lipid metabolism, with some cytokines acting by similar mechanisms, some by different mechanisms, some exhibiting synergistic interactions, and some cytokines inhibiting the action of other cytokines.

TNF does not affect the activity of the enzymes involved in esterification of fatty acids to glycerol[27] indicating that the TNF-induced increase in hepatic triglyceride production is primarily driven by the availability of fatty acid substrate. The effect of other cytokines on esterification has not been investigated. Whether increased de novo fatty acid synthesis in the liver or increased lipolysis in adipose tissue is the primary source of fatty acids depends on the specific cytokine studied and the state of the animal. IL-1 increases hepatic triglyceride secretion solely by increasing fatty acid synthesis in the liver[3]. In chow-fed animals, TNF increases hepatic triglyceride secretion by stimulating both lipolysis and hepatic fatty acid synthesis while in sucrose-fed animals, TNF does not stimulate lipolysis but markedly increases hepatic fatty acid synthesis, which is the source of fatty acids for hepatic triglyceride secretion[27]. These results demonstrate the importance of nutritional status in modulating the mechanisms by which cytokines regulate lipid metabolism.

It is possible that under different experimental conditions (higher doses of cytokines, different species, different time points of study, etc.) other mechanisms, such as inhibition of lipoprotein lipase activity and decreased lipoprotein clearance, could play a role in the cytokine-induced increase in serum triglyceride levels. We have recently shown that while low doses of endotoxin (100 ng/100 g body weight) rapidly increase serum triglyceride levels in rats primarily by stimulating hepatic lipoprotein secretion, high doses of endotoxin (50 μg/100 g body weight) do not stimulate hepatic lipoprotein secretion but rather inhibit the clearance of triglyceride rich lipoproteins and decrease lipoprotein lipase activity[40]. TNF-α, IL-1, IL-6, LIF and IFN-α and -γ decrease the activity of adipose tissue lipoprotein lipase in vivo 16h following administration[7,23–25,41]. In muscle, IL-1 and IFN-γ decrease lipoprotein lipase activity but TNF-α, LIF and IFN-α have no effect[24,42]. The effect of these late changes in lipoprotein lipase activity on lipoprotein metabolism need to be addressed further.

Cytokine induced changes in apolipoprotein levels could also play a role in the hypertriglyceridaemia. For example, endotoxin administration decreases serum levels of apolipoprotein CII[43], a key endogenous activator of lipoprotein lipase. Decreased apolipoprotein CII levels could result in a decrease in lipoprotein lipase activity and delayed clearance of triglyceride-rich lipoproteins. The effect of cytokines on apolipoprotein CII levels have not been addressed. Infection and inflammation also decrease apolipoprotein E levels in VLDL[44,45]. Recent studies by our laboratory have demonstrated that the combination of TNF and IL-1 decreases apolipoprotein E mRNA levels in the liver[46]. Apolipoprotein E is an important determinant of receptor-mediated uptake of VLDL and decreased apolipoprotein E levels could result in decreased triglyceride clearance, thereby contributing to hypertriglyceridaemia. Thus, in addition to altering lipid metabolism, cytokines could alter either the production and/or degradation of apolipoproteins that play crucial roles in the metabolism of triglyceride-rich lipoproteins.

EFFECTS OF CYTOKINES ON CHOLESTEROL METABOLISM

TNF and IL-1 increase serum cholesterol levels in rodents[2,14,46,47]. The increase is delayed in onset, occurring 7–8h following cytokine administration, and is primarily due to an increase in LDL cholesterol[2,13]. In contrast, HDL cholesterol levels decrease following TNF or IL-1 administration in hamsters[46]. In primates, cytokines decrease rather than increase serum cholesterol levels: the underlying mechanism for these interspecies differences are unknown[48].

In rodents, the increase in serum cholesterol levels appears to be due to an increase in hepatic production. TNF-α, lymphotoxin (TNF-β), IL-1 and IFN-γ but not IFN-α, increase cholesterol synthesis in the liver[2,33,47]. Incorporation of acetate but not mevalonate into cholesterol is stimulated following cytokine treatment, indicating that the increase in hepatic cholesterogenesis is localized to the early steps of cholesterol synthesis[2]. Cytokines also increase the activity of HMG CoA reductase, the rate limiting enzyme in cholesterol synthesis[2,47]. TNF and IL-1 increase hepatic HMG CoA reductase mRNA levels, which could account for the increase in activity[46]. Neither TNF nor IL-1 decrease hepatic LDL receptor mRNA levels, suggesting that decreased clearance of LDL is unlikely to account for the increase in LDL cholesterol levels[46].

Infection and endotoxin administration are also associated with increases in serum cholesterol levels and in hepatic cholesterol synthesis[49]. Pretreatment with antibodies that neutralize TNF activity result in a marked inhibition of the ability of endotoxin to increase serum cholesterol levels, hepatic cholesterol synthesis and hepatic HMG CoA reductase activity[47]. This indicates that TNF is an important in vivo mediator of the effect of endotoxin on cholesterol metabolism in the liver.

ACUTE PHASE PROTEINS AND LIPID METABOLISM

The hepatic synthesis of certain proteins increase during infection or inflammation. These acute phase proteins are believed to play an important homeostatic role in host defence, and the increase in the synthesis of these proteins is mediated by cytokines such as TNF, IL-1 and IL-6. Of note is that several of the 'classic' acute phase proteins are known to interact with lipoproteins. Serum amyloid A (SAA) levels increase during infection and inflammation and hepatic mRNA levels of SAA are increased by cytokines[50–53]. SAA binds to HDL, displacing apolipoprotein A1, and SAA-rich HDL are rapidly cleared from the circulation[54]. Increased SAA levels could thereby contribute to a reduction in HLD levels following cytokine treatment. Moreover, SAA-rich HDL have a lower affinity for hepatocytes than normal HDL but increased affinity for macrophages, suggesting that SAA-rich HDL may be directed towards macrophages[55].

The acute phase protein C-reactive protein binds to lipoproteins[56,57], and recent studies have demonstrated that C-reactive protein enhances the uptake of LDL by macrophages[58]. Thus, as is the case for SAA, C-reactive protein may also play a role in redirecting lipoproteins to macrophages.

Recent studies by our laboratory have shown that apolipoprotein J mRNA levels markedly increase in the liver following TNF or IL-1 administration[59].

Cytokine administration also increases serum apolipoprotein J levels and apolipoprotein J is primarily associated with HDL[59]. The effect of increased apolipoprotein J on HDL metabolism remains to be elucidated.

POTENTIAL DELETERIOUS EFFECTS OF CYTOKINE-INDUCED CHANGES IN LIPID METABOLISM

The changes in lipid metabolism induced by cytokines are likely to affect the host in a variety of ways. Whether these changes are beneficial or deleterious is likely to depend on a number of factors including the duration of cytokine release, the magnitude of the change, the interactions between different cytokines and the metabolic state of the animal.

One potential harmful side-effect of the alterations in lipid metabolism is cachexia. Cytokine-induced changes in lipid metabolism may contribute to cachexia in a number of different ways. First, the induction of hepatic fatty acid synthesis, triglyceride production, and VLDL secretion by cytokines uses energy which may be wasteful at times when the body needs to conserve energy. Second, the catabolic effects of cytokines on adipocytes, which includes the inhibition of LPL activity, increased lipolysis and decreased fatty acid synthesis, may decrease fat storage in adipose tissue. Finally, the simultaneous lipolytic and lipogenic effects of cytokines may result in cycling of fatty acids from adipose tissue to liver and back to adipose tissue which 'wastes' energy. Thus, a number of the effects of cytokines on lipid metabolism may play a role in cachexia, although these changes are not likely to be the sole cause. Studies by our laboratory have shown that the chronic administration of TNF can produce hypertriglyceridaemia without resulting in weight loss[19]. Cachexia is complex and most likely results from additive or synergistic effects of numerous cytokines acting on many different tissues.

POTENTIAL BENEFICIAL EFFECTS OF CYTOKINE-INDUCED CHANGES IN LIPID METABOLISM

As described above, cytokines alter lipid metabolism in many tissues, leading to hyperlipidaemia. This increase in serum lipid and lipoprotein levels produced by cytokines can be considered part of the acute phase response. It is believed that the acute phase response proteins are beneficial in host defence[60,61]. For example, C-reactive protein and C_3 help in the opsonization of bacteria and other foreign particles, protease inhibitors such as α_1-antitrypsinase may limit proteolysis to sites of inflammation, and fibrinogen and similar proteins may restore or maintain serum levels of clotting factors[60,61].

The hyperlipidaemia caused by cytokines may be beneficial in a number of ways. The increase in serum lipid levels could result in the enhanced delivery of lipids to cells that are activated during the immune response and the cells involved in tissue repair. As noted above, increases in SAA and C-reactive protein may direct HDL and LDL respectively, to macrophages. Additionally, decreases in adipose tissue lipoprotein lipase activity may decrease the delivery of nutrients to adipose tissue and allow for other tissues to consume these fuels. That the cytokine-induced hyperlipidaemia can be beneficial is also suggested by numerous in vitro studies that have demonstrated that lipoproteins bind endotoxin[62-68]. Moreover, the ability of LPS to cause death can be prevented by preincubating endotoxin with either HDL, LDL, VLDL, or chylomicrons prior to administration[68]. Furthermore, the infusion of large quantities of chylomicrons, which markedly increases serum triglyceride levels, prior to endotoxin administration also protects from endotoxin-induced death[69]. Similarly, data indicate that transgenic mice which overproduce apolipoprotein A1 and have elevated HDL levels are also protected from endotoxin toxicity[70]. Lipoproteins diminish the ability of endotoxin to stimulate macrophage cytokine production in vitro[71,72]. In vivo, the increase in serum TNF levels that follows endotoxin administration is blunted by infusion of lipoproteins[69].

It is now well recognized that many of the adverse effects of endotoxin are mediated by the overproduction of cytokines and it is therefore possible that one mechanism by which lipoproteins may protect from endotoxin toxicity is to direct the clearance of endotoxin away from macrophages towards other sites. Studies by our laboratory have shown that endotoxin complexed with lipoproteins is preferentially cleared by hepatocytes and secreted into the bile[69,73]. The diminished uptake of endotoxin by macrophages when administered with lipoproteins is likely to be the cause of the decreased cytokine production and reduced toxicity. Thus, binding of endotoxin to lipoproteins may blunt the ability of endotoxin to stimulate macrophages and redirect the endotoxin away from macrophages and towards other cells where the endotoxin may be safely processed.

In addition to detoxifying endotoxin, lipoproteins can bind a variety of viruses and thus reduce their toxic effects[74-78]. Lipoproteins also induce the lysis of the parasite *Trypanosoma brucei*[79,80] and bind urate crystals, reducing the inflammatory response induced by these crystals[81]. Lastly, recent studies have shown that certain viruses are taken up by cells via the LDL receptor pathway; therefore LDL is a competitive inhibitor of uptake[82,83] and elevated LDL levels might be beneficial in decreasing viral toxicity. Lipoproteins may therefore represent a non-specific immune response that can decrease the toxicity of a variety of harmful biological and chemical agents. Considered in this light it makes sense that multiple different cytokines are capable of altering lipid metabolism in a variety of different tissues in a manner that leads to an increase in serum lipid levels.

REFERENCES

1. Kurrock R, Rhode MF, Quesada JR et al. Recombinant gamma interferon induces hypertriglyceridemia and inhibits post-heparin lipase activity in cancer patients. J Exp Med. 1986;164:1093–101.
2. Feingold KR, Grunfeld C. Tumor necrosis factor alpha stimulates hepatic lipogenesis in the rat in vivo. J Clin Invest. 1987;80:184–90.
3. Olsen EA, Lichtenstein GR, Wilkinson WE. Changes in serum lipids in patients with condylomata acuminata treated with interferon alpha-n1 (Wellferon). J Am Acad Dermatol. 1988;19:286–9.
4. Malmendier CL, Lontie J-F, Sculier JP, Dubois DY. Modifications of plasma lipids, lipoproteins

and apolipoproteins in advanced cancer patients treated with recombinant interleukin-2 and autologous lymphokine-activated killer cells. Atherosclerosis. 1988;73:173–80.

5. Starnes HF Jr, Warren RS, Jeevanandam M et al. Tumor necrosis factor and the acute metabolic response to tissue injury in man. J Clin Invest. 1988;82:1321–5.

6. Sherman ML, Spriggs DR, Arthur KA, Imamura K, Frei E, III, Kufe DW. Recombinant human tumor necrosis factor administered as a five-day continuous infusion in cancer patients: Phase I toxicity and effects on lipid metabolism. J Clin Oncol. 1988;6:344–50.

7. Chajek-Shaul T, Friedman G, Stein O, Shiloni E, Etienne J, Stein Y. Mechanism of the hypertriglyceridemia induced by tumor necrosis factor administration to rats. Biochim Biophys Acta. 1989;1001:316–24.

8. Argiles JM, Lopez-Soriano FJ, Evans RD, Williamson DH. Interleukin-1 and lipid metabolism in the rat. Biochem J. 1989;259:673–8.

9. Kurzrock R, Feinberg B, Talpaz M, Saks S, Guterman JU. Phase I study of a combination of recombinant tumor necrosis factor alpha and recombinant interferon gamma in cancer patients. J Interferon Res. 1989;9:435–44.

10. Wilson DE, Birchfield GR, Hejazi JS, Ward JH, Samlowski WE. Hypocholesterolemia in patients treated with recombinant interleukin-2: Appearance of remnant-like lipoproteins. J Clin Oncol. 1989;7:1573–7.

11. Ettinger WH, Miller LD, Albers JJ, Smith TK, Parks JS. Lipopolysaccharide and tumor necrosis factor cause a fall in plasma concentration of lecithin: cholesterol acyltransferase in cynomolgus monkeys. J Lipid Res. 1990;31:1099–107.

12. Rosenzweig IB, Wiebe DA, Hank JA et al. Effects of interleukin-2 (IL-2) on human plasma lipid, lipoprotein and C-reactive protein. Biotherapy. 1990;2:193–8.

13. Krauss RM, Grunfeld C, Doerrler W, Feingold KR. Tumor necrosis factor acutely increases plasma levels of very low density lipoproteins of normal size and composition. Endocrinology. 1990;127:1016–21.

14. Feingold KR, Soued M, Adi S et al. Effect of interleukin-1 on lipid metabolism in the rat: Similarities to and differences from tumor necrosis factor. Arteriosclerosis Thrombosis. 1991;11:495–500.

15. Ruiz-Moreno M, Carreno V, Rua MJ et al. Increase in triglycerides during alpha interferon treatment of chronic viral hepatitis. J Hepatol. 1992;16:384–8.

16. Berruti A, Gorzegno G, Vitetta G, Tampellini M, Dogliotti L. Hypertriglyceridemia during long-term interferon alpha therapy: efficacy of diet and gemfibrosil treatment. A case report. Tumori. 1992;78:353–5.

17. Sweep CGJ, Hermus ARMM, van der Meer MJM et al. Chronic intraperitoneal infusion of low doses of tumor necrosis factor alpha in rats induces a reduction in plasma triglyceride levels. Cytokine. 1992;4:561–7.

18. Hermus ARMM, Sweep CGJ, Demacker PNM, van der Meer MJM, Kloppenborg PWC, van der Meer JWM. Continuous infusion of interleukin-1 beta in rats induces a profound fall in plasma levels of cholesterol and triglycerides. Arteriosclerosis and Thrombosis. 1992;12:1036–43.

19. Grunfeld C, Wilking H, Neese R et al. Persistence of the hypertriglyceridemic effect of tumor necrosis factor despite development of tachyphylaxis to its anorectic/cachectic effect in rats. Cancer Res. 1989;49:2554–60.

20. Kawakami M, Pekala PH, Lane MD, Cerami A. Lipoprotein lipase suppression in 3T3-L1 cells by an endotoxin-induced mediator from exudate cells. Proc Natl Acad Sci USA. 1982;82:912–6.

21. Patton JS, Shepard HM, Wilking H et al. Interferons and tumor necrosis factors have similar catabolic effects on 3T3-L1 cells. Proc Natl Acad Sci USA. 1986;83:8313–17.

22. Price SR, Mizel SB, Pekala PH. Regulation of lipoprotein lipase synthesis and 3T3-L1 adipocyte metabolism by recombinant interleukin-1. Biochim Biophys Acta. 1986;889:374–81.

23. Semb H, Peterson J, Tavernier J, Olivecrona T. Multiple effects of tumor necrosis factor on lipoprotein lipase in vivo. J Biol Chem. 1987;262:8390–4.

24. Grunfeld C, Gulli R, Moser AH, Gavin LA, Feingold KR. The effect of tumor necrosis factor administration in vivo on lipoprotein lipase activity in various tissues of the rat. J Lipid Res. 1989;30:579–85.

25. Feingold KR, Soued M, Staprans I et al. The effect of TNF on lipid metabolism in the diabetic rat: Evidence that inhibition of adipose tissue lipoprotein lipase activity is not required for TNF induced hyperlipidemia. J Clin Invest. 1989;83:1116–21.

26. Feingold KR, Serio MK, Adi S, Moser AH, Grunfeld C. Tumor necrosis factor stimulates hepatic lipid synthesis and secretion. Endocrinology. 1989;124:2336–42.
27. Feingold KR, Adi S, Staprans I et al. Diet affects the mechanisms by which TNF stimulates hepatic triglyceride production. Am J Physiol. 1990;259:E177–84.
28. Van der Poll T, Romijn JA, Endert E, Borm JJJ, Buller HR, Sauerwein HP. Tumor necrosis factor mimics the metabolic response to acute infection in healthy humans. Am J Physiol. 1991;261:E457–65.
29. Memon RA, Feingold KR, Moser AH, Doerrler W, Grunfeld C. In vivo effects of interferon alpha and interferon gamma on lipolysis and ketogenesis. Endocrinology. 1992;131:1695–702.
30. Kawakami M, Murase T, Ogawa H et al. Human recombinant TNF suppresses lipoprotein lipase activity and stimulates lipolysis in 3T3-L1 cels. J Biochem. 1987;101:331–8.
31. Ogawa H, Nielsen S, Kawakami M. Cachectin/tumor necrosis factor and interleukin-1 show different modes of combined effect on lipoprotein lipase activity and intracellular lipolysis on 3T3-L1 cells. Biochim Biophys Acta. 1989;1003:131–5.
32. Feingold KR, Doerrler W, Dinarello CA, Fiers W, Grunfeld C. Stimulation of lipolysis in cultured fat cells by tumor necrosis factor, interleukin-1 and the interferons is blocked by inhibition of prostaglandin synthesis. Endocrinology. 1992;130:10–16.
33. Feingold KR, Soued M, Serio MK, Moser AH, Dinarello CA, Grunfeld C. Multiple cytokines stimulate hepatic lipid synthesis in vivo. Endocrinology. 1989;125:267–74.
34. Grunfeld C, Adi S, Soued M, Moser AH, Fiers W, Feingold KR. Search for mediators of the lipogenic effects of tumor necrosis factor: Potential role for interleukin-6. Cancer Res. 1990;50:4233–8.
35. Grunfeld C, Dinarello CA, Feingold KR. Tumor necrosis factor alpha, interleukin-1, interferon alpha stimulate triglyceride synthesis in HepG2 cells. Metab Clin Exp. 1991;40:894–8.
36. Feingold KR, Soued M, Serio MK, Adi S, Moser AH, Grunfeld C. The effect of diet on tumor necrosis factor stimulation of hepatic lipogenesis. Metabolism. 1990;39:623–32.
37. Grunfeld C, Verdier JA, Neese R, Moser AH, Feingold KR. Mechanisms by which tumor necrosis factor stimulates hepatic fatty acid synthesis in vivo. J Lipid Res. 1988;29:1327–35.
38. Grunfeld C, Soued M, Adi S, Moser AH, Dinarello CA, Feingold KR. Evidence for two classes of cytokines that stimulate hepatic lipogenesis: Relationships among tumor necrosis factor, interleukin-1 and interferon alpha. Endocrinology. 1990;127:46–54.
39. Grunfeld C, Soued M, Adi S et al. Interleukin-4 inhibits stimulation of hepatic lipogenesis by tumor necrosis factor, interleukin-1 and interleukin-6 but not by interferon alpha. Cancer Res. 1991;51:2803–7.
40. Feingold KR, Staprans I, Memon RA et al. Endotoxin rapidly induces changes in lipid metabolism that produce hypertriglyceridemia: Low doses stimulate hepatic triglyceride production while high doses inhibit clearance. J Lipid Res. 1992;33:1765–76.
41. Greenberg AS, Nordan RP, McIntosh J, Calvo JC, Scow RO, Jablons R. Interleukin-6 reduces lipoprotein lipase activity in adipose tissue of mice in vivo and in 3T3-L1 adipocytes: a possible role for interleukin-6 in cancer cachexia. Cancer Res. 1992;52:4113–6.
42. Feingold KR, Marshall M, Gulli R, Moser AH, Grunfeld C. The effect of endotoxin and cytokines on lipoprotein lipase activity in mice. Arteriosclerosis Thrombosis. 1994;14:1866–72.
43. Sakaguchi S. Metabolic disorders of serum lipoproteins in endotoxin-poisoned mice: The role of high density lipoprotein (HDL) and triglyceride-rich lipoproteins. Microbiol Immunol. 1982;26:1017–34.
44. Cabana VG, Siegel JN, Sabesin SM. Effects of the acute phase response on the concentration and density distribution of plasma lipids and apolipoproteins. J Lipid Res. 1989;30:39–49.
45. Lanza-Jacoby S, Wong SH, Tabares A, Baer D, Schneider T. Disturbances in the composition of plasma lipoproteins during gram-negative sepsis in the rat. Biochim Biophys Acta. 1992;1124:233–40.
46. Hardardottir I, Moser AH, Memon RA, Grunfeld C, Feingold KR. Effects of TNF, IL-1 and the combination of both cytokines on cholesterol metabolism in Syrian hamsters. Lymphokine Cytokine Res. 1994;13:161–6.
47. Memon RA, Grunfeld C, Moser AH, Feingold KR. Tumor necrosis factor mediates the effects of endotoxin on cholesterol and triglyceride metabolism in mice. Endocrinology. 1993;132:2246–53.
48. Hardardottir I, Grunfeld C, Feingold KR. Effects of endotoxin and cytokines on lipid metabolism. Curr Opin Lipidol. 1994;5:207–15.

49. Feingold KR, Hardardottir I, Memon R et al. Effect of endotoxin on cholesterol biosynthesis and distribution in serum lipoproteins in Syrian hamsters. J Lipid Res. 1993;34:2147–58.
50. Hofman JS, Benditt EP. Changes in high density lipoprotein content following endotoxin administration in the mouse. J Biol Chem. 1982;257:10510–7.
51. Ramador G, Sipe JD, Dinarello CA, Mizel SB, Colten HR. Pretranslational modulation of acute phase hepatic protein synthesis by murine recombinant interleukin-1 (IL-1) and purified human IL-1. J Exp Med. 1985;162:930–42.
52. Sipee JD, Vogel SN, Douches S, Neta R. Tumor necrosis factor/cachectin is a less potent inducer of serum amyloid A synthesis than interleukin-1. Lymphokine Res. 1987;6:93–101.
53. Dowton SB, Peters CN, Jestus JJ. Regulation of serum amyloid A gene expression in Syrian hamsters by cytokines. Inflammation. 1991;15:391–7.
54. Hoffman JS, Benditt EP. Plasma clearance kinetics of the amyloid-related high density lipoprotein apoprotein, serum amyloid protein (Apo SAA), in the mouse. Evidence for rapid Apo SAA clearance. J Clin Invest. 1983;71:926–34.
55. Kisilevsky R, Subrahamanyan L. Serum amyloid A changes high density lipoprotein's cellular affinity. A clue to serum amyloid A's principal function. Lab Invest. 1992;66:778–85.
56. Pepys M, Rowe I, Baltz M. C-reactive protein binding to lipids and lipoproteins. Int Rev Exp Pathol. 1985;27:83–111.
57. Saxena U, Nagpurkar A, Dolphin P, Mookarjea S. A study of the selective binding of apoprotein B and E containing human plasma lipoproteins to immobilized rat serum phosphorylcholine binding protein. J Biol Chem. 1987;262:3011–6.
58. Mookerjea S, Francis J, Hunt D, Yang CY, Nagpurkar A. Rat C-reactive protein causes a charge modification of LDL and stimulates its degradation by macrophages. Arteriosclerosis Thrombosis. 1994;14:282–7.
59. Hardardottir I, Kunitake ST, Moser AH et al. Endotoxin and cytokines increase hepatic mRNA levels and serum concentrations of apolipoprotein J (clusterin) in Syrian hamsters. J Clin Invest. 1994;94:1304–9.
60. Kushner I. The phenomenon of the acute phase response. Ann NY Acad Sci. 1982;389:39–48.
61. Richards C, Galdie J, Baumann H. Cytokine control of acute phase protein expression. Eur Cytokine Net. 1991;2:89–98.
62. Ulevitch RJ, Johnston AR. The modification of the biophysical and endotoxic properties of bacterial lipopolysaccharide by serum. J Clin Invest. 1978;62:1313–24.
63. Ulevitch RJ, Johnston AR, Weinstein DB. New function for high density lipoproteins: Their participation in intravascular reactions of bacterial lipopolysaccharides. J Clin Invest. 1979;64:1516–24.
64. Ulevitch RJ, Johnson AR, Weinstein DB. New function for high density lipoproteins: Isolation and characterization of a bacterial lipopolysaccharide-high density lipoprotein complex formed in rabbit plasma. J Clin Invest. 1981;67:827–37.
65. Munford RS, Hall CL, Lipton JM, Dietschy JM. Biological activity, lipoprotein binding behavior and in vivo disposition of extracted and native forms of *Salmonella typhimurium* lipopolysaccharides. J Clin Invest. 1982;70:877–88.
66. Van Lenten BJ, Fogelman AM, Haberland ME, Edwards PA. The role of lipoproteins and receptor-mediated endocytosis in the transport of bacterial lipopolysaccharide. Proc Natl Acad Sci USA. 1986;83:2704–8.
67. Navab M, Hough GP, Van Lenten BJ, Berliner JA, Fogelman AM. Low density lipoproteins transfer bacterial lipopolysaccharides across endothelial monolayers in a biologically active form. J Clin Invest. 1988;81:601–5.
68. Harris HW, Grunfeld C, Feingold KR, Rapp JH. Human VLDL and chylomicrons can protect against endotoxin induced death in mice. J Clin Invest. 1990;86:696–701.
69. Harris HW, Grunfeld C, Feingold KR et al. Chylomicrons alter the fate of endotoxin decreasing tumor necrosis factor release and preventing death. J Clin Invest. 1993;91:1028–34.
70. Levine DM, Parker TS, Donnelly TM, Wals A, Rubin AL. In vivo protection against endotoxin by plasma high density lipoprotein. Proc Natl Acad Sci USA. 1993;90:12040–4.
71. Flegel WA, Wolpl A, Mannel DW, Northoff H. Inhibition of endotoxin induced activation of human monocytes by human lipoproteins. Infect Immunol. 1989;57:2237–45.
72. Cavaillon JM, Fittin C, Cavaillon NH, Kirsch SJ, Warren HS. Cytokine response by monocytes and macrophages to free and lipoprotein bound lipopolysaccharide. Infect Immunol. 1990;58:2375–82.

73. Read TE, Harris HW, Grunfeld C et al. Chylomicrons enhance endotoxin excretion in bile. Infect Immun. 1993;61:3496–502.
74. Shortridge KR, Ho WK, Oya A, Kobayashi M. Studies on the inhibitory activities of human serum lipoproteins for Japanese encephalitis virus. *SE Asian J Trop Med Public Health.* 1975;6:461–6.
75. Leong JC, Kane JP, Oleszko O, Levy JA. Antigen specific nonimmunoglobulin factor that neutralizes xenotropic virus is associated with mouse serum lipoproteins. Proc Natl Acad Sci USA. 1977;74:276–80.
76. Seganti L, Grassi M, Matromarino P, Pana A, Superti F, Orsi N. Activity of human serum lipoproteins on the infectivity of rhabdoviruses. Microbiology. 1983;6:91–9.
77. Sernatinger J, Hoffman A, Harmon D, Kane JP, Levy JA. Neutralization of mouse xenotropic virus by lipoproteins involves binding to virons. J Gen Virol. 1988;69:2651–61.
78. Heumer HP, Menzel HJ, Portratz D et al. Herpes simplex virus binds to human serum lipoproteins. Intervirology. 1988;29:68–76.
79. Rifkin MR. Identification of the trypanocidal factor in normal human serum: High density lipoprotein. Proc Natl Acad Sci USA. 1978;75:3450–4.
80. HajdUk SL, Moore DR, Vasudevacharya J et al. Lysis of trypanosoma bruceii by a toxic subspecies of human high density lipoprotein. J Biol Chem. 1989;264:5210–7.
81. Terkettaub R, Curtiss LK, Tenner AJ, Ginsberg MH. Lipoproteins containing apoprotein B are a major regulator of neutrophil responses to monosodium urate crystals. J Clin Invest. 1984;72:1719–30.
82. Bates P, Young JA, Varmus H. A receptor for subgroup A Rous sarcoma virus is related to the low density lipoprotein receptor. Cell. 1993;74:1043–51.
83. Hofer F, Gruenberger M, Kowalski H et al. Members of the low density lipoprotein receptor family mediate cell entry of a minor-group common cold virus. Proc Natl Acad Sci USA. 1994;91:1839–42.

Section VII
Liver transplantation

17
Cytokines in liver transplantation and alcoholic liver disease

R. G. THURMAN, E. SAVIER, Y. ADACHI, S. I. SHEDLOFSKY,
J. J. LEMASTERS, W. GAO, B. U. BRADFORD, Z. ZHONG,
K. T. KNECHT, W. QU, R. T. CURRIN, S. LICHTMAN,
J. WANG and M. GOTO

INTRODUCTION

Kupffer cells are vital to host defence mechanisms; however, they also produce mediators, including cytokines, prostaglandins and oxygen radicals, which play a role in inflammation, immune responses, modulation of hepatocyte metabolism[1] and hepatic injury. Previous studies from our laboratory demonstrated the involvement of Kupffer cells in mechanisms of pathophysiology following liver transplantation; therefore, we investigated whether cytokines and free radicals released from activated Kupffer cells play a role in reperfusion injury following transplantation.

Liver transplantation is performed routinely in children and adults, but primary non-function still occurs in 5–15% of cases[2,3]. Primary non-function can compromise postoperative recovery and necessitate retransplantation. Although the mechanism is not clearly understood, Kupffer cells, the hepatic macrophages, are activated following cold storage and reperfusion[4]. Activated Kupffer cells release toxic mediators including cytokines such as tumour necrosis factor (TNF) as well as eicosanoids[5]. We asked whether hepatic injury following transplantation involves release of TNF and whether TNF release can be modulated by a calcium channel blocker. Interleukin 6 (IL-6) also may influence postoperative outcome since it is involved in the acute phase response[6] as well as in regulation of the immune system[7]. Therefore, we investigated the time course of release of TNF and IL-6 following liver transplantation.

Reports in the literature support the idea that chronic exposure to alcohol leads to activation of Kupffer cells. For example, alcohol affects phagocytosis, bactericidal activity and cytokine production by Kupffer cells[8,9], and serum TNF levels are increased in alcoholics[10], consistent with the idea that Kupffer cells of patients with alcoholic liver disease are activated since TNF is produced exclusively by the monocyte-macrophage lineage, which is represented largely by Kupffer cells[11]. Furthermore, Ca^{2+} activates Kupffer cells[5], and chronic ethanol treatment makes Ca^{2+} channels in Kupffer cells easier to open[12]. Thus, we wondered whether Kupffer cells participate in the mechanism of early alcohol-induced liver injury.

Kupffer cells participate in hepatic injury associated with sepsis by releasing chemical mediators and free radicals[13,14]. In sepsis, the major cause of activation of Kupffer cells is endotoxin originating from the cell wall of Gram-negative bacteria[15]. Plasma endotoxin levels increase in rats on an enteral feeding protocol as well as in the chronic alcoholic[16,17], and levels correlate well with pathology[18]. Accordingly, it was hypothesized that endotoxin derived from intestinal bacteria affects alcohol-induced liver injury and that Kupffer cell activation by endotoxin is involved in the mechanism of pathophysiology. This hypothesis was tested by blocking endotoxin production by intestinal sterilization using antibiotics.

MATERIALS AND METHODS

Orthotopic liver transplantation

Inbred Lewis rats (180–220 g, female) were used to exclude immunological rejection and were transplanted according to procedures described by Zimmermann[19] and Kamada[20]. Rats were anaesthetized lightly with ether, and surgery was performed under clean conditions. The explantation procedure included incision of the skin, sectioning of the hepatic ligaments, insertion of a splint (polyethylene tubing , PE 10) into the bile duct and dissection of the portal vein and inferior vena cava. The portal vein was then clamped and the liver was rinsed with 10 ml of Ringer's solution at 4°C followed by 15 ml of Euro-Collins solution at 4°C. Livers were then removed and immersed in Euro-Collins solution at 1°C and cuffs were placed on the portal vein and inferior hepatic vena cava before storage under survival or non-survival conditions. Implantation was performed by connecting the suprahepatic vena cava with a running suture, inserting cuffs into the appropriate vessels, and anastomosing the bile duct with an intraluminal splint. Grafts were rinsed with 5 ml of Ringer's solution at 21°C before reperfusion, and effluent was collected. Gut ischaemia due to clamping the portal vein did not exceed 20 minutes. Ringer's solution (5 ml) was infused via the tail vein during implantation to maintain blood pressure.

Blood sample collection and cytokine assays

The rat was anaesthetized lightly with ether, the right external jugular vein was exposed and a glass micropipette (Corning) was inserted into the superior vena cava via the jugular vein to collect blood (400 μl) at 60, 150, 210 and 300 min after graft reperfusion. The protease inhibitor aprotinin (3 U/ml) was added to effluent and blood samples, and sera were stored at −70°C until assay. Cytotoxicity of TNF was assayed in L-M fibroblasts incubated with serum or effluent in the presence of 1 μg/ml actinomycin D as described elsewhere[21] or with an enzyme-linked immunosorbent assay (ELISA). Interleukin 6 (IL-6) was measured using the growth stimulation of B-9 cells as described by Aarden[22]. Results from unknown samples were compared with curves prepared using authentic standards.

Enteral feeding model

Male Wistar rats, weighing about 300 g, were used in the enteral feeding model. An intragastric cannula was implanted into the stomach of rats as described by Tsukamoto and French[23], and diet was infused continuously for up to 4 weeks.

A liquid diet was prepared according to Thompson and Reitz[24], containing corn oil as fat (37% of total calories), protein (23%), carbohydrate (5%), minerals and vitamins, plus ethanol or isocaloric maltose dextrin (35%). Ethanol levels in the diet were adjusted daily for each rat (e.g. 26–35%) based on the urine alcohol concentration. Where indicated, $GdCl_3$ (10 mg/kg) was administered via the tail vein twice weekly beginning on the day of the operation to destroy Kupffer cells[25].

Antibiotic treatment

Polymyxin B and neomycin[26] were added to the liquid diet of rats on the enteral feeding protocol to prevent bacterial growth, the main source of endotoxin in the gastrointestinal tract. Based on the results of preliminary experiments, 150 mg/kg/day of polymyxin B and 450 mg/kg/day of neomycin were administered via the liquid diet.

Blood collection and asparate aminotransferase (AST) assay

Blood was collected via the tail vein once a week and centrifuged. Serum was stored at −20ºC in a microtube until assayed for AST by standard enzymatic procedures[27].

Pathological evaluation

Rats underwent biopsy after 2 and 3 weeks of ethanol exposure. Livers were formalin-fixed, embedded in paraffin, and stained with haematoxylin and eosin to assess inflammation and necrosis and with osmium to identify lipid. Liver pathology was scored using a system described by Nanji et al.[28].

Liver surface oxygen tension measurement

Following anaesthesia with methoxyflurane, the abdomen was opened and a Clark-type platinum oxygen electrode was placed gently on the liver surface to determine oxygen tension[29]. Since the portal venule terminates 200 μm from the liver surface, this value largely reflects oxygen tension in pericentral regions of the hepatic lobule.

Free radical detection

Male Wistar rats (300–320 g) were infused continuously with a high-fat liquid diet for at least 2 weeks. Rats were anaesthetized with Nembutal (75 mg/kg). Ethanol was given to rats fed a high-fat diet or chow control diet to make ethanol levels of all animals comparable, and animals were breathalysed. Blood was collected from the tail vein, centrifuged, and stored frozen as serum for later AST analysis. Bile ducts were cannulated with PE10 tubing, rats were given the spin trap POBN (100 mg/kg), and bile samples were collected for 15 min intervals into 30 μl of a solution of desferroxamine mesylate (5 mM) to prevent ex vivo radical formation. Samples were frozen immediately on dry ice and stored at − 70°C until EPR analysis. Bile samples were thawed and placed in a quartz flat cell, and a Varian E-109 EPR spectrometer equipped with a TM110 cavity was used. Instrument conditions were as follows: 20 mW microwave power, 0.53-G modulation amplitude, 80-G scan width, 16 min time scan, and 1 s time constant. Data were collected with an IBM-type computer interfaced to the spectrometer. Simulations and double integrations of spectra to determine amplitude were carried out with a computer program.

Low-flow, reflow perfusion model

Reperfusion injury to the liver was studied in a low-flow reflow reperfusion model. Livers from female Sprague-Dawley rats (125–150 g) were perfused at low flow rates of 1 ml/g/min to cause anoxia in pericentral regions. When normal flow rates (4 ml/g/min) were restored for 40 min, an oxygen-dependent reperfusion injury occurred. Lactate dehydrogenase (LDH) was measured in the effluent perfusate.

TNF release in isolated Kupffer cells

Female Sprague-Dawley rats (200–250 g) treated chronically with ethanol were fed an ethanol-containing Lieber-DeCarli diet for 4 weeks with appropriate controls. Rats treated acutely with ethanol received ethanol intragastrically (5 g/kg) 24 h prior to isolation of cells. Nonparenchymal cells were isolated by centrifugation through Percoll gradients following collagenase digestion. Kupffer cells were purified by seeding non-parenchymal cells on 96 well microtiter plates for 1 h. Following culture in RPMI with 20% FCS for 24 h, adherent Kupffer cells were stimulated with LPS (*E. coli* 055:B5) for 4 h and supernatants were assayed for TNF by ELISA.

Statistics

Data are presented as mean±SEM. Statistical analyses were performed using Student's *t*-test or ANOVA, as indicated. For comparison of pathological scores, the Kruskal–Wallis ANOVA for ranks was used. The criterion for significance for all experiments was $p < 0.05$.

RESULTS

Effect of nisoldipine on release of cytokines following transplantation

Following transplantation under survival conditions, blood levels of TNF and IL-6 were measured at various time points during the first 5 h postoperatively (Fig. 1). Under these conditions, TNF levels were detectable but low (< 4 U/ml) in samples of rinse effluent and sera from livers in both control and nisoldipine-treated groups (Fig. 1A). IL-6 was undetectable in effluent, but reached levels between 150 and 1500 U/ml 300 min after graft reperfusion (Fig. 1B). However, under these conditions, there were no statistical differences between the groups. Following sham operation, levels of TNF and IL-6 release were similar to those observed after control transplantation of livers stored under survival conditions for 4 h in Euro-Collins. TNF reached maximal values 60 min following the operation while IL-6 reached 366 ± 72 U/ml at 150 min.

Only three of eight liver transplant recipients survived when grafts were stored for 10 h prior to surgery (non-survival conditions). Under these conditions, TNF in the blood increased slowly after transplantation, beginning 90 min following graft reperfusion and reaching values around 15 U/ml at 150 min before declining to basal levels at 210 min (Fig. 2A). Nisoldipine prevented this increase. Five hours following transplantation, IL-6 release reached values around 10 000 U/ml, a phenomenon which was also minimized by nisoldipine (Fig. 2B).

The effect of transplantation on serum TNF from control and alcohol-treated donors was examined. Treatment with a large dose of alcohol (5 g/kg) 24 h prior to serum collection did not appreciably elevate serum TNF (Fig. 3). Following transplantation of both control and alcohol-treated rats, however, TNF in the serum was elevated from values of around 50 to around 200 pg/ml in less than 2 h. There did not appear to be any differences between the groups (Fig. 3).

Effect of inactivation of Kupffer cells on early alcohol-induced liver injury

To determine whether Kupffer cells are involved in early alcohol-induced liver injury, they were inactivated by twice weekly treatment with gadolinium chloride ($GdCl_3$), a selective Kupffer cell toxicant. When rats were exposed to ethanol continuously by intragastric feeding using an enteral feeding model (i.e. the Tsukamoto-French model), AST levels reached 192 ± 13 and 244 ± 56 IU/l in rats treated with ethanol for 2 and 4 weeks, respectively (Fig. 4), compared with control values of 88 ± 7 IU/l. $GdCl_3$ treatment prevented this injury almost completely (Figure 4). In addition, fatty changes, inflammation and necrosis, along with elevated rates of ethanol elimination, were all minimized by $GdCl_3$ treatment[25].

Effect of antibiotics on liver injury and oxygen tension

Following treatment with polymyxin B and neomycin, Gram-negative bacteria in the intestinal tract were almost completely absent. After 2 and 3 weeks of

SURVIVAL CONDITIONS

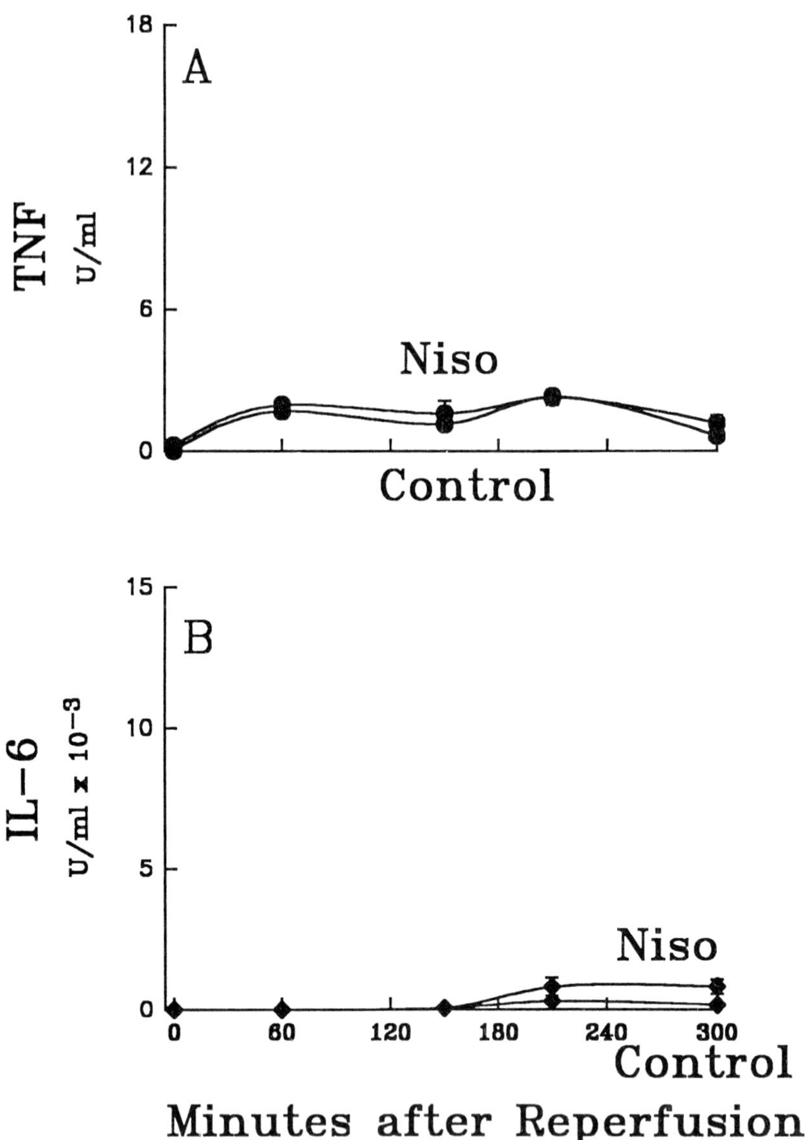

Fig. 1 Effect of nisoldipine on TNF and IL-6 release following transplantation. Livers were stored for 4h in cold Euro-Collins solution and transplanted as described in Methods. TNF and IL-6 were measured in the effluent collected after storage (0 min) and in recipient rat serum collected at various times. Rats were randomly placed in an untreated control group or a nisoldipine-treated group. Nisoldipine (1.4 μM) in DMSO was added to Ringer's and Euro-Collins solutions during explantation and storage. Reperfusion was initiated by opening the portal vascular clamp. Mean $\pm$ SEM; $p < 0.05$; $n = 3-6$ per group

NONSURVIVAL CONDITIONS

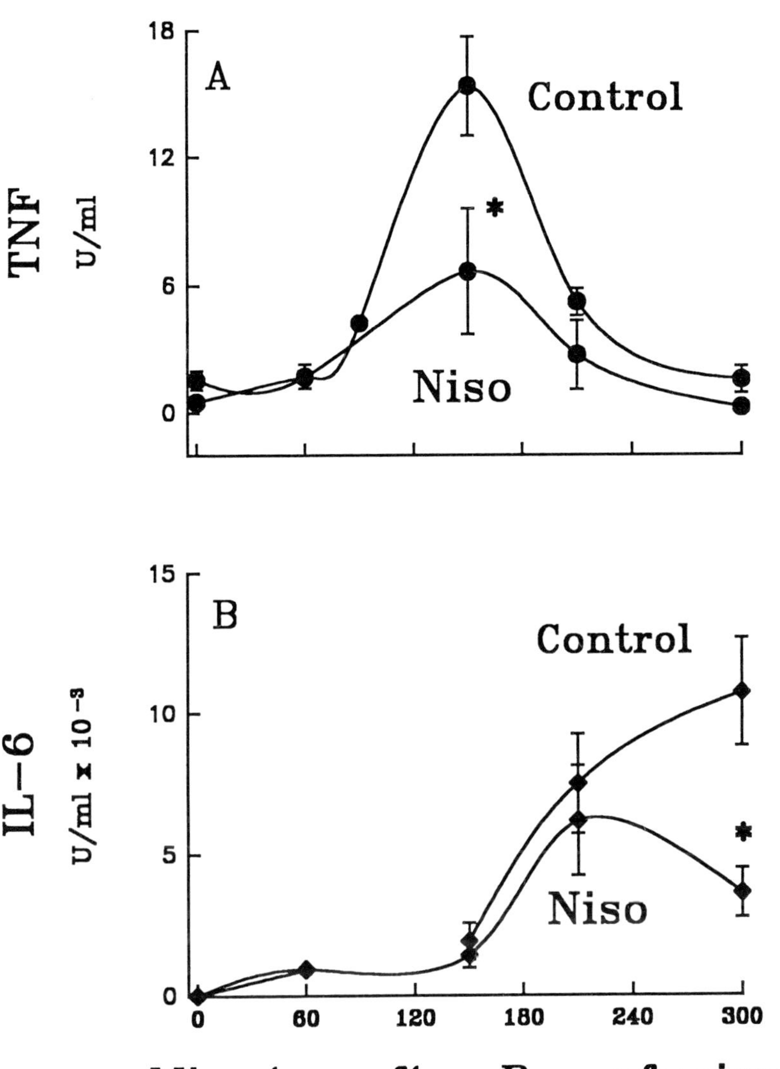

Minutes after Reperfusion

Fig. 2 Effect of nisoldipine on TNF and IL-6 release following transplantation. Livers stored for 10h in cold Euro-Collins solution were transplanted, and TNF and IL-6 were measured postoperatively as described in Methods and in the legend of Fig. 1. Mean±SEM, *$p<0.05$; **$p<0.01$ ($n=4–5$ per group)

treatment, AST levels in the serum of ethanol-fed rats increased gradually and reached levels of 185 ± 14 and $205\pm24\,IU/l$ (Fig. 5), levels which were significantly higher than in untreated rats or rats fed a high-fat control diet

SERUM TNF

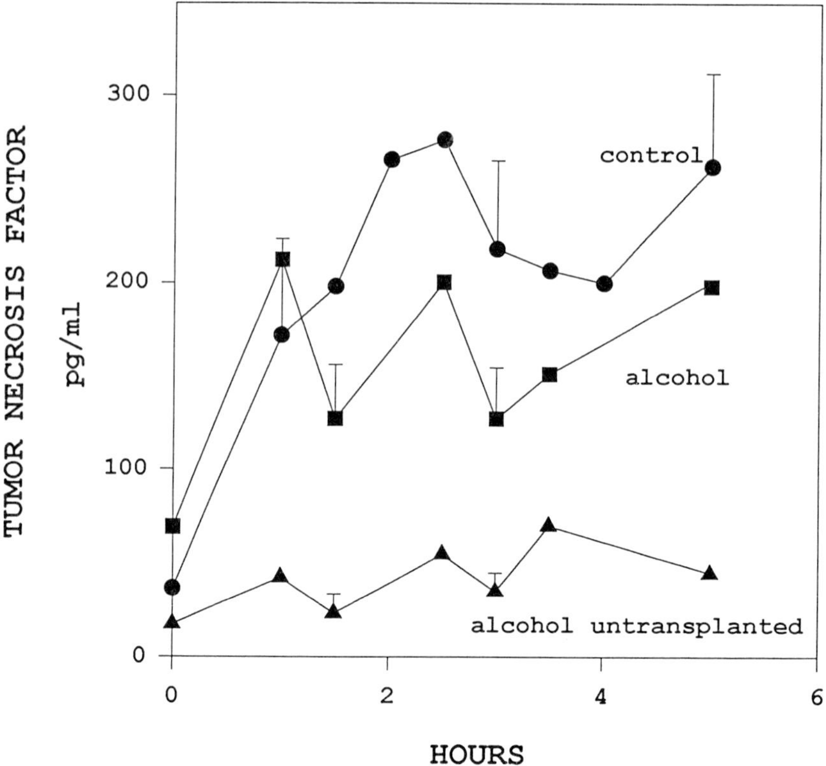

Fig. 3 Effect of alcohol on TNF release following transplantation in vivo. Rats were treated with a single dose of ethanol (5 g/kg i.g.). Twenty-four hours later, livers were removed, stored for 48 h in cold UW solution, and transplanted as described in Methods. One control group was treated with alcohol but not transplanted. TNF was measured in the effluent as described in Methods ($n = 5-7$ per group)

without ethanol. Treatment with antibiotics reduced this elevation significantly to 101 ± 8 and 126 ± 17 IU/l. Moreover, oxygen tension on the surface of the liver was significantly lower in rats treated with ethanol for 3 weeks than in untreated rats or rats fed a high-fat liquid diet without ethanol. Antibiotic treatment prevented this decrease in oxygen tension (Fig. 6).

Possible role of free radicals in alcoholic liver disease

It is hypothesized that elevated levels of endotoxin, which activate Kupffer cells to release cytokines, also increase levels of deleterious free radicals. Recently, we detected a free radical in bile from rats exposed to ethanol via the Tsukamoto-French model of intragastric ethanol administration (Fig. 7)[30]. When Kupffer

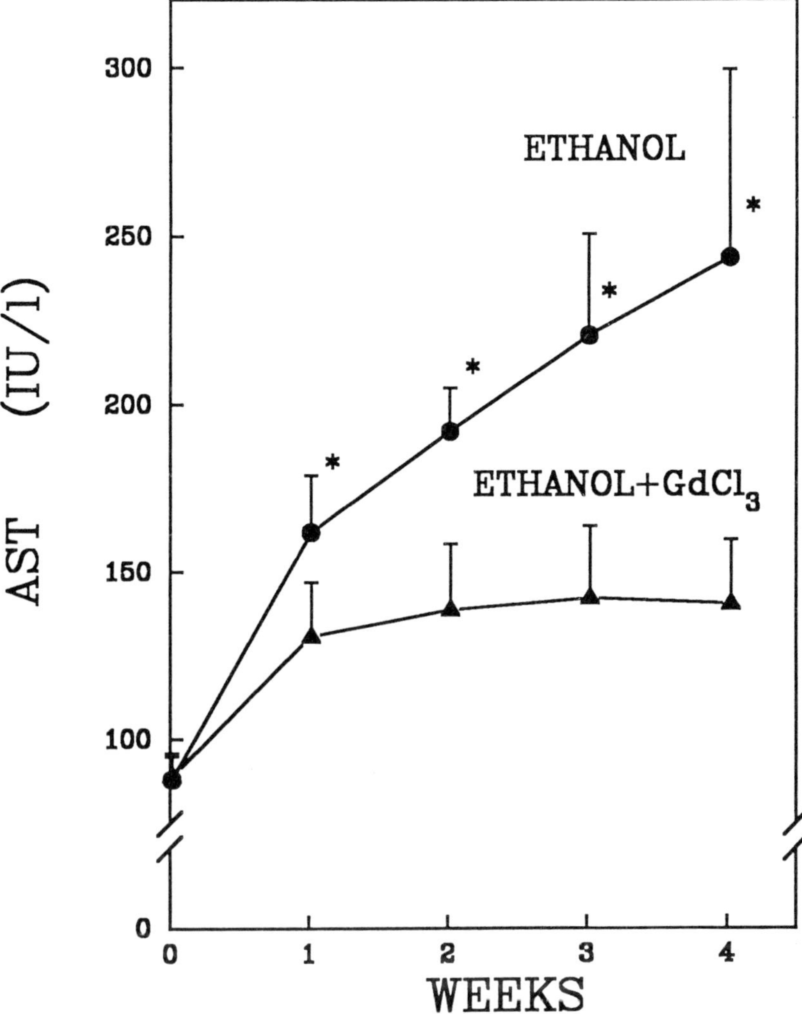

Fig. 4 Effect of ethanol and GdCl₃ treatment on serum AST levels. Blood was collected from the tail vein once a week and AST was determined as described in Methods. Data represent mean ± SEM ($n = 4-8$). *$p < 0.01$ compared with control value

cells were eliminated with GdCl₃, this radical signal was diminished by >50%. In addition, a six-line radical adduct spectrum was detected in the bile of rats treated with an ethanol-containing, high-fat diet but not in bile from chow-fed animals. The free radical adducts had hyperfine coupling constants characteristic of lipid-derived free radical products. Therefore, free radical formation can be detected in the bile of Tsukamoto-French rats treated intragastrically with a high-fat and ethanol-containing diet.

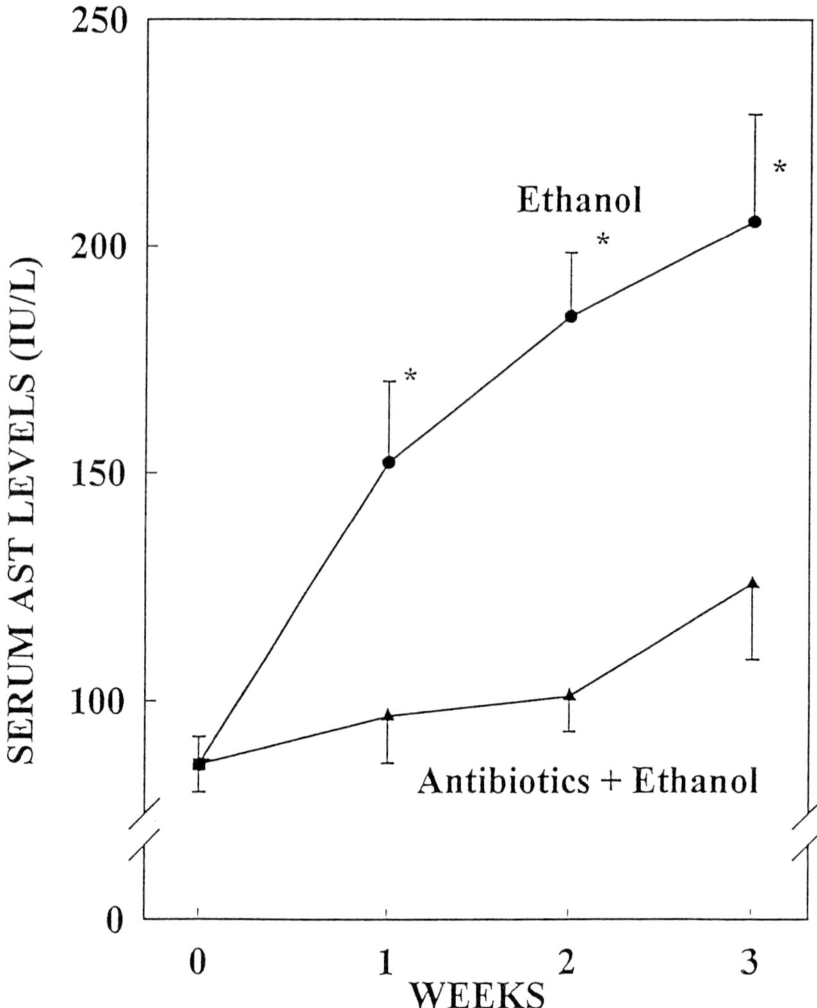

Fig. 5 Effect of ethanol and antibiotic treatment on serum AST levels. Blood was collected from the tail vein once a week and AST was determined as described in Methods. Data represent mean $\pm$ SEM ($n = 5 - 10$). *$p < 0.05$ compared with other values

Role of Kupffer cells in reperfusion injury in ethanol-induced fatty liver

The low-flow, reflow perfusion model was used to study the effect of ethanol on reperfusion injury in livers from lipid-loaded, ethanol-treated rats where blood elements are absent. During reperfusion, maximal release of LDH was around 17 IU/g/h in control rats but was increased by ethanol treatment to 37 IU/g/h. Thus, reperfusion injury was exacerbated by alcohol treatment. $GdCl_3$ treatment minimized release of LDH during reperfusion to 5 and 8 IU/g/h in control and

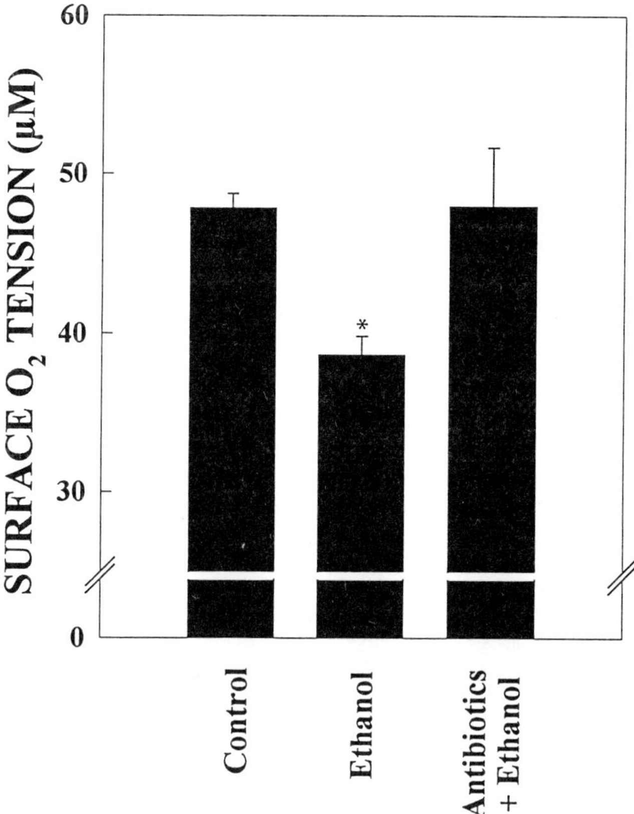

Fig. 6 Effect of ethanol and antibiotics on surface oxygen tension of the liver. Oxygen tension was measured after 3 weeks of treatment with a Clark-type oxygen electrode as described in Methods. Mean ± SEM, $n = 4–5$. *$p < 0.05$ compared with other values

ethanol-treated rats, respectively (Fig. 8), implicating Kupffer cells in reperfusion injury due to ethanol.

Effect of chronic ethanol treatment on endotoxin-stimulated TNF release by Kupffer cells

Rats were fed an ethanol-containing diet for 4 weeks or were treated acutely with ethanol, then Kupffer cells were isolated and incubated with LPS, and the supernatant was assayed for TNF. With 100 ng/ml LPS, TNF production was increased significantly in the acute treatment group. In contrast, values were diminished significantly by chronic ethanol treatment compared with corn oil-treated controls (Table 1).

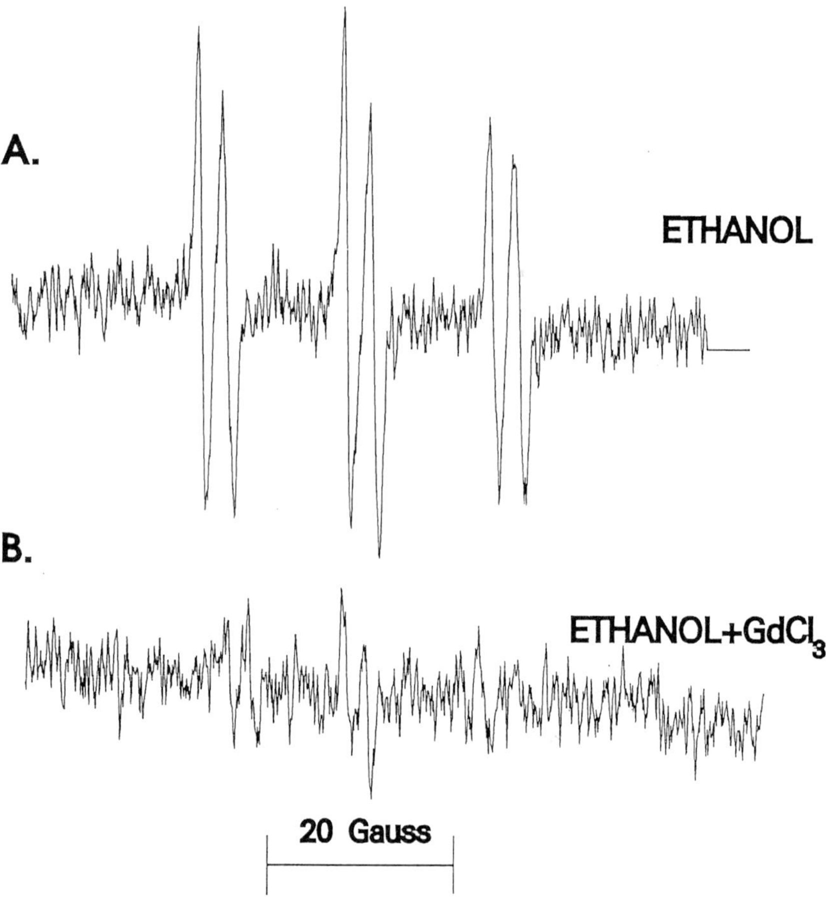

Fig. 7 Destruction of Kupffer cells prevents free radical adduct formation due to chronic enteral ethanol exposure. Representative EPR spectra of radical adducts in bile from rats treated for at least 2 weeks with continuous intragastric infusion of an ethanol-containing, high-fat diet (**A**) or an ethanol diet administered to GdCl$_3$-treated rats (**B**). Bile ducts were cannulated under Nembutal anaesthesia and the spin trap POBN (100 mg/kg) was administered i.p. Bile samples were collected into vials containing desferal (50 mM) in order to prevent ex vivo free radical formation for 3–4 h, frozen on dry ice, and analysed for free radical adducts with EPR spectroscopy as described in Methods. Typical experiments

DISCUSSION

Kupffer cells are involved in mechanisms of pathophysiology following liver transplantation[31] as well as in hepatic injury caused by ethanol[25]. It is possible that alcoholics exhibit a mild form of sepsis involving cytotoxic cytokines which is more severe following major transplantation surgery.

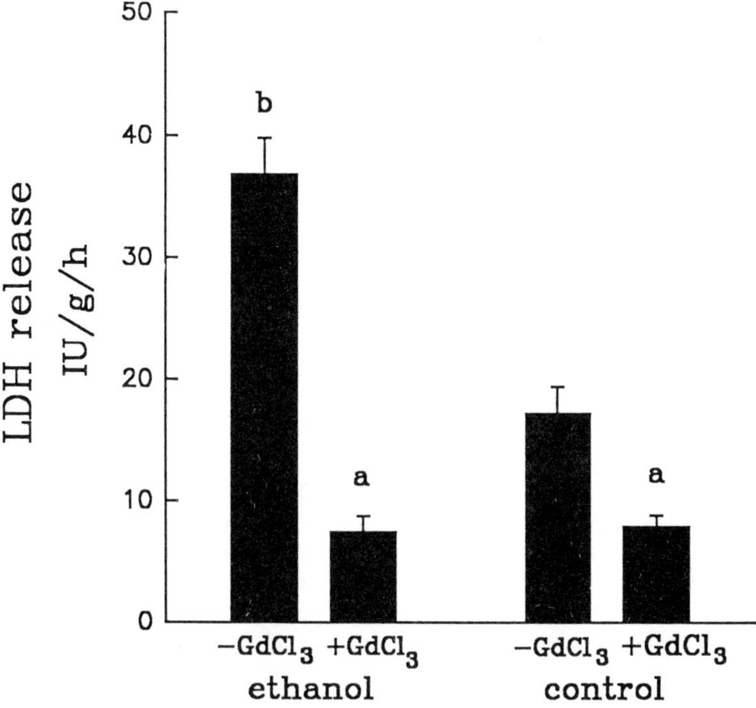

Fig. 8 Effect of GdCl$_3$ on maximal release of LDH during reperfusion in livers from control and ethanol-treated rats. Livers were perfused as described in Methods. GdCl$_3$ (20 mg/kg) was injected intravenously 24 h prior to perfusion experiments. Values are mean±SEM. $n=5-7$. [a]$p<0.05$ compared with low-flow period; [b]$p<0.05$ compared with control group. Data were analysed using ANOVA

Release of TNF following transplantation and chronic ethanol treatment

Liver transplantation and chronic treatment with ethanol stimulated release of TNF, a toxic mediator present in the blood during pathological states[32]. TNF was released a few hours (Fig. 2A) following liver transplantation under non-survival conditions. A possible factor influencing TNF release after reperfusion of the graft is explantation time in the donor. During explantation of the liver, manipulation of the gut may increase release of bacteria and endotoxin (LPS) into the portal blood, activating TNF production[32]. Therefore, time of explantation could increase hepatic exposure to LPS in the transplant model, leading to elevated TNF release after storage and reperfusion (Fig. 2A). Indeed, a dose-dependent release of TNF occurred in vivo following injection of LPS[33]. Therefore, LPS release into blood during explantation probably contributes to TNF release following transplantation (Fig. 9).

Duration of cold storage could also influence TNF release after graft reperfusion. When cold storage time was increased but explantation time was kept constant, TNF release was elevated dramatically (Figs 1A and 2A).

Table 1 TNF production (pg/ml) in endotoxin-stimulated Kupffer cells isolated from rats treated acutely or chronically with ethanol

LPS (ng/ml)	Untreated control	Acute ethanol	Corn oil control	Chronic ethanol
0	27±8	33±7	34±25	36±39
1	117±55[a]	407±68[a,b]	110±44	50±19[a]
100	148±47[a]	526±62[a,b]	320±60	100±33[a,b]

Rats were given intragastric ethanol (5 g/kg 24h before incubation; acute) or were fed an ethanol-containing diet for 5–6 weeks (chronic), and Kupffer cells were isolated as described in Methods. Kupffer cells were stimulated with LPS for 4h and supernatants were assayed for TNF by ELISA. Values are mean±s.d. of five rats/group.
[a]$p < 0.05$ compared with appropriate control; [b]$p < 0.05$ when acute and corresponding chronic ethanol groups are compared

Nisoldipine decreased TNF and IL-6 release (Fig. 2) and has been shown to decrease liver and lung injury following liver transplantation[34]. The protective effect is thought to involve prevention of Kupffer cell activation, thereby blocking TNF release.

Furthermore, chronic ethanol treatment decreased LPS-stimulated TNF release, whereas acute treatment had the opposite effect (Table 1). This may be due to changes in intracellular signal pathways, specifically by increasing PGE_2, and may represent an adaptive response to elevated endotoxin due to ethanol exposure. However, in vivo serum TNF was not elevated by ethanol. Thus, one must interpret data from cultured Kupffer cells cautiously.

Antibiotics prevent alcohol-induced liver injury

The role of endotoxin in the pathophysiology of alcohol-induced liver injury is supported by our results demonstrating that antibiotic treatment prevented the early injury to the liver caused by ethanol. Elevated serum AST after exposure to ethanol was prevented completely by antibiotic treatment (Fig. 5), and all components of the hepatic pathology score were also reduced significantly (data not shown). Polymyxin B and neomycin were used to sterilize the intestinal tract because they are not absorbed and they prevent growth of Gram-negative bacteria[26]. Moreover, polymyxin B binds endotoxin avidly, preventing its biological effect[35]. Thus, it is concluded that antibiotic treatment prevented alcohol-induced liver injury by diminishing endotoxin levels. Other reports suggest that acute and chronic exposure to alcohol is a major cause of endotoxaemia, which is thought to participate in alcoholic liver injury[18,36,37]. Both increased Gram-negative bacterial flora, a major source of endotoxin[38], and altered permeability of the gut membrane could increase endotoxin in the portal circulation (Fig. 9).

Role of Kupffer cells in alcohol-induced liver injury and in reperfusion injury to fatty livers from ethanol-treated rats

Endotoxin activates Kupffer cells and triggers the release of a number of potent effectors and cytokines (Fig. 9). Most of the biological effects of endotoxin are

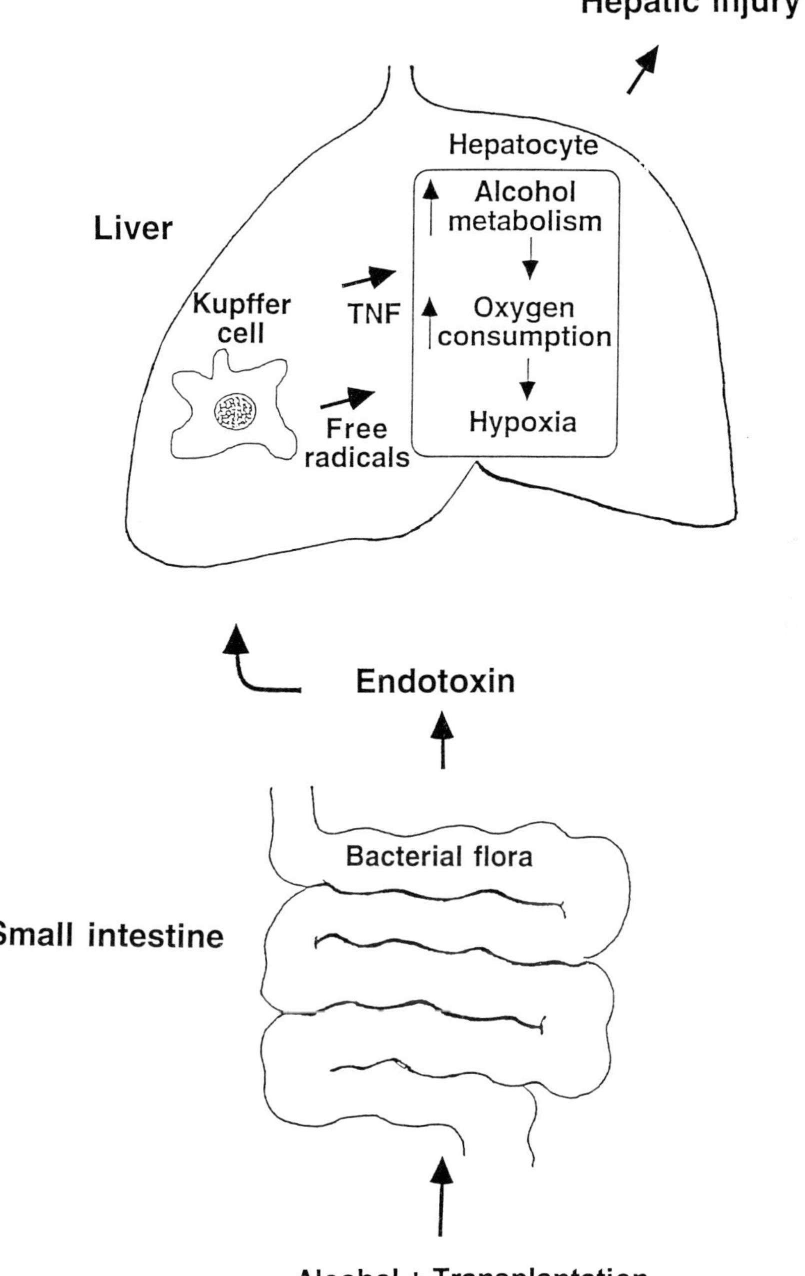

Fig. 9 Scheme depicting the possible involvement of Kupffer cells, endotoxin, hypoxia, and free radicals in the mechanism of alcohol-induced liver injury

probably mediated by these chemical factors, including chemoattractants (leukotrienes and TNF), procoagulants, cytotoxic factors (reactive oxygen free radicals, lysosomal enzymes), and vasoactive eicosanoids (leukotrienes, prostaglandins). Furthermore, since 90% of endotoxin injected intravenously is scavenged in the liver by Kupffer cells[39], most endotoxin derived from the intestine should also be removed by the liver. The production of mediators from activated Kupffer cells may lead directly to parenchymal cell injury[14,40].

Early injury to the liver caused by ethanol was prevented by inactivation of Kupffer cells with $GdCl_3$. Kupffer cells are probably activated by ethanol exposure[41], and endotoxin could be involved (Fig. 9). Levels of endotoxin in the peripheral blood of chronic alcoholics with liver disease are elevated[17]. In addition, plasma levels of endotoxin in rats infused continuously with an ethanol-containing diet increased in 1–2 weeks and a close correlation was seen between plasma endotoxin levels and severity of liver injury[28]. $GdCl_3$ also blocked the hypermetabolic state seen following liver transplantation[42], further supporting the link between mechanisms of alcohol- and transplantation-induced injury.

Further, in perfused livers from lipid-loaded, ethanol-treated rats, ethanol treatment exacerbated reperfusion injury, which occurs when oxygen is reintroduced to previously anoxic regions. This injury was minimized when Kupffer cells were inactivated (Fig. 8). Thus, Kupffer cells are involved in both alcohol-induced liver injury and in reperfusion injury in fat-loaded livers from ethanol-treated rats.

Possible mechanisms of Kupffer cell participation in liver injury

Kupffer cells activated by ethanol treatment may participate in liver injury through several possible mechanisms, including hypoxia, release of toxic mediators, and free radical formation (Fig. 9). Indeed, links between hypoxia and alcohol-induced liver injury exist[43–46]. In support of this idea, oxygen tension on the surface of the liver was increased significantly by ethanol treatment and was prevented by antibiotics (Fig. 6). Kupffer cells may participate in alcohol-induced liver injury by stimulating oxygen uptake, thus contributing to pericentral hypoxia. Alternatively, Kupffer cells activated by ethanol could release mediators which are directly toxic to liver cells or which attract cytotoxic neutrophils into the liver. TNF and interleukin-1, two of the mediators known to be released from activated Kupffer cells[8], are cytotoxic. In addition, both mediators stimulate neutrophil migration and activation as well as protease and oxygen radical release[47]. Cellular infiltration of activated neutrophils, which secrete oxygen radicals and other toxic mediators, may enhance the inflammatory response and lead to cell injury and death, and inflammatory cell infiltration due to ethanol has been shown to be blocked by $GdCl_3$[25]. Microcirculatory disturbances due to vasoconstrictive mediators released from Kupffer cells and neutrophils could potentiate hypoxia and lead to a vicious cycle of pathophysiology.

Free radicals have been implicated in hepatic injury following liver transplantation[48], and release of free radicals from Kupffer cells activated following ethanol administration is likely to be a factor in the hepatotoxicity of ethanol

(Fig. 9). We detected free radical adducts in the bile of rats treated intra-gastrically with a high-fat, ethanol-containing diet (Fig. 7), and antioxidant-insensitive free radicals have also been detected in livers of alcohol-treated rats after transplantation[49]. Although the precise pathway responsible for formation of free radicals in alcohol-treated rats remains unclear, since the EPR signal was reduced by $GdCl_3$, a strong possibility is oxygen radical production by the NADPH oxidase system in resident Kupffer cells and neutrophils. However, a reperfusion injury following hypoxia and free radical formation via the xanthine – xanthine oxidase system in parenchymal cells cannot be ruled out.

CONCLUSION

We propose that the pathophysiology of alcoholic hepatitis and liver transplantation of fatty grafts from alcohol-consuming donors is similar, differing only in magnitude. The mechanisms involve endotoxin and release of cytokines and eicosanoids from Kupffer cells which, directly or indirectly, lead to parenchymal cell death (Fig. 9).

Acknowledgements

Supported, in part, by grants AA-09156 from NIAAA and DK-37034 from NIH.

References

1. Nolan JP. Endotoxin, reticuloendothelial function, and liver injury. Hepatology. 1981;1:458–65.
2. Kahn D, Esquivel CO, Makowka L et al. Causes of death after liver transplantation in children treated with cyclosporine and steroids. Clin Transplant. 1989;3:150–5.
3. Greig PD, Woolf GM, Sinclair SB et al. Treatment of primary liver graft nonfunction with prostaglandin E_1. Transplantation. 1989;48:447–53.
4. Thurman RG, Cowper KB, Marzi I, Currin RT, Lemasters JJ. Activation of Kupffer cells by storage of the liver in Euro-Collins solution. Hepatology. 1988;8:261.
5. Decker K. Biologically active products of stimulated liver macrophages (Kupffer cells). Eur J Biochem. 1990;192:245–61.
6. Heinrich PC, Castell JV, Andus T. Interleukin-6 and the acute phase response. Biochem J. 1990;265:621–36.
7. Akira S, Hirano T, Taga T, Kishimoto T. Biology of multifunctional cytokines: IL 6 and related molecules (IL 1 and TNF). FASEB J. 1990;4:2860–7.
8. Martinez F, Abril ER, Earnest DL, Watson RR. Ethanol and cytokine secretion. Alcohol. 1992;9:455–8.
9. Yamada S, Mochida S, Ohno A et al. Evidence for enhanced secretory function of hepatic macrophages after long-term ethanol feeding in rats. Liver. 1991;11:220–4.
10. Stahnke LL, Hill DB, Allen JI. $TNF\alpha$ and IL-6 in alcoholic liver disease. In: Wisse E, Knook DL, McCuskey RS, editors. Cells of the hepatic sinusoids, 3rd edn. Leiden: Kupffer cell foundation, 1991:472–5.
11. Decker T, Lohmann-Matthes ML, Karck U, Peters T, Decker K. Comparative study of cytotoxicity, tumor necrosis factor, and prostaglandin release after stimulation of rat Kupffer cells, murine Kupffer cells, and murine inflammatory liver macrophages. J Leukocyte Biol. 1989;45:39–46.
12. Goto M, Lemasters JJ, Thurman RG. Activation of voltage-dependent calcium channels in Kupffer cells by chronic treatment with alcohol in the rat. J. Pharmacol Exp Ther. 1993;267:1264–8.

13. Monden K, Arii S, Itai S et al. Enhancement and hepatocyte-modulating effect of chemical mediators and monokines produced by hepatic macrophages in rats with induced sepsis. Res Exp Med. 1991;191:177–87.

14. Monden K, Arii S, Itai S et al. Enhancement of hepatic macrophages in septic rats and their inhibitory effect on hepatocyte function. J Surg Res. 1991;50:72–6.

15. Keller GA, West MA, Cerra FB, Simmons RL. Multiple system organ failure modulation of hepatocyte protein synthesis by endotoxin activated Kupffer cells. Ann Surg. 1985;201:87.

16. Bode C, Kugler V, Bode JC. Endotoxemia in patients with alcoholic and non-alcoholic cirrhosis and in subjects with no evidence of chronic liver disease following acute alcohol excess. J Hepatol. 1987;4:8–14.

17. Fukui H, Brauner B, Bode JC, Bode C. Plasma endotoxin concentrations in patients with alcoholic and non-alcoholic liver disease: reevaluation with an improved chromogenic assay. Hepatology. 1991;12:162–9.

18. Nanji AA, Khettry U, Sadrzadeh SMH, Yamanaka T. Severity of liver injury in experimental alcoholic liver disease. Correlation with plasma endotoxin, prostaglandin E_2, leukotriene B_4, and thromboxane B_2. Am J Pathol. 1993;142:367–73.

19. Zimmermann FA, Butcher GW, Davies HS, Brons G, Kamada N, Türel O. Techniques of orthotopic liver transplantation in the rat and some studies of the immunologic response to fully allogeneic liver grafts. Transplant Proc. 1979;1:571–7.

20. Kamada N, Calne RY. Orthotopic liver transplantation in the rat. Technique using cuff for portal vein anastomosis and biliary drainage. Transplantation. 1979;28:47–50.

21. Kramer SM, Carver ME. Serum-free in vitro bioassay for the detection of tumor necrosis factor. J Immunol Methods. 1986;93:201–206.

22. Aarden LA, De Groot ER, Schaap OL, Lansdorp PM. Production of hybridoma growth factor by human monocytes. Eur J Immunol. 1987;17:1411–6.

23. Tsukamoto H, Reiderberger RD, French SW, Largman C. Long-term cannulation model for blood sampling and intragastric infusion in the rat. Am J Physiol. 1984;247:R595–9.

24. Thompson JA, Reitz RC. Effects of ethanol ingestion and dietary fat levels on mitochondrial lipids in male and female rats. Lipids. 1978;13:540–50.

25. Adachi Y, Bradford BU, Gao W, Bojes HK, Thurman RG. Inactivation of Kupffer cells prevents early alcohol-induced liver injury. Hepatology. 1994;20:453–60.

26. Satoh H, Guth PH, Grossman MI. Role of bacteria in gastric ulceration produced by indomethacin in the rat: cytoprotective action of antibiotics. Gastroenterology. 1983;84:483–9.

27. Bergmeyer HU. Methods of enzymatic analysis. New York: Academic Press, 1988.

28. Nanji AA, Mendenhall CL, French SW. Beef fat prevents alcoholic liver disease in the rat. Alcohol Clin Exp Res. 1989;13:15–19.

29. Adachi Y, Bradford BU, Gao W, Thurman RG. Mechanisms of alcohol-induced liver injury: Hypoxia and role of Kupffer cells. Toxicologist. 1994;14:369.

30. Knecht KT, Adachi Y, Thurman RG. Detection of free radical adducts in the bile of rats treated chronically with intragastric alcohol. Hepatology. 1993;18:270A.

31. Thurman RG, Bunzendahl H, Lemasters JJ. Role of sinusoidal lining cells in hepatic reperfusion injury following cold storage and transplantation. Semin Liver Dis. 1993;13:93–100.

32. Beutler B, Cerami A. The history, properties, and biological effects of cachectin. Biochemistry. 1988;27:7575–82.

33. Mathison JC, Wolfson E, Ulevitch RJ. Participation of tumor necrosis factor in the mediation of gram negative bacterial lipopolysaccharide-induced injury in rabbits. J Clin Invest. 1988;81:1925–37.

34. Savier E, Shedlofsky SI, Swim AT, Lemasters JJ, Thurman RG. The calcium channel blocker nisoldipine minimizes the release of tumor necrosis factor and interleukin-6 following rat liver transplantation. Transplant Int. 1992;5:S398–402.

35. Lopes J, Iniss WE. Electron microscopy of effect of polymyxin B on E. coli lipopolysaccharide. J Bacteriol. 1969;100:1128–30.

36. Bode JC. Alcohol and the gastrointestinal tract. In: Frick HP, Harnack GA, Martini GA, Prader A, editors. Advances in Internal Medicine and Pediatrics. Heidelberg: Springer-Verlag, 1980: 1–75.

37. Remmer H. Die Wirkungen des Alkohols. Alkoholwirkungen. 1981;17:1–11.

38. Bode JC, Bode C, Heidelbach R, Durr H-K, Martini GA. Jejunal microflora in patients with chronic alcohol abuse. Hepato-gastroenterol. 1984;31:30–4.

39. Arii S, Monden K, Itai S, Sasaoki T, Shibagaki M, Tobe T. The three different phases of reticuloendothelial system phagocytic function in rats with liver injury. J Surg Res. 1988;45: 314–9.
40. Wendell GD, Thurman RG. Effect of ethanol concentration on rates of ethanol elimination in normal and alcohol-treated rats in vivo. Biochem Pharmacol. 1979;28:273–9.
41. D'Souza NB, Bagby GJ, Lang CH, Deaciuc IV, Spitzer JJ. Ethanol alters the metabolic response of isolated, perfused rat liver to a phagocytic stimulus. Alcohol Clin Exp Res. 1993;17:147–54.
42. Qu W, Savier E, Thurman RG. Stimulation of monooxygenation and conjugation following liver transplantation in the rat: involvement of Kupffer cells. Mol Pharmacol. 1992;41:1149–54.
43. Videla L, Bernstein J, Israel Y. Metabolic alteration produced in the liver by chronic alcohol administration. Increased oxidative capacity. Biochem J. 1973;134:507–14.
44. Bernstein J, Videla L, Israel Y. Metabolic alterations produced in the liver by chronic ethanol administration. Changes related to energetic parameters of the cell. Biochem J. 1973;134: 515–21.
45. Ji S, Lemasters JJ, Thurman RG. Intralobular hepatic pyridine nucleotide fluorescence: evaluation of the hypothesis that chronic treatment with ethanol produces pericentral hypoxia. Proc Natl Acad Sci USA. 1982;80:5415–9.
46. Yuki T, Thurman RG. The swift increase in alcohol metabolism. Time course for the increase in hepatic oxygen uptake and the involvement of glycolysis. Biochem J. 1980;186:119–26.
47. Thiele DL. Tumor necrosis factor, the acute phase response and the pathogenesis of alcoholic liver disease. Hepatology. 1989;9:497–9.
48. Connor HD, Gao W, Nukina S, Lemasters JJ, Mason RP, Thurman RG. Free radicals are involved in graft failure following orthotopic liver transplantation: An EPR spin trapping study. Transplantation. 1992;54:199–204.
49. Gao W, Connor HD, Lemasters JJ, Mason RP, Thurman RG. Primary non-function of transplanted livers produced by ethanol is associated with new antioxidant insensitive free radicals. Transplantation. 1995; in press.

18
Role of cytokines in the regulation of cell – cell and cell – matrix adhesion molecules in human liver transplants

G. STEINHOFF

INTRODUCTION

A large number of cell contact molecules that regulate membrane bound intercellular contact and signalling as well as the specific binding of cell membrane receptors to matrix molecules have been identified[1-4]. These are classified according to molecular structure into immunoglobulin supergene, integrin, selectin, cadherin and CD44 molecular families[1]. Table 1 gives a survey of the respective receptor–ligand interactions. The identification of these molecules forms a major basis for the understanding of processes by which differentiated cell types make contact in various organ systems. Intercellular membrane contact processes mediated by adhesion molecules are of general importance for immunological reactions to pathogens and target cells in different organs. The organ-specific and systemic regulation of these processes is probably dependent on the local presence of endothelial adhesion ligand molecules for leukocyte receptors in the vascular stream bed of inflamed organs and mainly mediated by soluble chemoattractants such as cytokines. Moreover, the result of inflammatory cytokine-induced cell activation is mainly executed by specific membrane adhesion receptor molecules mediating cell migration and phagocytosis. Organ-specific variations in intravascular endothelial activation and adhesion molecule expression are of major importance for the local appearance of leukocyte mediated inflammatory processes. As well as activation of inflammatory cells by direct receptor-mediated intercellular membrane contact a second pathway of cell activation is most likely exerted by membrane receptor interaction with soluble or bound matrix molecules.

Table 1 Overview on receptor–ligand combinations of cell–cell and cell–matrix adhesion molecules

Adhesion molecule	Receptor/ligand
Immunoglobulin supergene family	
CD2	LFA-3
ICAM-1	LFA-1, Mac-1/CD18
ICAM-2	LFA-1
ICAM-3	LFA-1, ?
VCAM-1	VLA-4 (CS-1; LDV-peptide)
CD31 (PECAM)	?
CD56 (NCAM)	Heparane sulphate, NCAM
CD4	MHC II
CD8	MHC I
MHC Class I	TCR, CD8
MHC Class II	TCR, CD4
Integrin family	
CD11a (LFA-1) β1(CD18)-Integrin	ICAM-1-3
CD11b (Mac-1) β1-Integrin	C3bi, Factor X, fibrinogen, ICAM-1
CD11c (p150,95) β1-Integrin	?
CD49a (VLA-1) β2(CD29)-Integrin	Laminin, Collagen (RGD-Peptide)
CD49b (VLA-2) β2-Integrin	Laminin, Collagen (RGD)
CD49c (VLA-3) β2-Integrin	Fibronectin, Laminin, Collagen (RGD)
CD49d (VLA-4) β2-Integrin	Fibronectin, Thrombospondin (RGD)
	M-Addressin/Madcam, VCAM-1 (CS-1)
CD49e (VLA-5) β2-Integrin	Fibronectin (RGD)
CD49f (VLA-6) β2-Integrin	Laminin (RGD)
CD51 β2-Integrin	Fibronectin (RGD)
CD51 β3(CD61)-Integrin	Vitronectin, Fibrinogen, vWF, Thrombospondin
Selectin-family	
L-Selectin	CD34, Madcam-1, Glycam-1
E-Selectin	Sialyl Lewis X, PSGL-1
P-Selectin	Sialyl Lewis X, PSGL-1, Glycam-1
C44 (isovariants)	Hyaluronic acid

INDUCTION OF ADHESION MOLECULES BY CYTOKINES IN HUMAN LIVER TRANSPLANTS

According to current knowledge from in vitro and in vivo studies the adherence of leukocytes to endothelial cells requires a particular sequence of adhesion receptor binding to result in firm binding and transendothelial diapedesis. The sequence of adhesion molecule induction, however, is dictated by the presence of cytokines. Table 2 shows the presumed role of early (histamine, thrombin) and late [interleukin-1 (IL-1), tumor necrosis factor (TNF) and interferon-γ (IFN-γ)] cytokines in regulation of respective ligand molecule expression on endothelial cells. From in vivo studies in transplanted livers it is clear that endothelial cells inside the organ stream bed of the liver differ in their basal expression of adhesion ligand molecules necessary to facilitate leukocyte contact[5–7]. Both the sequence of induction after transplantation and the pattern of later induced adhesion ligand molecules (ICAM-1) support a concept of a stepwise expression regulated by cytokines[7]. A survey of the expression of adhesion molecules on liver endothelia and parenchyma cells during rejection and inflammatory

Table 2 Role of cytokines in adhesion molecule induction on endothelial cells

	Adhesion molecule	*Cytokine*
Immediate phase of adhesion (leukocyte rolling) (5 – 30 min)	P-Selectin	Histamine, thrombin, LTC4
Intermediate phase of adhesion (1 – 6 h)	E-selectin	IL-1, TNF
	ICAM-1	IL-1, TNF
Late phase of adhesion (12 – 48 h)	ICAM-1	IL-1, TNF, IFN-γ
	VCAM-1	IL-4, IFN-γ
Leukocyte extravasation and transmigration (all phases)	PECAM-1 (CD31)	
	VCAM-1	IL-8, PAF

complications after transplantation is given in Table 3[7]. Comparative analysis of the distribution of cytokines and adhesion molecules in human liver grafts demonstrated that local differences in ICAM-1 expression on endothelia relates to local concentrations of the respective inducing cytokines (IL-1, TNF-α) in sinusoidal endothelia and Kupffer cells[8]. A major point of relevance to the organ-specific appearance of leukocyte infiltration could be the resistance of sinusoidal lining endothelia to express selectin receptors[6,7]. It is clear now that the essential start signal to intravascular leukocyte and thrombocyte adherence is the binding of selectin receptors to oligosaccharides (sialyl Lewis X) and additional ligand molecules such as CD34, PSGL-1, Glycam-1, Madcam-1[9–11]. The selectin-dependent physiological adherence process of leukocytes is described as 'rolling'[12] and is necessary for the initiation of sequential binding of β1- and β2-integrin receptors of leukocytes[13,14]. The lack of selectins in the liver sinusoid therefore may prohibit a full activation and firm adhesion of leukocytes.

Following the selectin-induced 'rolling' of leukocytes on endothelial membrane glycoproteins a cascade of adhesion steps leading to firm leukocyte binding and transendothelial migration is effective. This involves mainly the β1-integrin receptors (CD11 a – c) and the β2-integrin VLA-4 (CS-1 peptide binding site) in binding to the ligand molecules ICAM-1, ICAM-2, VCAM-1 and CD31 expressed or induced on endothelial cells[7]. Adhesion of the RGD-binding site of the VLA-4 leukocyte β2-integrin receptor to matrix molecules probably becomes effective at the level of subendothelial basal membrane glycoproteins and during interstitial migration. RGD-dependent stimulation of β2-integrin receptors, however, may also be initiated intravascularly by circulating soluble matrix molecules as fibrinogen, fibronectin, laminin and procollagen. This binding may lead to the intracellular gene activation of leukocytes, resulting in increased integrin receptor expression and the stimulation of cytokine production for IL-1, IL-6 and TNF-α[15,16]. This interaction of soluble matrix molecules with integrin receptors may form a potent mechanism of intravascular leukocyte stimulation prior to their contact to liver endothelia during inflammation. The liver, as a site of production of soluble matrix molecules and of cytokines capable of inducing adhesion receptor expression, may therefore regulate systemic intravascular adhesiveness of leukocytes.

Table 3 Patterns of adhesion molecule expression on resident liver cells in acute and chronic transplant inflammation

Cell type	Normal liver	Organ reperfusion	Acute rejection	Irreversible and chronic rejection	Sepsis, cholangitis, viral infection
Endothelial cells					
Portal artery	ICAM-2	ICAM-2, CD62 ELAM-1	ICAM-2, CD62, VCAM-1, ELAM-1 ICAM-1, LFA-3	ICAM-2, CD62 VCAM-1, ELAM-1 ICAM-1, LFA-3	ICAM-2, CD62 VCAM-1, ELAM-1 ICAM-1, LFA-3
	VLA-1,3,5,6	VLA-1,2,3,5,6	VLA-1,2,3,5,6	VLA-1,2,3,5,6	VLA-1,2,3,5,6
Portal vein	(ELAM-1)	CD62, ELAM-1	CD62, ELAM-1 ICAM-1, VCAM-1 LFA-3	CD62, ELAM-1 ICAM-1, VCAM-1 LFA-3	CD62, ELAM-1 ICAM-1, VCAM-1 LFA-3
	VLA-1,2,3,5,6 CD51	VLA-1,2,3,5,6 CD51	VLA-1,2,3,5,6 CD51	VLA-1,2,3,5,6 CD51	VLA-1,2,3,5,6 CD51
Sinusoidal endothelium	ICAM-1, ICAM-2 LFA-3 CD-4, CD51 VLA-1,(3,4),5	ICAM-1, ICAM-2 LFA-3 CD-4, CD51 VLA-1,(3,4),5	ICAM-1, ICAM-2 LFA-3, (VCAM-1) CD-4, CD51, CD44 VLA-1,3,4,5,6	ICAM-1, ICAM-2 LFA-3, VCAM-1, NCAM CD-4, CD51, CD44 VLA-1,3,4,5,6	ICAM-1, ICAM-2 LFA-3, VCAM-1 CD-4, CD51, CD44 VLA-1,3,4,5,6
Central vein	VLA-1,5	VLA-1,5 (CD62)	VLA-1,5 CD62, ELAM-1 (VAM-1, LFA-3)	VLA-1,2,5 CD62, ELAM-1 VCAM-1, LFA-3 ICAM-1	VLA-1,5 CD62, ELAM-1 VCAM-1, LFA-3 ICAM1
Epithelial cells					
Bile duct	VLA-2,3,6	VLA-2,3,6	VLA-2,3,6 ICAM-1, NCAM LFA-3, CD51	VLA-2,3,6 ICAM-1, NCAM LFA-3, CD51	VLA-2,3,6 ICAM-1, NCAM LFA-3, CD51
Hepatocytes	VLA-1,5 (HECA452)	VLA-1,5 ICAM-1 (HECA452)	VLA-1,2,3,5,6 ICAM-1, LFA-3 CD-51,HECA452	VLA-1,5,6;HECA452 ICAM-1, LFA-3 (CD-51, CD31, VCAM-1)	VLA-1,5,(6) ICAM-1;HECA452 (CD-51)

Intravascular cytokine effects on leukocyte adhesion receptors

A prerequisite for the induction of leukocyte integrin receptor binding is a cytokine-induced change of receptor affinity. Alteration in receptor conformation that leads to higher affinity for the ligand can be induced either by the systemic cytokine levels in the blood stream (IL-1, TNF-α) or at the endothelial contact site. The intravascular change in intercellular affinity of leukocytes following cytokine stimulation is probably a consequence of changes in the conformation of the extracellular domain of the LFA-1 heterodimer, either by physical association with the actin-based cytoskeleton or by direct biochemical modification of the cytoplasmic domains. The first measurable event in this context is the multi-step activation of Ca^{2+}-dependent protein kinase[17] C combined with a temporary increase in intracellular Ca^{2+} concentration. In connection with this, a network of protein kinase C-dependent phosphorylations of a variety of substrates in addition to the LFA-1 heterodimer may cause a change in affinity of this molecule. The cytoskeleton-associated isoforms of LFA- and other integrins undergo changes in the conformation of their extracellular domain, with the creation of neo-epitopes[18,19] and the loss of other epitopes that exist in heterodimers, but are not associated with the cytoskeleton. Polarization of a cell resulting from the new arrangement of the cytoskeleton may help to direct the secretory part of the leukocyte toward the cell-bound. This may allow effector functions to be performed with the secretion of soluble mediators in a very efficient paracrine form. Lastly, adhesion receptor diffusion or lateral mobility of the receptors is an important factor that determines the fate of the interaction between a receptor and its ligand. The observed event is probably a mechanism caused by a high lateral mobility of glycosyl-phosphatidyl-inositol bound forms that accumulate soluble or transmembranous ligands in the area of cellular attachment[20]. This is supported by the fact that adhesion to transmembranous forms of the ligand is less efficient when they are expressed at a lower density. Localization of various ligand isoforms in certain areas of the cell membrane[21] suggests that sequential leukocyte adhesion to different isoforms of these molecules is related to a mechanistic movement from the site of initial contact (apical) to areas of transmigration (basement membrane).

The activation-dependent interaction of leukocyte integrin receptors is stable for minutes under physiological shear stress conditions, but seems to be a reversible event[22]. As a consequence of this reversibility, extravasation is not obligatory following endothelial cell binding. The progress from temporary endothelial binding of leukocytes may depend on a second signal that may originate from extravascular stimulants such as chemoattractive substances. This second signal may be a requirement for the initiation of diapedesis and tissue migration. If, however, the second permissive signal is derived from the endothelial cell itself, extravascular chemoattractants may then function for the initiation of extravasation. Thus in several situations, and probably in organ-specific sites, the kind of extravascular signals and chemoattractive substances released determine whether an endothelial bound leukocyte is able to emigrate or to be released to the circulation again[14].

CYTOKINE EFFECTS ON ORGAN-SPECIFIC EXPRESSION OF CELL ADHESION MOLECULES

Organ-specific differences in the immunological susceptibility to the rejection response in transplanted livers can be explained by the patterns of basal or induced expression of intercellular adhesion molecules on different organ cell types. The expression of MHC- and other adhesion molecules including cell matrix receptors is clearly cell type specific[23]. Despite major differences in the patterns of ligand molecules and their inducibility by cytokines it can be generally postulated that almost all cell types can be immunologically recognized by immune cells upon induction of the main ligand molecules, allo-MHC (class I) and ICAM-1. This induction of ligand molecules, however, requires the local release of cytokines such as IL-1 and TNF-α by tissue macrophages, endothelial cells or infiltrating leukocytes. A relative resistance against immunological recognition can result from deficient basal expression (for instance on hepatocytes and myocytes) or from a relative resistance to cytokine-mediated induction (myocytes). This may be explained in part by a differential distribution of cytokine receptors on different cell types. The composition of an organ with cell types of different immunocompetence with regard to adhesive binding capacity of infiltrating leukocytes most likely determines its susceptibility to the immune assault. Generally, a minor basal expression of adhesion ligand molecules or an incomplete ligand pattern can be overcome by the action of locally released cytokines from infiltrating leukocytes or tissue macrophages. Susceptibility to cytokine stimulation of different cell types may also determine patterns of adhesion ligand molecules induced in a specific organ. Therefore the regulation of the anti-alloantigenic immune response and its manifestation may depend on organ-specific intravascular stimulation (in vascularized organ transplants). On the other hand, the localization and mode of interstitial infiltration may depend on the organ-specific composition of adhesion ligands and cell matrix molecules, allowing differences in the stimulation and manifestation of immune reactivity. The local cellular sensitivity to immune recognition – mainly determined by expression of MHC and other adhesion ligand molecules – may determine the organ-specific differences in cytokine-mediated effector mechanisms and the extent of organ destruction by the rejection response.

The tissue-specific immunogenicity of the transplanted liver is probably determined by the specific patterns of adhesive ligand molecules on endothelial cells in the organ stream bed of the liver. This expression differs in arterial, venous and sinusoidal endothelial cells of normal liver and liver transplants during rejection[5–7]. This fact could explain differing vascular adhesiveness and activation of leukocytes inside the vascular bed. A special regulation of lymphocyte adhesion has to be assumed for the liver sinusoid. Differences in susceptibility of epithelial and mesenchymal cell types to the immune response can be explained by the degree of basal expression and cytokine-dependent inducibility of immunological ligand molecules. Organ-specific peculiarities exist in the intravascular or perivascular distribution of cells possessing major immunocompetence by expression of adhesion molecules and other cell functions (interstitial dendritic cells, Kupffer cells).

A central regulator of the antigen specific reaction of $CD4^+$ T-helper lymphocytes is the tissue expression of allo-class II (HLA-DR) MHC molecules in transplants. These are present or may be induced by cytokines on many cell types of liver transplants. The stimulation of T-lymphocytes by the various cell types, however, may have different effects. This could have a basis in the fact that additional co-stimulatory ligand molecules such as B7 (BB7 ligand to CD28), LFA-3, ICAM-1 and -2, and VCAM-1 have a variable expression on different cell types and are co-expressed in high density mainly on the 'immunocompetent' interstitial dendritic cells and monocytes/macrophages. Therefore the order in which different cell types react to T-lymphocytes may depend on the presence of a panel of adhesion ligand molecules. In addition, these cell types are capable of producing stimulatory cytokines such as IL-1 and IFN-γ upon binding of T-lymphocytes. Intracellular functions such as the cleavage and presentation of antigenic peptides with MHC molecules determine their immunological interactivity. For $CD8^+$ cytotoxic lymphocytes to interact with target cells and cause cytolysis, the presence of the target antigen, alloantigenic MHC molecules, is also a prerequisite. However, additional binding co-structures such as ICAM-1 and LFA-3 may also be necessary to induce a cascade reaction leading to cytolysis. Therefore the presence, or rather the inducibility, of certain immune ligand molecules mainly by IL-1, IL-6, IFN-γ and TNF-α in an organ transplant is a precondition for the sensitization of alloantigen-directed T-lymphocytes and the manifestation of an effector reaction.

ADHESION MOLECULES AND TRANSPLANT INFLAMMATION

The existence of a membrane-bound local regulation of leukocyte and lymphocyte reactivity by the activation of the transplant endothelium and the possible systemic immune activation by the secretion of soluble adhesion molecules (MHC, ICAM-1, ICAM-2, ELAM-1) and cytokines (IL-1, TNF-α) by the transplant endothelia places immunological changes of an organ transplant in the centre of the regulation of the immune response. The endothelial cell, and in the liver the Kupffer cell, probably play a previously unrecognized active role in the modification of immune reactions. These functions are probably only partially influenced by the immunosuppression given. Organ-specific and general conclusions about the regulation of rejection and other inflammatory reactions can be drawn with new insight. An important factor for the generation of tissue inflammation is the key role of LFA-1/MAC-1 binding to ICAM-1 and binding of VLA-4 to VCAM-1. This could explain the synergistic inflammatory actions of different leukocyte subpopulations. Furthermore, it is of importance that different pathological stimuli, such as for instance viral infection (of leukocytes or transplant cells) or transplant rejection, may influence each other by the use of identical inflammatory pathways. This may be of particular relevance for chronic inflammatory transplant disease due to different causes.

The analysis of adhesion molecules in the transplant could be of clinical diagnostic interest. The agreement of induction phenomena in different rejection- and non-rejection-related inflammatory reactions shows general mechanisms of the inflammatory response. Additional information about the kind of pathological stimulus cannot therefore be expected from such an analysis. Information about the inflammatory state of the transplant, can, however, be drawn. An example of this is the expression and induction of vascular adhesion ligand molecules. These may point to subclinical and clinical pathological activation states. The activation of only sinusoidal endothelial cells without co-activation of hepatocytes, for instance, may point to a systemic stimulus. Such information may help to assess the risk situation of an organ transplant as a result of endothelial activation (viral infection, chronic rejection). This may influence the immunosuppressive and anti-inflammatory drug regimen. A prospect for anti-inflammatory intervention is a direct approach of adhesion molecules by oligosaccharide or peptide receptor blockade. In the near future a close connection between diagnosis of cellular changes of adhesion molecules or their excretion in soluble form in the serum and therapeutic modulation can be expected. Further advances may result from knowledge about the induction of cell matrix integrin receptors on transplant cells during inflammation. This could be a way to diagnose and interfere with fibrogenetic changes in the transplant. At the present time it is unclear which cytokines or inducers change integrin receptor expression on the different cell types and how this relates to fibrogenetic inflammatory activity. Further investigation, however, may reveal the fibro-genetic activity of different cell types such as hepatocytes, endothelia or Kupffer cells. Further in vitro studies may clarify the interaction of cytokine-induced fibrogenesis and membrane or intracellular changes in different transplant cell types mediated by cell matrix integrin receptors.

References

1. Springer TA. Adhesion receptors of the immune system. Nature. 1990;346:425–34.
2. Hogg N, Harvey J, Cabanas C, Landis RC. Control of leukocyte integrin activation. Am Rev Resp Dis. 1993;148:55–9.
3. Springer TA, Lasky TA. Sticky sugars for selectins. Nature. 1991;349:196.
4. Hynes RO. Integrins: Versatility, modulation and signaling in cell adhesion. Cell. 1992;69:11–25.
5. Steinhoff G. Cell adhesion molecules in human organ transplants. Austin: RG Landes Co. 1993:1–110.
6. Steinhoff G, Behrend M, Schrader B, Duijvestijn AM, Wonigeit K. Expression patterns of leucocyte adhesion ligand molecules on human liver endothelia: lack of ELAM-1 and CD62 inducibility on sinusoidal endothelia and distinct distribution of VCAM-1, ICAM-1, ICAM-2, and LFA-3. Am J Pathol. 1993;142:481–8.
7. Steinhoff G, Behrend M, Schrader B, Pichlmayr R. Intercellular immune adhesion molecules in human liver transplants – overview on expression patterns of leukocyte receptor and ligand molecules. Hepatology. 1993;18:440–53.
8. Hoffmann MW, Wonigeit K, Steinhoff G, Herzbeck H, Flad HD, Pichlmayr R. Production of cytokines (TNF-α, IL-1β) and endothelial cell activation in human liver allograft rejection. Transplantation. 1993;55:329–35.
9. Sako D, Chang XJ, Barone KM et al. Expression cloning of a functional glycoprotein ligand for P-selectin. Cell. 1993;75:1179–86.
10. Baumheter S, Singer MS, Henzel W et al. Binding of L-selectin to the vascular sialomucin CD34. Science. 1993;262:436–8.
11. Imai Y, Lasky LA, Rosen SD. Sulphation requirement for GlyCAM-1, an endothelial ligand for L-selectin. Nature. 1993;361:555–7.
12. Lawrence MB, Springer TA. Leukocytes roll on a selectin at physiologic flow rates: distinction from and prerequisite for adhesion through integrins. Cell. 1991;65:859–73.

13. Lindbohm L, Xie X, Raud J, Hedqvist P. Chemoattractant-induced leukocyte adhesion to vascular endothelium in vivo is critically dependent on initial leukocyte rolling. Acta Physiol Scand. 1992;146:415–21.
14. Butcher EC. Leukocyte-endothelial cell recognition: three (or more) steps of specificity and diversity. Cell. 1991;67:1033–6.
15. Yurochko AD, Liu DY, Eierman D, Haskill S. Integrins as a primary signal transduction molecule regulating monocyte immediate-early gene induction. Proc Natl Acad Sci USA. 1992;89:9034–8.
16. Dayer JM, Isler P, Nicad LP. Adhesion molecules and cytokine production. Am Rev Resp Dis. 1993;148:70–4.
17. Dustin ML, Springer TA. Role of lymphocyte adhesion receptors in transient interactions and cell locomotion. Annu Rev Immunol. 1991;9:27–66.
18. van Kooyk Y, Weder P, Hogervorst F et al. Activation of LFA-1 through a Ca^{2+}-dependent epitope stimulates lymphocyte adhesion. J Cell Biol. 1991;112:345–54.
19. Altieri DC, Edgington TS. A monoclonal antibody reacting with distinct adhesion molecules defines a transition in the state of the receptor CD11b/CD18 (Mac-1). J Immunol. 1988;141:2656–60.
20. Chan BMC, Kassner PD, Schiro JA, Byers HR, Kupper TS, Hemler ME. Distinct cellular functions mediated by different VLA-integrin a subunit cytoplasmic domain. Cell. 1992;68:1051–60.
21. Powell SK, Cunningham BA, Edelman GM, Rodriguez-Boulan E. Targeting of transmembrane and GPI-anchored forms of N-CAM to opposite domains of a polarized epithelial cell. Nature. 1991;353:76–77.
22. Lo SK, Detmers PA, Levin SM, Wright SD. Transient adhesion of neutrophils to endothelium. J Exp Med. 1989;169:1779–93.
23. Steinhoff G, Wonigeit K, Pichlmayr R. Analysis of sequential changes in major histocompatibility complex expression in human liver grafts after transplantation. Transplantation. 1988;45:394–401.

19
Cytokines in liver allograft rejection

A. S. GAWECO and W. J. HOFMANN

INTRODUCTION

Substantial progress in our understanding of transplantation immunology has made solid organ transplantation a clinical reality for the treatment of several end-stage disorders. Orthotopic liver transplantation (OLTX) remains the only therapeutic procedure for end-stage liver disease. However, allograft rejection still imposes a constant threat to the patient and graft. In the event of an acute rejection transplant recipients require anti-rejection therapy with high-dose steroids and OKT3, associated with a high degree of toxicity and a high incidence of infections in the short term, and development of lympho-proliferative disorders in the long term. Recently, acute rejection episodes have been implicated in the development of chronic rejection, the most common cause of late graft loss following orthotopic liver transplantation[1,2]. Thus, under-standing the mechanisms of the acute rejection process is of crucial importance in the optimal control of graft acceptance.

Following grafting, incompatible major histocompatibility complex (MHC) antigens (Ag) of the foreign graft are presented to the host by antigen-presenting cells (APC) of donor and recipient origin. The foreign antigens, presented directly or indirectly, are recognized by CD4$^+$ T-cells through the T-cell receptor (TCR)–CD3 complex. Engagement of the TCR during T cell activation initiates a series of events leading to activation of effector mechanisms mediating both cellular and humoral responses. Allograft rejection involves an intricate interaction between Ag-specific and non-specific effector cells with the foreign allograft which is critically regulated by their elaborated cytokines. The immunosuppressive effects of drugs currently used in maintenance immunosuppression, such as CsA and FK 506, are known to arise from inhibition of cytokine production[3,4]. Studying the cytokine interactions following organ transplantation in an immunomodulated host system may lead to a better understanding of the complex graft rejection process. These may help to optimize immunosuppressive strategies and raise the possibility of detecting cytokines as an additional immunological monitoring parameter to complement the diagnosis of rejection from other post-transplant complications.

CYTOKINE DETECTION

Attempts have been made to correlate systemic cytokine levels measured in body fluids following organ transplantation with the immunological events within the allograft. Several studies assessing the possible application of detecting cytokines in correlating ongoing acute rejection crises have been without success. Detection of systemic cytokine levels may not be an accurate measure of the presence of these factors within the graft during an acute rejection episode. The transient and brief production of small amounts of cytokines in the graft may already mediate in the destructive graft effector mechanisms in an autocrine and paracrine manner. Levels in the periphery may only be detected and measured if high amounts are produced where the immunological events are taking place, i.e. within the graft, reflecting the tip of the iceberg. In addition to its low sensitivity, the lack of specificity of commercially available assays may lead to inaccurate and misleading results[5,6].

Studies involving samples from human allografts are greatly restricted because of the limited amount of material available for investigation. Liver biopsy samples processed by formalin fixation for routine diagnosis necessitate priority. Such material is, however, not suitable for further translational and transcriptional analysis following fixation because of protein degradation and the extreme instability of cytokine mRNAs due to the presence of AU-rich consensus sequences in their 3′ untranslated region[7,8]. Studying the local intragraft events in the host–graft interplay provides an accurate picture of the immunological activities within the graft, as shown by the superior results of local against systemic immunosuppression[9]. The advantage of morphological studies employing immunohistochemistry and in situ hybridization, particularly important in identifying the source of the elaborated cytokines of an immunological event in study, has limitations because of its low sensitivity. Localizing the cellular source of cytokine message transcription using in situ PCR which combines the sensitivity of PCR and localizing abilities of in situ hybridization, although still in a developing stage, holds promise in the future.

Given the limited amount of snap-frozen biopsy material available from liver transplant patients, cytokine studies require techniques with a high degree of sensitivity without compromising specificity. An approach to the analysis of cytokine patterns is at the mRNA transcript level. The Northern blot technique however, requires the presence of at least 10^5-10^6 molecules per sample to produce a positive signal for the mRNA transcript in question[10]. With the rapid development in molecular biological techniques, cytokine patterns could be successfully studied employing minimal amount of clinical material based on cytokine gene activity using solution-phase reverse-transcriptase polymerase chain reaction (RT-PCR). RT-PCR has many advantages including direct analysis of allograft sample biopsies. However, optimized PCR conditions for each primer pair have to be established, since amplification under suboptimal PCR conditions could otherwise lead to false positive and negative results (Gaweco et al., unpublished observations). Qualitative information regarding cytokine expression obtained using semi-quantitative solution-phase RT-PCR has its limitations, since obtaining quantitative information from conventional PCR can be difficult if not inconsistent. Further refinements of quantitative competitive RT-PCR may solve this problem.

The relative ease of RT-PCR has prompted several transplant centres, including ours, to approach cytokine analysis based on mRNA transcript detection using this method. mRNA expression patterns of several cytokines in human liver, kidney, pancreas, heart and lung allografts have been investigated in attempts to correlate the cytokine profile with the immunological status of the transplant allograft.

CYTOKINES IN ALLOIMMUNITY

Following grafting of a foreign tissue, the recipient will reject the foreign graft unless the host immune response is suppressed. In clinical transplantation, graft rejection is prevented by potent immunosuppressive agents which selectively inhibit host effector mechanisms that would otherwise lead to the destruction of the allograft. These processes are tightly regulated by the complex interaction of elaborated cytokines during allograft rejection. Indeed, the profound immuno-suppressive effects of these agents are thought to arise from its inhibitory effects on cytokine production.

Graft destruction during the acute rejection process is primarily mediated by cellular effector mechanisms through cytotoxic T lymphocyte (CTL) activity by CD8[+] CTL and delayed-type hypersensitivity (DTH) responses by activated macrophages. Initially described in mice[11,12], human CD4[+] T lymphocytes can be subdivided into two subsets based on cytokine production and its effector functions[13-15]. CD4[+] T helper type 1 (TH$_1$) cells produce interleukin-2 (IL-2), interferon (IFN-γ) and lymphotoxin promoting cellular responses through DTH and CTL activity, while T helper type 2 (TH$_2$) cells produce IL-4, IL-5, IL-6, IL-10 and IL-13 mediating humoral responses. Both subsets are counter-regulatory, inhibiting each others' function and proliferation following elaboration of their characteristic cytokines[16,17]. From the CD4[+] paradigm, it can be speculated that TH$_1$ cytokines principally mediate damage to the graft by promoting cell-mediated responses. Not surprisingly, TH$_1$ cytokines are readily demonstrated in acute rejecting allografts but not in the absence of clinical rejection[18-25]. Data from experimental models show that in addition to the downregulation of TH$_1$ cytokine expression, expression of TH$_2$ cytokines is enhanced in a state of hyporesponsiveness following alloantigen-specific induced peripheral tolerance[18,22,26]. These data suggest that TH$_2$ responses promote a tolerant state through the inhibitory effects of TH$_2$ cytokines on TH$_1$ functions. This concept may seem attractive since both subsets cross-regulate each others' function. However, while the 'immunosuppressive' properties of TH$_2$ cytokines have been emphasized, their immunodestructive properties have been ignored. Data obtained from animal and human models of allograft rejection by several groups, including ours, show no delineation in TH cytokine responses but, rather, an upregulation of certain key TH cytokines correlating with acute rejection.

ROLE OF THE TH CYTOKINES IN ACUTE (CELLULAR) REJECTION

The importance of IL-2 in allograft rejection is well documented. Recently, there has been increasing evidence for the immunoregulatory role of the TH_2 cytokine IL-4 in transplant graft rejection. IL-2-deficient mice display intact in vivo immune responses, suggesting that other cytokines such as IL-4 may equally play a critical function in T-cell activation[27]. In fact, IL-4 transcripts could be readily detected in acute rejecting pancreatic allografts in a murine IL-2 knockout model (T. Strom, personal communication). In several experimental models, IL-4 expression correlated with rejection in both allografts[28–30] and xenografts[31–33]. In humans, these observations could be confirmed by our own data in acute rejecting hepatic allografts[23–25] (Gaweco et al., manuscript in preparation) and from several centres demonstrating IL-4 expression in rejecting kidney[34], liver[35,36], heart[37,38] and lung[39] allografts.

IL-4 regulates both T- and B-cell functions that could be involved in the destructive cellular and humoral effector mechanisms leading to graft rejection. IL-4 is a potent helper factor for alloreactive T cell proliferation and CTL activity[40]. The importance of antibody-mediated mechanisms in acute rejection critically implicates IL-4 as a principal mediator of TH_2 humoral responses. IL-4 also has several proinflammatory properties, including upregulation of MHC class II[41] and co-stimulatory[42,43] molecules, and stimulation of the production of inflammatory mediators[44–46]. The critical importance of IL-4 in transplant rejection can be clearly shown in experiments demonstrating in vivo immuno-suppressive effects following blockade of IL-4 activity[47,48].

Thus, both IL-2 and IL-4, selectively produced by human TH_1 and TH_2 cells respectively[13], appear to play a critical role in the acute rejection process. Our extensive analysis of cytokine expression patterns in rejecting human hepatic allografts provide evidence that both IL-2 and IL-4 are upregulated during acute (cellular) rejection, in contrast to properly selected non-rejecting control allografts with no evidence of infection (Fig. 1)[23,24] (Gaweco et al., manuscript in preparation). These findings are strongly supported by our recent data describing the same patterns of IL-2 and IL-4 upregulation during acute (cellular) rejection during administration of different immunosuppressive agents known to differentially inhibit cytokine production[25]. The concomitant upregulation of IL-2 and IL-4 expression during acute rejection was first demonstrated by Dallman et al. in a murine allograft transplant model[49]. Similar observations have also recently been confirmed in human cardiac[38] and lung[39] allografts and in graft infiltrating cells (GIC) propagated from endomyocardial[50] and renal allograft biopsies[51] during an acute rejection episode. In vivo studies have implicated the deleterious combination of IL-2 and IL-4 in acute rejection and steroid resistance. Both cytokines reciprocally augment proliferative T cell responses to alloantigen, and these are hardly affected by CsA[52,53]. In addition, the inhibitory effects of CsA on CTL effector activity are bypassed in the presence of both cytokines, leading to a synergistic amplification of CTL responses[54]. The specific impairment of T cell responses to glucocorticoids (GC) through reduction of GC receptor binding affinity could be of critical importance in the pathogenesis of steroid-resistant rejection[55]. Therefore, both cytokines may act synergistically not only to contribute to efficient graft destruction but also to develop resistance

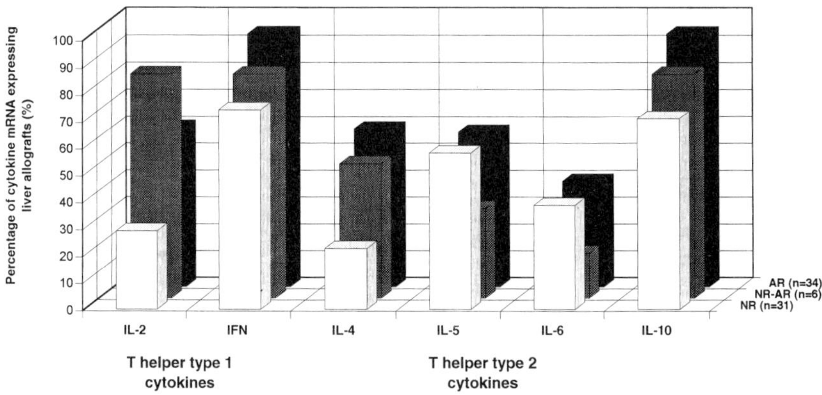

Fig. 1 TH_1 and TH_2 cytokine mRNA expression patterns within the graft evaluated by RT-PCR from biopsies of transplanted livers during stable graft function without evidence of rejection or infection (NR, □), during acute rejection (AR, ■) and in impending acute rejection (NR-AR, ▨). Positive biopsies for the different cytokine mRNA are given as percentage of all biopsies from the respective group. Only the differences for IL-2 and IL-4 mRNA expression are statistically significant between groups

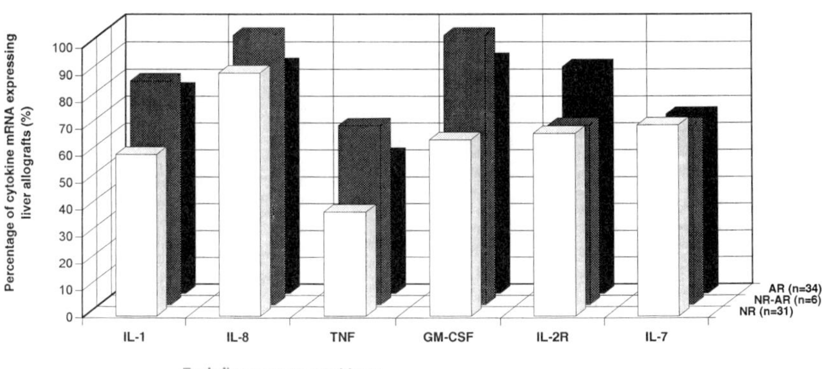

Fig. 2 Proinflammatory cytokine mRNA expression patterns within the graft evaluated by RT-PCR from biopsies of transplanted livers during stable graft function without evidence of rejection or infection (NR, □), during acute rejection (AR, ■) and in impending acute rejection (NR-AR, ▨). Positive biopsies for the different cytokine mRNA are given as percentage of all biopsies from the respective group. No statistically significant differences for any cytokine could be observed between the different groups

mechanisms, bypassing immunosuppressive effects of current therapeutic agents.

Data from our centre show no correlation between the expression patterns of the other TH_1 (IFN-γ) and TH_2 (IL-5, IL-6 and IL-10) cytokines (Fig. 1), proinflammatory cytokines IL-1β, TNF-α, GM-CSF, the chemokine IL-8, including IL-2R and IL-7, in non-rejecting and acute rejecting hepatic allografts (Fig. 2). Detection of the proinflammatory cytokines in non-rejecting liver allografts is not surprising since most of these cytokines are endogenously produced in normal tissue, including hepatocytes and non-parenchymal cells in the liver[56–58]. The previously reported correlation of IL-5 mRNA expression with acute rejection in liver allografts[59] was not observed in our study. We found the same pattern of IL-5 expression in both acute rejecting and non-rejecting allografts from patients receiving CsA immunosuppression; data confirmed by the Sydney group[35]. The discrepancy between our findings and those of the San Francisco group could be explained by a steroid-dosage effect on IL-5 synthesis. Since glucocorticoids have been reported to have an inhibitory effect on IL-4 production[60], the higher total cumulative steroid dosage used in the immuno-suppressive regimen by the San Francisco group could account for the downregulated IL-5 expression in immunologically stable allografts.

In summary, the data presented provide compelling evidence that the TH cytokines dominate, showing no preferential TH_1/TH_2 responses based on cytokine patterns during acute (cellular) rejection of human hepatic allografts. The critical role of the TH_2 cytokine IL-4, as well as the TH_1 cytokine IL-2 in the acute rejection process is strongly implicated. These findings are clearly supported by the common pattern of IL-2 and IL-4 dysregulation observed under the effects of different immunosuppressive agents. These may have important implications in developing optimal immune intervention strategies that could result in less acute rejection episodes and allow for more effective control of transplant rejection and in the potential monitoring of intragraft cytokine expression as an additional diagnostic marker of allograft rejection.

References

1. Backman L, Gibbs J, Levy M, et al. Causes of late graft loss after liver transplantation. Transplantation. 1993;55:1078–82.
2. Basadonna GP, Matas AJ, Gillingham KJ et al. Early versus late acute renal allograft rejection: impact on chronic rejection. Transplantation. 1993;55:993–5.
3. Schreiber SL, Crabtree GR. The mechanism of action of cyclosporin A and FK506. Immunol Today. 1992;13:136–42.
4. Liu J. FK506 and cyclosporin, molecular probes for studying intracellular signal transduction. Immunol Today. 1993;14:290–5.
5. Chirmule N, Oyaizu N, Kalyanaraman VS, Pahwa S. Misinterpretation of results of cytokine bioassays. J Immunol Methods. 1991;137:141–4.
6. James K, Milne I, Cunningham A, Elliot SF. The effect of alpha 2 macroglobulin in commercial cytokine assays. J Immunol Methods. 1994;168:33–7.
7. Shaw G, Kamen R. A conserved AU sequence from the 3′ untranslated region of GM-CSF mRNA mediates selective mRNA degradation. Cell. 1986;46:659–67.
8. Caput D, Beutler B, Hartog K, Thayer R, Brown Shimer S, Cerami A. Identification of a common nucleotide sequence in the 3′-untranslated region of mRNA molecules specifying inflammatory mediators. Proc Natl Acad Sci USA. 1986;83:1670–4.
9. Gruber SA. Locoregional immunosuppression of organ transplants. Immunol Rev. 1992;129:5–30.
10. Bouaboula M, Legoux P, Pessegue B et al. Standardization of mRNA titration using a polymerase chain reaction method involving co-amplification with a multispecific internal control. J Biol Chem. 1992;267:21830–8.
11. Mosmann TR, Cherwinski H, Bond MW, Giedlin MA, Coffman RL. Two types of murine helper T cell clone. I. Definition according to profiles of lymphokine activities and secreted proteins. J Immunol. 1986;136:2348–57.
12. Mosmann TR, Coffman RL. TH1 and TH2 cells: different patterns of lymphokine secretion lead to different functional properties. Annu Rev Immunol. 1989;7:145–73.
13. Romagnani S. Human TH1 and TH2 subsets: doubt no more. Immunol Today. 1991;12:256–7.

14. Yamamura M, Uyemura K, Deans RJ et al. Defining protective responses to pathogens: cytokine profiles in leprosy lesions. Science. 1991;254:277–9.
15. Yssel H, Shanafelt MC, Soderberg C, Schneider PV, Anzola J, Peltz G. *Borrelia burgdorferi* activates a T helper type 1-like T cell subset in Lyme arthritis. J Exp Med. 1991;174:593–601.
16. Fernandez Botran R, Sanders VM, Mosmann TR, Vitetta ES. Lymphokine-mediated regulation of the proliferative response of clones of T helper 1 and T helper 2 cells. J Exp Med. 1988;168:543–58.
17. Mosmann TR, Moore KW. The role of IL-10 in crossregulation of TH1 and TH2 responses. Immunol Today. 1991;12:A49–53.
18. Hancock WW, Sayegh MH, Kwok CA, Weiner HL, Carpenter CB. Oral, but not intravenous, alloantigen prevents accelerated allograft rejection by selective intragraft Th2 cell activation. Transplantation. 1993;55:1112–8.
19. Salom RN, Maguire JA, Hancock WW. Mechanism of a clinically relevant protocol to induce tolerance of cardiac allografts. Perioperative donor spleen cells plus cyclosporine suppress IL-2 and interferon-gamma production. Transplantation. 1993;56:1309–14.
20. Bugeon L, Cuturi MC, Hallet MM, Paineau J, Chabannes D, Soulilou JP. Peripheral tolerance of an allograft in adult rats – characterization by low interleukin-2 and interferon-gamma mRNA levels and by strong accumulation of major histocompatibility complex transcripts in the graft. Transplantation. 1992;54:219–25.
21. Dallman MJ, Shiho O, Page TH, Wood KJ, Morris PJ. Peripheral tolerance to alloantigen results from altered regulation of the interleukin-2 pathway. J Exp Med. 1991;173:79–87.
22. Takeuchi T, Lowry RP, Konieczny B. Heart allografts in murine systems. The differential activation of Th2-like effector cells in peripheral tolerance. Transplantation. 1992;53:1281–94.
23. Gaweco A, Otto G, Otto HF, Geisse T, Hofmann WJ. Kinetics of sequential intragraft cytokine gene activity following orthotopic liver transplantation reveals 'early' IL-2 and 'late' IL-4 mRNA overexpression in acute cellular rejection. Hepatology. 1994;19:691.
24. Gaweco A, Otto G, Otto HF, Geisse T, Hofmann WJ. Cyclosporine (CsA) versus FK 506 primary immunosuppression reveals distinct intragraft gene expression patterns in acute cellular rejection following orthotopic liver transplantation. Gastroenterology. 1994;106:A897.
25. Gaweco A, Otto G, Otto HF, Meuer S, Geisse T, Hofmann WJ. Common and sequential overexpression patterns of the T helper cytokines during acute (cellular) rejection, and correlation of the proinflammatory cytokine expression with chronic (ductopenic) rejection of human liver allografts: A study under CsA, FK 506, and quadruple BT 563 immunosuppression. Transplant Proc. 1995; in press.
26. Abramowicz D, Durez P, Gerard C, et al. Neonatal induction of transplantation tolerance in mice is associated with in vivo expression of IL-4 and -10 mRNAs. Transplant Proc. 1993;25:312–3.
27. Kundig TM, Schorle H, Bachmann MF, Hengartner H, Zinkernagel RM, Horak I. Immune responses in interleukin-2-deficient mice. Science. 1993;262:1059–61.
28. Wang SC, Tweardy DJ, Ford HR, Hoffman RA, Simmons RL. Cytokine products of T-helper 2 (Th2) cells are present in rejecting sponge matrix allografts. Transplant Proc. 1991;23:809–10.
29. Abramowicz D, Doutrelepont JM, Lambert P, Van der Vorst P, Bruyns C, Goldman M. Increased expression of Ia antigens on B cells after neonatal induction of lymphoid chimerism in mice: role of interleukin 4. Eur J Immunol. 1990;20:469–76.
30. Gaweco AS, Dufter C, Terness P et al. Lack of preferential TH1/TH2 cytokine gene expression patterns in both α/β T cell tolerance and rejecting rat cardiac allografts. Transplant Proc. 1995; in press.
31. Bruck W, Bruck Y, Maruschak B, Friede RL. Macrophage properties during peripheral nervous tissue rejection in vitro. J Neuropathol Exp Neurol. 1994;53:51–60.
32. Thai NL, Wang SC, Valdivia LA et al. Cytokine messenger RNA profiles in hamster-to-rat liver xenografts. Transplant Proc. 1993;25:444–5.
33. Wren SM, Wang SC, Thai NL et al. Evidence for early Th2 T cell predominance in xenoreactivity. Transplantation. 1993;56:905–11.
34. Krams SM, Falco DA, Villanueva JC et al. Cytokine and T cell receptor gene expression at the site of allograft rejection. Transplantation. 1992;53:151–6.
35. Bishop GA, Rokahr KL, Napoli J, McCaughan GW. Quantitation of cytokine mRNA expression in biopsies from human liver allografts by a novel reverse transcriptase/polymerase chain reaction (RT/PCR) method. XVth World Congress of the Transplantation Society 1994; 708.
36. Martinez OM, Krams SM, Sterneck M et al. Intragraft cytokine profile during human liver allograft rejection. Transplantation. 1992;53:449–56.

37. van Emmerik N, Baan C, Vaessen L et al. Cytokine gene expression profiles in human endomyocardial biopsy (EMB) derived lymphocyte cultures and in EMB tissue. Transpl Int. 1994;7(Suppl. 1):623–6.
38. Cunningham DA, Dunn MJ, Yacoub MH, Rose ML. Local production of cytokines in the human cardiac allograft. A sequential study. Transplantation. 1994;57:1333–7.
39. Whitehead BF, Stoehr C, Wu CJ et al. Cytokine gene expression in human lung transplant recipients. Transplantation. 1993;56:956–61.
40. Widmer MB, Grabstein KH. Regulation of cytolytic T-lymphocyte generation by B-cell stimulatory factor. Nature. 1987;326:795–8.
41. Noelle R, Krammer PH, Ohara J, Uhr JW, Vitetta ES. Increased expression of Ia antigens on resting B cells: An additional role for B-cell growth factor. Proc Natl Acad Sci USA. 1984;81:6149–53.
42. Stack RM, Lenschow DJ, Gray GS, Bluestone JA, Fitch FW. IL-4 treatment of small splenic B cells induces costimulatory molecules B7-1 and B7-2. J Immunol. 1994;152:5723.
43. Galea P, Valentin JF, Lebranchu Y. Lymphocyte adhesion to allogeneic endothelium involves at least four different pathways. Transplant Proc. 1993;25:146–8.
44. Rollins BJ, Pober JS. Interleukin-4 induces the synthesis and secretion of MCP-1/JE by human endothelial cells. Am J Pathol. 1991;138:1315–9.
45. Moutabarrik A, Ishibashi M, Namiki M et al. Disparate regulation of interleukin-6 secretion from blood monocytes and vascular endothelial cells by interleukin-4. Transplant Proc. 1992;24:2898–9.
46. Orlofsky A, Lin EY, Prystowsky MB. Selective induction of the beta chemokine C10 by IL-4 in mouse macrophages. J Immunol. 1994;152:5084–91.
47. Maliszewski CR, Morrissey PJ, Fanslow WC, Sato TA, Willis C, Davison B. Delayed allograft rejection in mice transgenic for a soluble form of the IL-4 receptor. Cell Immunol. 1992;143:434–48.
48. Fanslow WC, Clifford KN, Park LS et al. Regulation of alloreactivity in vivo by IL-4 and the soluble IL-4 receptor. J Immunol. 1991;147:535–40.
49. Dallman MJ, Larsen CP, Morris PJ. Cytokine gene transcription in vascularised organ grafts: analysis using semiquantitative polymerase chain reaction. J Exp Med. 1991;174:493–6.
50. Daane CR, van Besouw NM, van Emmerik NEM et al. Discrepancy between mRNA expression and production of IL-2 and IL-4 by cultured graft infiltrating cells propagated from endomyocardial biopsies. Transplant Proc. 1994;7(Suppl. 1):627–8.
51. Kirk AD, Ibrahim MA, Bollinger RR, Dawon DV, Finn OJ. Renal allograft-infiltrating lymphocytes. A prospective analysis of in vitro growth characteristics and clinical relevance. Transplantation. 1992;53:329–38.
52. Akbar AN, Salmon M, Ivory K, Taki S, Pilling D, Janossy G. Human CD4+CD45RO+ and CD4+CD45RA+ T cells synergize in response to alloantigens. Eur J Immunol. 1991;21:2517–22.
53. Bohjanen PR, Okajima M, Hodes RJ. Differential regulation of interleukin 4 and interleukin 5 gene expression: a comparison of T-cell gene induction by anti-CD3 antibody or by exogenous lymphokines. Proc Natl Acad Sci USA. 1990;87:5283–7.
54. Heeg K, Gillis S, Wagner H. IL-4 bypasses the immune suppressive effect of cyclosporin A during the in vitro induction of murine cytotoxic T lymphocytes. J Immunol. 1988;141:2330–4.
55. Kam JC, Szefler SJ, Surs W, Sher ER, Leung DY. Combination IL-2 and IL-4 reduces glucocorticoid receptor-binding affinity and T cell response to glucocorticoids. J Immunol. 1993;151:3460–6.
56. Thornton AJ, Ham J, Kunkel SL. Kupffer cell-derived cytokines induce the synthesis of a leukocyte chemotactic peptide, interleukin-8, in human hepatoma and primary hepatocyte cultures. Hepatology. 1991;14:1112–22.
57. Magilavy DB, Rothstein JL. Spontaneous production of tumor necrosis factor alpha by Kupffer cells of MRL/lpr mice. J Exp Med. 1988;168:789–94.
58. Tovey MG, Gugenheim J, Guymarho J et al. Genes for interleukin-1, interleukin-6, and tumor necrosis factor are expressed at markedly reduced levels in the livers of patients with severe liver disease. Autoimmunity. 1991;10:297–310.
59. Martinez OM, Villanueva JC, Lake J, Roberts JP, Ascher JL, Krams SM. IL-2 and IL-5 gene expression in response to alloantigen in liver allograft recipients and in vitro. Transplantation. 1993;55:1159–66.
60. Rolfe FG, Hughes JM, Armour CL, Sewell WA. Inhibition of interleukin-5 gene expression by dexamethasone. Immunology. 1992;77:494–9.

Index

AAR-interleukin-8 (IL-8) 7
acetaldehyde 76, 77
acetyl-CoA carboxylase, citrate-activated, and
    fatty acid synthesis 173
α_1-acid glycoprotein 165, 167
activin, and liver generation 95–6
acute phase proteins
  classification 14, 25
  hepatic expression, cytokine regulation
    164–70
  hepatocyte 14
  and host defence 176
  and lipid metabolism 175–6
acute phase response, anti-inflammatory 164
acute phase response element (APRE) 15
acute phase response factor (APRF) 15–22
  binding sequences 15
  binding sites, GAF binding site sequence
    comparisons 19
  gp130 association 20, 21
  interferon-γ activated factor binding
    17–19
  phosphorylation by tyrosine 16–17, 20
  phosphotyrosine/phosphoserine 20
  post-translational activation, in cytoplasm
    16
  purification 16
adenovirus vectors, and cytokine gene transfer
    168–70
adhesion molecules
  cell-matrix, sinusoidal epithelial cell
    expression 52–4
  and cytokines 37–44
  molecular families 204
  oligosaccharide/peptide receptor blockade
    211
  organ-specific expression, cytokine effects
    209–10
  receptor–ligand interactions 204, 205
  regulation by cytokines, in transplants
    204–211
  vascular ligand, and transplant inflammation
    211
  see also individual molecules and families
alcoholic liver disease
  blood collection, and AST assay 187
  cytokine production 128–31
  cytokine-related therapy 133–5
  enteral feeding model 187
  free radicals 186, 188, 192–3, 196, 199,
    200–1
  and hypoxia 199, 200
  isolated Kupffer cells, TNF release 188
  Kupffer cell activation 185–6
  Kupffer cell inactivation effects 189, 193,
    200
  liver surface oxygen tension 187, 189,
    191, 192, 195, 200
  pathological evaluation 187
  transplantation, and cytokines 185–201
cAMP, intrastellate cell level 85, 88–9
amyloid A, serum levels, inflammation/
    infection effects 175
anaphylatoxin C5a 5
anti-muscle antibody (AMA), profiles, in PBC
    147, 150
antibiotic therapy, effect on liver injury and
    oxygen tension 189, 191–2, 194, 195,
    198
antibiotic treatment, for intestinal sterilization
    186, 187
antinuclear antibodies (ANA), AIH type I
    138, 139
AP-1, activation in Kupffer cells 31–5
apolipoproteins, serum levels, cytokine effects
    167, 175–6
arginase, catalytic activity, in hepatocyte
    conditioned medium 61
arginase, membrane-bound
  and cultured FSC 74–6
  hepatocellular damage 76
aspartate aminotransferase (AST), assay,
    alcoholic liver disease 187, 189, 193
autoantigens, regulation by cytokines 140–1
autoimmune hepatitis (AIH)
  and cytokines 138–43
  IL-5 activity 152, 153
  and interferons 139–40
  serum cytokine levels, PBC comparisons
    150, 151, 152

type I, TH2 cells   141
type II
  TH1 cells   141, 143
  and virus-induced autoimmunity   143
  types   138, 139
azathioprine, in autoimmune hepatitis   139

B lymphocytes, IgA production, alcoholic
  liver disease   131
basophils, action of CC chemokines   8–9
bone marrow stem cells, IL-6 gene
  overexpression induction   167–8
bromodeoxyuridine, incorporation into FSC
  61

C-MET binding   104
C-reactive protein, lipoprotein binding   175
Ca^{2+}
  intrastellate cell level   85, 87, 88
  Kupffer cell activation   185–6
cachexia, cytokine-associated   176
CAT gene, induction by interferon-gamma
  17
CC chemokines   5, 7–10
  activity comparisons   8
  and basophil/eosinophil leukocytes   8–9
  cDNA sequences   8
CD18 macrophages, endotoxin binding   116
CD4+ T-helper cells   141, 145
  antigen-specific reaction, and HLA-DR
    202
  and PBC   151–3
CD8+ cytotoxic T cells
  and alloantigenic MHC molecules   210
  and PBC   151
  and transplant rejection   215
chemokines   5–10
  myofibroblast expression   59
  pathophysiological implications   9–10
cholangitis, primary sclerosing (PSC)   146
  cytokine serum levels, PBC comparisons
    150, 151, 152
cholesterol
  hepatic synthesis, and cytokines   175
  metabolism, cytokine effects   175
chylomicrons   177
ciliary neurotrophic factor (CNTF)   15, 164
  overexpression induction   168
cirrhosis
  alcoholic
    bacterial infections, cytokine diagnostic
      markers   131, 133, 134
    cytokines   127–35
  primary biliary *see* primary biliary cirrhosis
    (PBC)
  and von Willebrand factor   55
citrate, hepatic levels, and fatty acid synthesis
  173
colchicine, in alcoholic liver disease   133

collagen gel method, long-lasting stellate cell
  contraction measurement   85, 87
collagenase   134
corticosterone, serum levels, and inflammation
  166–7
Corynebacterium parvum   128
CXC chemokines   5, 6–7
cyclosporin A, effects of IL-2/IL-4
  combination   216
cysteine proteinase inhibitor, serum levels, and
  inflammation   167
cytochrome P450 2D6
  herpes simplex virus cross-reactivity   143
  regulation by cytokines   140, 142
cytokine receptors, differential distribution,
  and cell types   209
cytokines
  and adhesion molecules   37–44
  fibrogenic   76
  inhibitors   134–5
  myofibroblast expression   59
  see also chemokines *and individual*
    cytokines
cytomegalovirus, IL-6 gene overexpression
  induction   167, 169
cytoskeletal proteins, immunofluorescent
  staining   62–3

desmin, immunoreactive   84
dexamethasone, AP-1 activation inhibition
  33
diabetes mellitus, insulin-dependent, TH1 cells
  145
diacetyl-LDL, uptake by sinusoidal epithelial
  cell   52
Disse space, extracellular matrix proteins   52
DNA, synthesis by HGF and TGF-α 106–7

ENA-78   6
encephalomyelitis, allergic experimental
  (EAE), and TH2-like cells   145
endogenous pyrogen *see* interleukin-1 (IL-1)
endothelial cells, hepatic
  adhesion molecule expression, and
    cytokines   205, 206
  immune reaction modification   210
endothelin (ET)   83
  stellate cell contraction   85, 86, 87, 90
  and stellate cell inositol-phosphate   87, 88
endotoxin
  biological effects, regulators   198, 200
  serum levels, in alcoholic hepatitis   43–4
eosinophils, action of CC chemokines   8–9
epithelial cells, recombinant adenovirus/IL-6
  gene infection, IL-6 production   168
extracellular matrix, components   58
extracellular matrix proteins
  and activated Ito cells   52
  Disse space   52

hepatic SEC role   54
immunofluorescent staining   62–3

F-actin, stellate cell-associated
   stress fibres, iloprost-induced
      de-aggregation   87
   TRITC-phalloidin staining   84
fat-storing cells (FSC)
   activation
      hepatocyte role   58–78
      pathways   59
      three step cascade model   76–8
   analytical procedures   63
   bromodeoxyuridine incorporation,
      measurement   61
   cultured, membrane-bound arginase
      74 –6
   and hepatocyte cell–cell contact loss
      74–6
   isolation/culture   59–60
   mitogenesis
      and hepatocyte-conditioned medium
         63–5
      Kupffer cell/hepatocyte synergism
         64–5
   paracrine activation inhibition   68–9, 70
      71
      by α_2-macroglobulin   62
   proliferation
      determination   60–1
      and IGF   71, 73–4
   proteoglycan synthesis
      determination   61
      and hepatocyte/Kupffer cell synergism
         65
   transformation to myofibroblasts   76
fatty acids
   esterification, and TNF   174
   hepatic synthesis, cytokine-stimulated
      173, 174
Fcα receptor, cross-linking   131
fibroblasts, recombinant adenovirus/IL-6 gene
      infection, IL-6 production   168
fibrogenesis
   cytokine-induced   211
   and fat-storing cells   58
fibronectin
   cellular, determination   62
   synthesis, α_2-macroglobulin effects   70, 72
fibrosis, hepatic
   and sinusoidal endothelial cells   51–5
   TGF-β_1 54–5
N-formylmethionyl peptides, microbial   5
free radicals, in alcoholic liver disease   186,
   188, 192–3, 196, 199, 200–1

gadolinium chloride, Kupffer cell inactivation,
   effects in alcoholic liver disease   189,
   193, 200

glucocorticoids
   in alcoholic liver disease   133
   in autoimmune hepatitis   139
glycosaminoglycans, and HGF binding   104
cGMP, intrastellate cell level   85, 89, 90
gp80, IL-6 binding, gp130 interaction   14
gp130
   APRF association   20, 21
   IL-6 gp80-bound, interaction   14
   and JAK1   22
granulocyte-monocyte-colony-stimulating
      factor (GM-CSF), and PBC   149, 150,
      152
granulocytosis, rebound, interleukin-8-induced
   6
GRO proteins   6
growth factors   164–70
   myofibroblast expression   59

H-7, protein kinase C inhibition   90
HDL cholesterol, serum levels, cytokine
   effects   175
hepatectomy, hepatocyte growth factor levels
   105
hepatectomy, partial
   decreased hepatic functional capacity   93
   HGF clearance/hepatic uptake   106–7
   liver and ectopic tissue regeneration   103–
   4
hepatitis
   aetiological classification   138, 139
   see also autoimmune hepatitis; liver
      inflammation
hepatitis C, associated autoimmunity,
      ALT/LKM-1 levels   139, 140
hepatocellular carcinoma
   and IGF-II   98
   and TGF-α inhibition   100
hepatocyte growth factor (HGF)
   binding sites   104
   DNA synthesis initiation   106–7
   and liver regeneration   103–8
   mitogenic targets   104
   and partial hepatectomy   105, 106–7
   posthepatectomy levels   105, 106–7
   receptor (MET)   104, 105
   tissue distribution/uptake   105
   uptake and processing in liver   106–7
hepatocytes
   acute phase proteins   14
   apoptosis, cytokine-induced   68, 69
   collagenase-treated, DNA synthesis   107
   conditioned medium
      FSC growth-promoting activity   63–5
      IGF and IGFBP   73, 74
      Kupffer cell conditioned medium
         synergism   64–5
      and LDH/AST activities   66–8
   preparation   60

and TGF-β-induced PC apoptosis 66–8
  Western ligand blotting 62
and cytokine-directed fat-storing cell
  activation 58–78
ethanol metabolism, acetaldehyde/lipid
  peroxide production 76
gene expression, and functional hepatic
  deficit 93–4
hyperplasia, and TGF-α overexpression
  97–8
IGF action modulation 71, 73–4
IGF-binding protein secretion 71, 73–4,
  75
isolation/culture 60
Kupffer cell-modified LPS processing 115
membrane-bound arginase, and cultured
  FSC 74–6
proliferation
  and TGF-α 97–8
  and toxic injury 94
toxin exposure 60
herpes simplex virus (HSV), cytochrome P450
  2D6 cross-reactivity 143
HMG-CoA reductase, activity, cytokine effects
  175
humoral immune response, and TH2 cells
  141
hyaluronic acid
  peripheral blood levels, in partial
    hepatectomy 107
  receptor (CD44) 53
hyperplasia, hepatocyte, TGF-α
  overexpression effects 97–8
hypersensitivity, delayed-type (DTH), and
  allograft rejection 215
hypoxia, and alcoholic liver disease 199, 200

I-309 8
ICAM-1 15, 139
  SEC expression of, in LPS-induced liver
    injury 41, 42
  serum levels, in alcoholic hepatitis 43–4
  TNF-α/IL-1-induced, expression on hepatic
    SEC 39–41
IgA, serum levels, and alcoholic liver disease
  131
IGF binding proteins (IGFBPs), IGF activity
  modulation 71, 73, 74
IgM, IL-6 gene overexpression induction
  167
iloprost
  F-actin stress fibre de-aggregation 87
  and intrastellate cell cAMP 89
  stellate cell contraction 85
immunosuppressive agents, cytokine inhibition
  215, 216–18
inflammation
  and chemokines 10

corticosterone serum levels 166–7
cysteine proteinase inhibitor, serum levels
  167
IL-6 serum levels 166–7
inositol phosphate, formation in stellate cells
  84–5, 87, 88
insulin-like growth factor-II (IGF-II), and
  hepatocarcinogenesis 97–8
insulin-like growth factors (IGF)
  action on FSC, and IGFBPs 71, 73–4, 75
  see also IGF binding proteins (IGFBPs)
integrins 52, 53–4
  cytoskeleton-associated, neo-epitope
    formation 208
  leukocyte binding 206
interferon regulatory factor-1 (IRF-1) 15
interferon-γ, APRF activation 17–19
interferon-γ activated factor (GAF)
  APRF binding site sequence comparisons
    9
  binding to APRE 17–19
  fibroblast/HeLa cells 19
  see also Stat91
interferons (INF)
  and autoimmune hepatitis 139 –140
  and SP 100 expression in PBC 140–1
interleukin-1 (IL-1) 164
  cytokine inducer 128
  expression on Kupffer cells 122–4
  ICAM-1 induction, and hepatic SEC 39–
    41
  inhibitors 128
  and lipopolysaccharide (LPS) 122
  and triglyceride serum levels 172–3
interleukin-2 (IL-2), and graft rejection 216–
  18
interleukin-4 (IL-4)
  and graft rejection 216–18
  and hepatic fatty acid synthesis 173
interleukin-5 (IL-5), and PBC 150, 152
interleukin-6 (IL-6) 14, 164, 165
  and acute phase proteins type 2 165–6
  and alcoholic liver disease 128–9, 15, 164
  APRF activation 15
  and APRF serine phosphorylation 22–3,
    25
  in bacterial infections and cirrhosis 133,
    134
  gene overexpression induction 167–8
  gp80-bound, gp130 interaction 14
  and hypergammaglobulinaemia 128
  post-transplantation release, nisoldipine
    effects 189, 190
  secretion, IgA-induced 131
  serum levels, and inflammation 166–7
  signal transduction, plasma membrane/
    nucleus 14–28
  target genes, induction, and serine/threonine
    kinases 22

interleukin-6 (IL-6) receptor   14
  soluble   169–70
interleukin-8 (IL-8)   5
  and alcoholic cirrhosis   131
  and alcoholic hepatitis   43–4, 129
  analogues   6
  carboxyl terminal sequence, receptor
    interaction   7
  ELR motif, receptor interaction   7
  glycosaminoglycan binding   10
  inflammation mediation   10
  lymphocyte attraction   6
  mode of action   6
  monomeric   6
interleukin-8 (IL-8) receptors   7
  cDNA cloning   7
  IL-8RA/8R1 and IL-8RB/8R2   7
interleukin-10 (IL-10)   127
  and alcoholic liver disease   130–1
interleukin-11 (IL-11)   15, 164
Ito cells, activated   51
  and extracellular matrix proteins   52
  see also stellate cells, hepatic

JAK1, and Gp130   22
JAK protein tyrosine kinases, IL-6-induced
    tyrosine phosphorylation   20, 22, 23, 24
JAK tyrosine kinases, and IL-6 signalling   22
junB   15

Kupffer cells
  activation, alcoholic liver disease   185–6
  AP-1 activation in   31–5
  bacterial LPS processing studies   115–24
    experimental animals   116
    Kupffer cell isolation   117
    LPS modification/radioiodination
      116–17
    LPS types   116
    materials and methods   116–19
    RNA extraction, Northern blot analysis
      118–19
    surface labelling   117
  and chronic gut-derived endotoxin exposure
    123–4
  conditioned medium
    and FSC mitogenesis   64–5
    preparation   60
  cytokine response to LPS   121
  and donor livers   185, 194
  electrophoretic mobility shift assay   31–2
  endotoxin binding proteins   123–4
  immune reaction modification   210
  inactivation by GdCl₃, effects in alcoholic
    liver disease   189, 193, 200
  NF-κB activation in   31–5
  reperfusion injury role, in ethanol-induced

    fatty liver   194–5, 197, 198–200, 201
  TNF-α synthesis inhibitors   33

lactate dehydrogenase, and FSC mitogenesis
  66–7
laminin   54
LDL
  cholesterol, serum levels, cytokine effects
    175
  diacetyl, uptake by sinusoidal epithelial
    cells   52
LDL receptors, virus uptake   177
leukaemia inhibitory factor (LIF)   15, 164
leukocytes
  diapedesis and tissue migration   208
  integrin receptors
    activation-dependent interaction   208
    and intravascular cytokines   208
  rolling, selectin-induced   206
  selectin-dependent adherence   206
  systemic intravascular adhesion   206
leukotriene B₄   5
leukotriene D₄   83
LFA-1α, PMN expression of   41, 42
lipid metabolism
  and acute phase proteins   175–6
  cytokine effects   172–7
    beneficial aspects   176–7
    deleterious aspects   176
lipid peroxides   76, 77
lipolysis, cytokine-stimulated, and fatty acid
  levels   173
lipopolysaccharide (LPS)
  ¹²⁵I-labelled, ligand blotting   118
  affinity column preparation   118
  albumin binding   121
  bacterial, Kupffer cell processing of   115–
    24
  binding protein isolation   118
  E. coli, APRF activation   15
  and interleukin-1   122
  Kupffer cell NF-κB/AP-1 activation   32–5
  SASD complex, and Kupffer cell surface
    endotoxin binding   119–21
  and TNF-α   38, 39, 122
lipoprotein lipase, activity, cytokine effects
  173
lipoproteins
  clearance, and serum triglyeride levels   173
  endotoxin binding   177
  very low density (VLDL), serum levels,
    cytokine effects   172, 173
  virus binding   177
liver cell membranes, FSC activity effects
  74–6
liver, inflammation, IL-6-dependent reaction
  166
liver injuries, experimental, cytokines and
  adhesion molecules   41–2

liver kidney microsomal (LKM) antibodies, AIH type II 138, 139
liver regeneration
  and HGF 103–8
  and TGF-α 93–100
liver transplantation *see* transplantation
lymphocyte cultures, in PBC cytokine studies 146

Mac-1, PMN expression of 41, 42
α_2-macroglobulin
  FSC paracrine stimulation inhibition 62
  myofibroblast autocrine stimulation inhibition 62
  and proteoglycan synthesis inhibition 68–9, 72
  synthesis, interferon-γ-stimulated 17
  TGF-β scavenging 68–71, 72, 73
macrophages
  endotoxin uptake, and lipoproteins 177
  isolation, for LPS studies 117
  peritoneal, Kupffer cell cross-linking 119–21
  populations, cross-linking 117
matrix degradation, liver regeneration, and urokinase 107–8
MCP-1, histamine release 9
MCP-2 8
MCP-3 8
  histamine release 9
MET, HGF receptor protein 104, 105
metalloproteinases (MMPs) 58
  tissue inhibitors (TIMPs) 58
MHC expression, and immune recognition sensitivity 209
MIP-1α 8
  histamine release 9
MIP-1β 8
mitogenesis, FSC, hepatocyte-derived 63–5
  and Kupffer cell medium 64–5
  and LDH 66–7
  and TGF-β-induced apoptosis 66–8
  and toxic damage 66–8
myofibroblasts 58, 59
  autocrine stimulation inhibition, by α_2-macroglobulin 62

neomycin 187, 189, 198
neoplasia
  and TGF-α overexpression 97–8
  see also hepatocellular carcinoma
neutropenia, interleukin-8-induced 6
neutrophil-activating protein-2 (NAP-2) 6
neutrophils, IL-8 receptors 6–7
NF-κB, activation in Kupffer cells 31–5
  inhibition, TNF-α synthesis effects 33
nisoldipine, and TNF/IL-6 post-transplantation release 189, 200
nitric oxide

sinusoidal microcirculation regulation 83
stellate cell contraction 85, 90–1
2′,5′-oligoisodenylate synthetase 139
oncostatin M (OM; OSM) 15, 164
oxygen tension, liver surface 187, 189, 191, 192, 195, 200

PDTC
  Ap-1 induction 35
  NF-κB activation inhibition 33
  TNF-α synthesis inhibition 33, 34
peripheral blood monocytes (PBMCs)
  autoantigen stimulation, and cytokine release 151, 152
  culture supernatant cytokines, in PBC 149–52
pertussis, toxin-sensitive G protein 87
phosphatidylcholine, and Ito cell activation inhibition 134
phosphoserine, and APRF 20
phosphotyrosine, and APRF 20
plasmin, extracellular matrix glycoprotein degradation 55
plasminogen activation inhibitor, type 1 55
platelet-activating factor 5
platelet-derived growth factor (PDGF), and α_2-macroglobulin 76
polymerase chain reaction (PCR)
  reverse transcriptase (RT-PCR) 214–15
  in situ, and cytokine message transcription 214
polymorphoneutrophils
  IL-8 level correlation, in alcoholic hepatitis 43–4
  and LPS-induced liver injury 41
  SEC adhesion, TNF-α effects 40–1
polymyxin B 187, 189, 198
primary biliary cirrhosis (PBC)
  CD4$^+$ T-helper cells 151–3
  cytokine serum levels
    and immunological/histological activity 150
    other disease comparisons 150–1, 152–3
  cytokine studies
    AMA profiles 147, 150
    cytokine assays 146
    cytokine profiles 147, 148 –51
    and immunoreactivity 145–53
    lymphocyte cultures 146
    methods 146–7
    patients 146
    results 147–51
  PMBC culture supernatant, cytokine profiles 149
  Sp100 expression, IFN effects 140–1
  TH-related cytokines
    serum levels, healthy control comparisons 147–9

TH1/TH2 ratio   151–3
prostaglandin E$_2$ (PGE$_2$)
    and intrastellate cell cAMP   89
    stellate cell contraction   85
prostaglandin F$_{2\alpha}$ (PGF$_{2\alpha}$)   83
    stellate cell contraction   85
protein kinase C
    Ca^{2+}-dependent activation   208
    and endothelin-induced stellate cell
        contraction   90
proteoglycan synthesis
    α_2-macroglobulin effects   68–9, 72
    FSC, and hepatocyte/Kupffer cell synergism
        65

R-interleukin-8 (IL-8)   7
RANTES   8
    histamine release   9
reactive oxygen intermediates (ROIs) and NF-
    κB activation   34
reverse transcriptase-polymerase chain
    reaction (RT-PCR), cytokine detection
    214–15
rheumatoid arthritis, serum cytokine levels,
    PBC comparisons   150, 151, 152

SAA, levels, inflammation/infection effects
    175
scatter factor   104
selectins, receptors, oligosaccharide binding
    206
serine kinases, and IL-6 target gene induction
    22
sin-1, and intrastellate cell cGMP   89, 90
sinusoidal epithelial cells (SEC), hepatic
    and extracellular matrix protein synthesis
        54
    ICAM-1 expression   39–41
    and liver fibrosis   51–5
    TGF-β_1 expression   55
sinusoids, hepatic, collagenization
    (capillarization)   51–2
smooth muscle antibodies (SMA), AIH type I
    138, 139
sodium nitroprusside, and intrastellate cell
    cGMP   89, 90
soluble liver antigen antibody (SLA), AIH
    type III   138, 139
Sp100, in primary biliary cirrhosis, and IFN
    140–1
spleen
    and cytokines   37–8
    and liver injuries   37–8
splenectomy, TNF-α serum levels, LPS effects
    38, 39
splenocytes, and TNF release   122–3
Stat3, and APRF   16
Stat91, tyrosine phosphorylation, IL-6-induced
    20

staurosporin   90
stellate cells, hepatic
    cellular cAMP and cGMP measurement
        85, 88–9, 90, 91
    contraction measurement   84
    contraction/relaxation, and Kupffer cell-
        derived vasoctive agents   83–91
    cytosolic free Ca^{2+} 85, 87, 88, 89
    endothelin receptors   90
    isolation and culture   83–4
    long-lasting contraction   85, 87
    radiolabelled, [^{3}H]inositol phosphate
        measurement   84–5, 87
    see also Ito cells

T-helper cells
    antigen-specific response, cytokine effects
        141
    type 1
        related cytokines, TH2-related cytokine
            ratio, in PBC   151–3
    and transplant cell-mediated responses
        215
    type 2, immunosuppressive properties   215
    types, and cytokine production   141, 145
        215
    see also CD4$^+$ T-helper cells
T-lymphocytes, liver-infiltrating, and cytokines
    141, 143
threonine, and IL-6 target gene induction   22
thrombospondin receptor   53
toxic injury, and hepatocyte proliferation   94
transcription factors, activation, and liver
    regeneration initiation   94–7
transforming growth factor-α (TGF-α)
    antisense gene, tumour growth inhibition
        99–100
    DNA synthesis initiation   106–7
    and liver regeneration   96–7
    liver regeneration/growth initiation
        93–100
    overexpression, and hepatic hyperplasia
        97–8
    parenchymal cell apoptosis   68
transforming growth factor-β (TGF-β)
    active (determination)   62
        in conditioned media   70, 73
    and liver regeneration   95–6
    peripheral blood levels, in partial
        hepatectomy   107
    scavenging by α_2-macroglobulin   68–71,
        72, 73
transforming growth factor-β_1 (TGF-β_1)
    and parenchymal cell apoptosis   66–8, 69
    protein synthesis modulation   54–5
transplantation
    adhesion molecule induction by cytokines
        205–7